Undergraduate Manual of Clinical Cases in Obstetrics & Gynaecology

Undergraduate Manual of Clinical Cases in Obstetrics & Gynaecology

N. Hephzibah Kirubamani, MD, DGO, FRCOG, FICOG, PhD, DSc
Prof., Saveetha Medical College
Former Prof., Stanley Medical College
Chennai, Tamil Nadu, India

A.P. Nalini Alexander, MD, DGO
Prof., Chettinad Medical College
Former Prof., Stanley Medical College
Chennai, Tamil Nadu, India

R. Premalatha, MD, DGO, DNB, FRCOG, FICOG
Senior Consultant, Mehta's Hospital
Former Prof., Madras Medical College
Chennai, Tamil Nadu, India

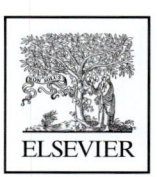

ELSEVIER   elsevier.com

ELSEVIER

RELX India Pvt. Ltd.
Registered Office: 818, 8th floor, Indraprakash Building, 21, Barakhamba Road, New Delhi-110001
Corporate Office: 14th Floor, Building No. 10B, DLF Cyber City, Phase II, Gurgaon-122002, Haryana, India

---

Undergraduate Manual of Clinical Cases in Obstetrics & Gynaecology, **1st Edition, N. Hephzibah Kirubamani, A.P. Nalini Alexander, R. Premalatha**

Copyright © 2017 by RELX India Pvt. Ltd.
All rights reserved.

ISBN: 978-81-312-4868-3
e-Book ISBN: 978-81-312-4923-9

No part of this publication may be reproduced or transmitted in any form or by any means, electronic or mechanical, including photocopying, recording, or any information storage and retrieval system, without permission in writing from the publisher. Details on how to seek permission, further information about the Publisher' permissions policies and our arrangements with organizations such as the Copyright Clearance Center and the Copyright Licensing Agency, can be found at our website: www.elsevier.com/permissions.

This book and the individual contributions contained in it are protected under copyright by the Publisher (other than as may be noted herein).

Notice

Knowledge and best practice in this field are constantly changing. As new research and experience broaden our understanding, changes in research methods, professional practices, or medical treatment may become necessary.

Practitioners and researchers must always rely on their own experience and knowledge in evaluating and using any information, methods, compounds, or experiments described herein. In using such information or methods they should be mindful of their own safety and the safety of others, including parties for whom they have a professional responsibility.

With respect to any drug or pharmaceutical products identified, readers are advised to check the most current information provided (i) on procedures featured or (ii) by the manufacturer of each product to be administered, to verify the recommended dose or formula, the method and duration of administration, and contraindications. It is the responsibility of practitioners, relying on their own experience and knowledge of their patients, to make diagnoses, to determine dosages and the best treatment for each individual patient, and to take all appropriate safety precautions.

To the fullest extent of the law, neither the Publisher nor the authors, contributors, or editors, assume any liability for any injury and/or damage to persons or property as a matter of product liability, negligence or otherwise, or from any use or operation of any methods, products, instructions, or ideas contained in the material herein.

Although all advertising material is expected to conform to ethical (medical) standards, inclusion in this publication does not constitute a guarantee or endorsement of the quality or value of such product or of the claims made of it by its manufacturer.

Please consult full prescribing information before issuing prescription for any product mentioned in this publication.

Content Strategist: Renu Rawat
Content Strategist (Digital): Nabajyoti Kar
Manager—Education Solutions (Digital): Smruti Snigdha
Sr Manager—Education Solutions: Shabina Nasim
Sr Content Development Specialist: Shivani Pal
Sr Project Manager: Anitha Rajarathnam
Sr Operations Manager: Sunil Kumar
Sr Production Executive: Ravinder Sharma
Sr Cover Designer: Milind Majgaonkar

Typeset by Thomson Digital

Printed by Rajkamal Electric Press, Kundli, Haryana.

*Dedicated to loving parents, supportive
spouse and encouraging children*

N. Hephzibah Kirubamani
A.P. Nalini Alexander
R. Premalatha

About the Book

Every student who aspires to become a doctor has to get through the exams before starting to practice the noble profession. He/she has to clear the theory and practical exam. I congratulate the authors Prof. N. Hephzibah Kirubamani, Prof. A.P. Nalini Alexander and Prof. Premalatha who have written 'Undergraduate Manual of Clinical Cases in Obstetrics & Gynaecology' to help the undergraduate to clear the clinical examination and viva voce in obstetrics and gynaecology. They individually have the experience of more than 35 years of teaching and practicing obstetrics and gynaecology and have been examiners for undergraduates and postgraduates for more than 25 years.

The manual is in two parts: Part 1 dealing with obstetrics and Part 2 dealing with gynaecology. 'Medicine is an Art and Science'—the art of history taking, especially getting the relevant history in its sequence and getting the confidence and trust of the woman to discuss her problems and the science of arriving at a diagnosis with relevant investigations and the art and science of discussing pros and cons of the management so that the patient gets the evidence-based best treatment available. Strong foundation is needed for any building—stronger the foundation better the high-rise buildings. History taking and clinical examination are the strong foundation that the medical student should learn and possess to go higher in any field of medicine. Hence the authors have dealt in detail the history taking and clinical examination in obstetrics and gynaecology. In other chapters, they have discussed the long cases with relevant history, clinical examination and appropriate investigations and have outlined the management in brief but to the point. Flow charts, tables, photographs of actual patients, diagrams, USG pictures and CTG tracings that accompany the subject will make it easy for the students to understand. The questions at the end of each chapter will help the students to prepare well.

In viva voce: specimens, instruments, charts, USG pictures, CTG tracings and drugs have been discussed with relevance to the examination. Anatomy of pelvis and foetal skull has been discussed in detail to enable the student to understand the mechanism of normal and abnormal labour. The steps of surgery for lower segment caesarean section, abdominal and vaginal hysterectomy have been included. I would recommend this book for medical students for whom it will be of immense help to succeed.

Prof. V. Madhini, MD, DGO, MNAMS
Former Director of Institute of Obstetrics & Gynaecology;
Prof. and HOD of Obstetrics & Gynaecology Department,
Madras Medical College, Chennai, Tamil Nadu, India

Table of Content

Foreword xi
Preface xiii
Abbreviations xv

PART 1 OBSTETRIC CASES

CASE 1 Obstetric History Taking and Examination 3
  Antenatal Examination 26

CASE 2 Normal Pregnancy 37
  Episiotomy Suturing 40

CASE 3 A Case of Anaemia Complicating Pregnancy 43

CASE 4 A Case of Hypertension in Pregnancy 53

CASE 5 A Case of Prolonged (Post-Term) Pregnancy 69

CASE 6 A Case of Pregnancy Following Caesarean Section 79
  How to Elicit Scar Tenderness in Previous LSCS Pregnancy 81

CASE 7 A Case of Heart Disease Complicating Pregnancy 87

CASE 8 A Case of Malpresentation 97

CASE 9 A Case of Multiple Pregnancy 107

CASE 10 A Case of Rh Negative Pregnancy 117

CASE 11 A Case of Cephalopelvic Disproportion 125

CASE 12 A Case of Diabetes Complicating Pregnancy 137

CASE 13 A Case of Recurrent Pregnancy Loss 147

CASE 14 A Case of Foetal Growth Restriction 155

CASE 15 Normal Puerperium and Postnatal Care 161

CASE 16 Viva Voce (Oral Exam) 171

PART 2 GYNAECOLOGICAL CASES

CASE 1 **Gynaec Case Sheet Writing** 217
    Palpating the Mass 224
    How to use Sim's Speculum 227
    How to use Cusco's Speculum 228

CASE 2 **A Case of Vaginal Discharge** 233

CASE 3 **Abnormal Uterine Bleeding** 241

CASE 4 **A Case of Genital Prolapse** 255
    Examination of Uterine Prolapse 257

CASE 5 **A Case of Fibroid Uterus** 265

CASE 6 **A Case of Cancer Cervix** 275
    How to do Papsmear 279

CASE 7 **A Case of Infertility** 289

CASE 8 **A Case of Primary Amenorrhoea** 299

CASE 9 **A Case of Secondary Amenorrhoea** 307

CASE 10 **A Case of Ovarian Tumour** 315

CASE 11 **A Case of Post-Menopausal Bleeding PV** 325

CASE 12 **A Case of Urinary Incontinence** 333

CASE 13 **Viva Voce Examination in Gynaecology** 339

Index 369

Follow the instruction on the front inner cover to access and view the videos( ) and the lecture ppts( ).

Foreword

Obstetrics and Gynaecology like every branch of Medical Science has grown in volume and complexity. This growth and development results in a state wherein teachers lose clarity in what is 'basic' that is to be taught to an undergraduate student of medicine and the student is perplexed about choosing sources or textbooks that will help to become knowledgeable and at the same time be found 'not wanting' by the examiners.

This handbook authored by Prof. N. Hephzibah Kirubamani, Prof. Nalini Alexander and Prof. R. Premalatha has been designed to satisfy the critical need.

The 'Undergraduate Manual of Clinical Cases in Obstetrics & Gynaecology' will be a ready reckoner for the MBBS students preparing for their final professional examination. I have no doubt that this book is useful and is bound to become popular as this has been designed to serve a long felt need of teachers and students alike.

Examinations are formidable even for the well prepared. The examinee could always be at loss to prepare for a clinical examination by senior teachers. This book with clinical examples accompanied by illustrations, tabulations and flow charts will be a welcome learning aid for the MBBS examinee. The online interactive access will be a very useful component to students and practitioners alike.

The authors deserve congratulations for their efforts in bringing out this companion volume to popular textbooks in obstetrics and gynaecology.

Dr T. Gunasagaran, MS, MCh (Onc), FRCS (Edin), MNAMS
Dean, Saveetha Medical College & Hospital,
Saveetha Nagar, Thandalam, Kanchipuram Dist.,
Chennai, Tamil Nadu, India

Preface

Our teachers were our source of inspiration and our motivation comes from our students.

Our aim in this book is to help students to understand the importance of history taking, physical examination and its relevance in making a provisional diagnosis.

This book also deals with relevant investigations based on provisional diagnosis. Presentation is kept very simple and concise. This book deals with common clinical conditions and is designed in such a way as to help students to prepare for their clinical and practical exams.

Photos of clinical importance, specimens, instruments and USG are incorporated in this book.

Case discussions and key points in each cases will help students to understand the subject easily. Frequently asked questions are also included after each chapter.

The symbols in the content list will help students to identify the online resources. Besides these, reader will get access to the complimentary e-book also.

N. Hephzibah Kirubamani
A.P. Nalini Alexander
R. Premalatha

Abbreviations

AFI	Amniotic fluid index
AFP	Alpha-foetoprotein
AGC	Atypical glandular cells
AIH	Artificial insemination—husband
AIS	Adenocarcinoma in situ
AMTSL	Active management of third stage of labour
APH	Antepartum haemorrhage
APLA	Anti-phospholipid antibody syndrome
APTT	Activated partial thromboplastin time
ARM	Artificial rupture of membranes
ART	Assisted reproductive technique
ASD	Atrial septal defect
AUB	Abnormal uterine bleeding
BBT	Basal body temperature
BMI	Body mass index
BOH	Bad obstetric history
BPD	Biparietal diameter
BRCA 1 and 2	Breast cancer gene 1 and 2
CCF	Congestive cardiac failure
CDC	Centers for Disease Control
CEA	Carcinoembryonic antigen
CGy	Centigray
CIN	Cervical intra-epithelial neoplasia
CPD	Cephalopelvic disproportion
CPT	Complete perineal tear
CRL	Crown–rump length
CT	Clotting time
CTG	Cardiotocograph
CVS	Cardiovascular system
DC	Differential count
DIPSI	Diabetes in Pregnancy Study Group India
DIVC	Disseminated intra-vascular coagulation
DNA	Deoxyribonucleic acid
DUB	Dysfunctional uterine bleeding
EDD	Expected date of delivery
Eff	Effacement
ESR	Erythrocyte sedimentation rate
FAQ	Frequently asked questions
FDG PET	Fluorodeoxyglucose positron emission tomography
FHR	Foetal heart rate
FOGSI	Federation of Obstetrics and Gynaecological Societies of India
FSH	Follicle-stimulating hormone
GA	Gestational age
GCT	Glucose challenge test

GnRHa	Gonadotropin-releasing hormone analogues
GTT	Glucose tolerance test
H/O	History of
H$_2$O	Water
Hb	Haemoglobin
HbA1C	Glycosylated haemoglobin, type A1C
HBsAg	Hepatitis B surface antigen
HC	Head circumference
HCG	Human chorionic gonadotropin
HELLP	Haemolysis, elevated liver enzymes, low platelet count
HIFU	High-intensity focused ultrasound
HIV	Human immunodeficiency virus
HPO	Hypothalamo pituitary ovarian
HPV	Human papilloma virus
HSG	Hysterosalpingogram
ICMR	Indian Council of Medical Research
ICSI	Intra-cytoplasmic sperm injection
IM	Intra-muscular
INR	International normalised ratio
IO chart	Intake output chart
ITP	Idiopathic thrombocytopenic purpura
IUCD	Intra-uterine contraceptive device
IUD	Intra-uterine death
IUGR	Intra-uterine growth restriction
IV	Intravenous
IVC	Inferior vena cava
IVF	In vitro fertilisation
IVP	Intravenous pyelogram
JVP	Jugular venous pressure
LBC	Liquid-based cytology
LBW	Low birth weight
LDH	Lactic dehydrogenase
LEEP	Loop electrosurgical excision procedure
LH	Luteinising hormone
LLETZ	Large loop excision of transformation zone
LMP	Last menstrual period
LPD	Luteal phase defect
LSA	Left sacroanterior
LSCS	Lower segment caesarean section
MAP	Mean arterial pressure
MBP	Modified bio physical profile
MAS	Meconium aspiration syndrome
MCA	Middle cerebral artery
MCDA	Monochrionic diamniotic twins
MCH	Mean corpuscular haemoglobin
MCHC	Mean corpuscular haemoglobin concentration
MCV	Mean corpuscular volume
MgSO$_4$	Magnesium sulphate

MRI	Magnetic resonance imaging
MS	Mitral stenosis
MTP	Medical termination of pregnancy
Na	Sodium
NETZ	Needle excision of transformation zone
NICE	National Institute for Health and Care Excellence
NICU	Neonatal intensive care unit
NO	Nitric oxide
NST	Non-stress test
NT	Nuchal translucency
NYHA	New York Heart Association
O_2	Oxygen
OCP	Oral contraceptive pill
PAPPA	Pregnancy-associated plasma protein A
PCOD	Polycystic ovarian disorder
PCOS	Polycystic ovarian syndrome
PCV	Packed cell volume
PE	Pre-eclampsia
PGE2	Prostaglandin E2
PGI2	Prostaglandin I2
PI	Pulsatility index
PID	Pelvic inflammatory disease
PIGF	Placental growth factor
PNMR	Perinatal mortality rate
POD	Pouch of Douglas
PPH	Post-partum haemorrhage
PPROM	Pre-term premature rupture of membranes
PR	Per rectal
PRL	Prolactin
PROM	Premature rupture of membranes
PT	Prothrombin time
PV	Per vaginal
RBC	Red blood corpuscle
Rh −ve	Rhesus negative
RI	Resistance index
RS	Respiratory system
RT	Radiotherapy
SERM	Selective oestrogen receptor modulator
SGA	Small for gestational age
SGOT	Serum glutamic oxaloacetic transaminase
SGPT	Serum glutamic pyruvic transaminase
SLE	Systemic lupus erythematosis
St.	Station
STI	Sexually transmitted infections
TAS	Transabdominal scan
TB	Tuberculosis
TC	Total white blood cell count
TIBC	Total iron-binding capacity

TO mass	Tubo-ovarian mass
TOF	Tetralogy of Fallot
TVS	Transvaginal scan
USG	Ultra sonogram
UTI	Urinary tract infection
VBAC	Vaginal birth after caesarean
VDRL	Venereal Disease Research Laboratory
VEGF	Vascular endothelial growth factor
VIA	Visual inspection with acetic acid
VILI	Visual inspection with Lugol's iodine
VSD	Ventricular septal defect
VVF	Vesicovaginal fistula
WHO	World Health Organisation

PART 1

OBSTETRIC CASES

1. OBSTETRIC HISTORY TAKING AND EXAMINATION 3
2. NORMAL PREGNANCY 37
3. A CASE OF ANAEMIA COMPLICATING PREGNANCY 43
4. A CASE OF HYPERTENSION IN PREGNANCY 53
5. A CASE OF PROLONGED (POST-TERM) PREGNANCY 69
6. A CASE OF PREGNANCY FOLLOWING CAESAREAN SECTION 79
7. A CASE OF HEART DISEASE COMPLICATING PREGNANCY 87
8. A CASE OF MALPRESENTATION 97
9. A CASE OF MULTIPLE PREGNANCY 107
10. A CASE OF RH NEGATIVE PREGNANCY 117
11. A CASE OF CEPHALOPELVIC DISPROPORTION 125
12. A CASE OF DIABETES COMPLICATING PREGNANCY 137
13. A CASE OF RECURRENT PREGNANCY LOSS 147
14. A CASE OF FOETAL GROWTH RESTRICTION 155
15. NORMAL PUERPERIUM AND POSTNATAL CARE 161
16. VIVA VOCE (ORAL EXAM) 171

OBSTETRIC HISTORY TAKING AND EXAMINATION

CASE 1

INTRODUCTION
History taking and clinical examination are essential skills for best clinical practice. Sound clinical knowledge is necessary in order to direct questions and it will help to shape presentation appropriately. Basic skills of history taking and physical examination can be easily acquired by examination of patients with different clinical conditions and sound theory knowledge.

GUIDELINES FOR OBSTETRIC HISTORY TAKING
Careful history taking is a clinical guide to perform physical examination that is to follow. Based on history, some signs may have to be elicited which is not done routinely. It is useful to have a checklist of what history is to be elicited, so that inadvertent omission of important details can be prevented and presentation will be in a logical sequence.

- Patient's Details
- History
- Physical Examination
  - *General Examination*
  - *Systemic Examination*
  - *Obstetric Examination*
- Summary of the case
- Provisional Diagnosis
- Differential Diagnosis

Patient's details
First introduce yourself and collect details.
   Following details are to be obtained:
   Name/Age/Address/Occupation/Socioeconomic Class...
   Gravida/Para/Booked/Unbooked .... Immunised—against tetanus .... LMP—last menstrual period/
   EDD—expected date of delivery

History
- H/O months of amenorrhoea/period of gestation with chief complaints, for example bleeding per vaginum, pain in abdomen etc.
- History of present illness

CASE 1 OBSTETRIC HISTORY TAKING AND EXAMINATION

- History of present pregnancy
- Menstrual history
- Marital history
- Past obstetric history
- Past medical history and drug history
- Past surgical history
- Family history
- Personal history

Discussion on patient details and it's importance
Name

Age

> Teenage pregnancy will have specific complications.

Maternal complications of teenage pregnancy
- Anaemia
- Abortion
- Cephalopelvic disproportion (CPD)/preeclampsia/abruption
- Pre-term delivery
- Psychological problems/failure of lactation

Foetal complications of teenage pregnancy
- Foetal growth restriction (FGR) (previous terminology—IUGR)
- Low birth weight
- Pre-term birth

> Elderly primi (35 years and above): pregnancy above 35 years will have specific complications.

Maternal complications of elderly primi
- Abortion
- CPD
- Diabetes
- Hypertension
- Pre-eclampsia/superimposed pre-eclampsia
- Abruptio placenta
- Exaggeration of existing medical problems
- Increased incidence of prolonged pregnancy
- Fibroid complicating pregnancy
- Prolonged labour due to anxiety
- Incoordinate uterine action during labour

- Increased chances for operative delivery (inelastic soft tissue of birth passage and impaired mobility of joints)
- Traumatic and atonic post-partum haemorrhage (PPH)
- Failure of lactation (sometimes)

Foetal complications of elderly primi
- FGR (previous terminology—IUGR)
- Low birth weight
- Pre-term birth
- Chromosomal anomalies, foetal anomalies

Address (urban, rural, slum, semi-urban)

Occupation

Socioeconomic class

Class 1	Executives
Class 2	Professionals
Class 3	Skilled
Class 4	Semi-skilled
Class 5	Unskilled

Specific problems based on low socioeconomic class:
- Anaemia
- Pre-eclampsia
- Abruptio placenta
- Pre-term delivery
- Premature rupture of membrane (PROM)
- Rheumatic heart disease
- Lack of antenatal care and family planning methods
- FGR/intra-uterine death (IUD)

Higher socioeconomic class is prone for:
- Hypertension
- Diabetes
- Obesity
- CPD
- Prolonged pregnancy
- Increased operative deliveries
- PPH
- Lactation failure
- Macrosomia

CASE 1 OBSTETRIC HISTORY TAKING AND EXAMINATION

TERMINOLOGY
Various terms used in obstetric history are given in Table 1.1.

Table 1.1 Terminology

Gravida	Number of pregnancies including present pregnancy irrespective of the outcome of pregnancy. Example: If a woman had delivered one term child, then delivered twins, had two abortions, and now if she is pregnant, she will be gravida 5.
Para	Previous number of deliveries, which has crossed the period of viability irrespective of outcome of pregnancy excluding present pregnancy. Example: If a woman had delivered one term child, then delivered twins, had two abortions, and now if she is pregnant, she will be para 2, living 3, abortion 2.
	For calculating gravida, abortion, ectopic gestation, vesicular mole, previous deliveries are included.
Abortion	Expulsion of the products of conception before period of viability, that is before 28 weeks or <1000 g in developing countries. Period of viability according to WHO—22 weeks, RCOG—24 weeks, weight—500 g.
Ectopic gestation	Pregnancy outside the uterine cavity.
Vesicular mole	It is an abnormal pregnancy where there is hydropic degeneration of chorionic villi.
Pre-term delivery	Delivery of foetus after 28 weeks and before 37 completed weeks of pregnancy.
Post-term delivery	Delivery after 42 completed weeks.
Nulligravida	Is one who is not pregnant now and never had been pregnant.
Nullipara	Is one who has never had a previous pregnancy, which has crossed the period of viability. She might or might not have aborted.
Primigravida	Is one who is pregnant for the first time.
Primipara	Is one who has delivered once beyond the period of viability.
Multigravida	Is one who has been pregnant previously.
Multipara	Is one who has delivered two or more deliveries beyond period of viability.
Grand multigravida	Is one who has been pregnant 5 times or more.
Grand multipara	Is one who has already had five or more deliveries beyond the period of viability.
Parturient	Is a woman in labour.
Puerpera	Is a woman who has just given birth.

Booking
Booking visit is the first antenatal visit when you register the patient for antenatal care.
Importance of booking
- To identify and assess risk factors, if present
- To give proper antenatal care

- To identify woman requiring multi-speciality care
- To diagnose women with asymptomatic disease
- To establish the correct gestational age
- To elicit past medical and surgical history
- To perform baseline investigations like Hb, blood group and Rh typing and urine analysis

Ideal antenatal booking
Antenatal booking in weeks is as follows:

Up to 28 weeks	Once in 4 weeks
28–36 weeks	Once in 2 weeks
36–40 weeks	Weekly

WHO Guidelines—four visits at specified intervals
WHO Guidelines at Specified Intervals

First	8–12 weeks	To confirm pregnancy, to calculate expected date of delivery (EDD), to classify women for basic four visits or more specialised care; screen, treat and give preventive measures; develop a birth and emergency plan; advice and counsel
Second	24–26 weeks	To assess maternal and foetal well-being; exclude PE and anaemia, can give preventive measures; review and modify birth and emergency plan; advice and counsel
Third	32 weeks	Assess maternal and foetal well-being, exclude anaemia, PE, multiple pregnancies, give preventive measures; review and modify birth and emergency plan; advice and counsel
Fourth	36–38 weeks	Assess maternal and foetal well being; exclude PE, anaemia, multiple pregnancy malpresentation; give preventive measures; review and modify birth and emergency plan; advice and counsel

Minimum antenatal booking

First Trimester	1
Second Trimester	1
Third Trimester	3

Immunisation
All pregnant women must be immunised with tetanus toxoid and it is mandatory.

First dose is given usually at the booking visit or at 16–20 weeks. Second dose is given at 4–6 weeks later. If woman becomes pregnant within 3 years, then single booster dose is given.

More than 3 years—re-immunize.

Immunisation against diphtheria

According to WHO guidelines: Two doses of tetanus toxoid or combined tetanus/diphtheria vaccine (Td) is given 1 month apart before delivery.

LMP: First day of the last menstrual period
- LMP is used to calculate EDD.
- *Naegele's rule*—Add 9 months and add 7 days or go back 3 months and add 7 days.
- Applicable when menstrual cycles are once in 28 days; only 4% will deliver on EDD.

- If the cycles are irregular, corrected EDD can be calculated by adding maximum of up to 14 days only.
- For example: If cycle are once in 40 days—then corrected EDD = calculated EDD + 12 days.

HISTORY
CHIEF COMPLAINTS TO BE NOTED IN CHRONOLOGICAL ORDER
- If there is no complaint, find out if she has come for regular antenatal check-up.
- Whether admitted for safe confinement in view of her past obstetric history.
- Whether admitted for investigations and management.

HISTORY OF PRESENT ILLNESS
Chief complaints should be elaborated with regard to following details:
- Onset
- Duration
- Severity
- Relieving and aggravating factors, if present
- Associated symptoms
- Medication used and any progress made

Example: Complaints of bleeding P/V
It is important to enquire into duration, amount of bleeding, association with pain and whether bleeding is continuing. History of precipitating factors like trauma, travel, coitus should be asked for and similar bleeding episodes in the past are to be enquired. If bleeding occurs in second or third trimester, history regarding perception of foetal movements should be asked for.

HISTORY OF PRESENT PREGNANCY
Chronological events that happen during each trimester should be precisely asked for:
- How long after marriage conception occurred?
- Whether conception occurred spontaneously.
- Any contraception practiced and if so, when it was stopped?
- If woman gives history of infertility, details regarding investigations for the same to be obtained.
- Whether conception occurred after induction of ovulation or other assisted reproductive technique.

History to be elicited in first trimester:
- How and when pregnancy was confirmed?
- H/O dating scan and findings, if available.
- Morning sickness, hyperemesis and treatment for the same.
- Fever with rashes, any other fever or infection, drug intake.
- Folic acid intake or any other drug intake.
- Exposure to irradiation.

HISTORY

- Bleeding PV.
- Investigations done and if any abnormality found.

History to be elicited in second trimester:
- Quickening.
- Immunisation.
- Anomaly scan and findings, if available.
- Intake of iron, folic acid and calcium.
- Glucose challenge test (GCT) and reports, if available.

History to be elicited third trimester:
- Perception of foetal movements.
- Growth scan.
- Discharge or draining PV, bleeding PV.
- Any other relevant history according to the respective case (Table 1.2).

In first trimester, date of confirmation of pregnancy by urine pregnancy test and dating scan is helpful in arriving at gestational age.

Details of laboratory tests like VDRL, Hb, blood group, Rh typing, HbsAg, HIV, blood sugar, GCT, HbA1C should be obtained.

> Organised, logical way of history taking is essential. Sometimes after physical examination we may have to go back for some more detailed history.

MENSTRUAL HISTORY

- Menstrual cycle—regularity, frequency, duration, amount of blood loss.
- LMP—is the first day of last menstrual period and by using this EDD is calculated. It is applicable only in 28 days regular cycle and prior to conception woman should have had three regular cycles and she should not have taken oral combined contraceptive pill 2 months before conception.

> Naegele's rule—add 9 months and add 7 days or go back 3 months and add 7 days to LMP to arrive at EDD.

- Applicable when menstrual cycles are once in 28 days. Only 4% will deliver on EDD.

Example: when LMP is 1st February, by adding 7 days, it becomes 8th and by adding 9 months, it comes to November 8th, which will be the EDD.

Corrected EDD (Knane's rule)
- When cycle is shorter or longer than 28 days, EDD will be corrected accordingly.
- Suppose if menstrual cycle is once in 21 days, the corrected EDD will be less by 7 days.
- If menstrual cycle is once in 40 days, for corrected EDD, add 12 days to calculated EDD. EDD can be corrected up to 14 days only.

Table 1.2 Relevance of History and Diagnosis

First Trimester, up to 12 Weeks	Second Trimester, 13–28 Weeks	Third Trimester, up to 40 Weeks
When and how pregnancy was confirmed (by urine test or USG) Morning sickness Excess vomiting means *hyperemesis gravidarum*	Swelling in the legs can be due to physiological oedema, which is seen in dependant parts, more towards evening and disappears after 12 h of rest	Swelling in the legs can be due to physiological oedema or pathological oedema
It can be due to vesicular mole, multiple pregnancy, metabolic causes, medical conditions like jaundice, gastritis, UTI to be ruled out in hyperemesis gravidarum	Pathological oedema seen in parts like face, dorsum of hand, (tightening of the ring) abdominal wall, lower limbs, vulva and pre-sacral area. It can be due to anaemia, pre-eclampsia, heart disease, renal disease, liver disease hypoproteinaemia	It can be due to same causes similar to second trimester
If bleeding occurs—it may be due to *threatened abortion, missed abortion, vesicular mole, inevitable abortion*	If bleeding PV occurs with or without pain—causes may be same as in first trimester bleeding up to period of viability	*If bleeding PV occurs—it may indicate* show/antepartum haemorrhage or lesions in cervix
If there is history of passage of products of conception, it denotes *incomplete abortion*	*After period of viability* abruptio placenta, placenta previa to be ruled out	*In painful bleeding PV*—rule out abruptio placenta *In painless bleeding PV*—rule out placenta previa
In missed abortion, symptoms of pregnancy subside	H/O immunisation against tetanus to be elicited	
In vesicular mole, history of passage of vesicles may be present *In ectopic gestation*, history of pain, syncope and fainting attack may be present *Lesions in the cervix to be ruled out*		
Vaginal discharge—may be due to *moniliasis*, which is common during pregnancy	Quickening—occurs in primi, around 20 weeks and in multi, between 16 and 18 weeks	If there is draining PV—it may be due to PPROM or PROM
History of taking folic acid to be elicited; history of any other drug intake—to rule out teratogenic effect on foetus	Whether iron, folic acid and calcium tablets were taken; history of any other drug intake	If woman has lower abdominal pain, it can be due to pre-term labour, false labour or true labour pains
Fever with rash—may indicate *measles and other viral infections*, which may have teratogenic effect	Enquire about foetal movements: excessive foetal movements may be due to *multiple pregnancy*	Enquire about foetal movements: excessive foetal movements may be due to *multiple pregnancy*
Exposure to radiation—may have teratogenic effect	Diminished foetal movements—may be due to *oligohydramnios, FGR*	Diminished foetal movements—may be due to *oligohydramnios, FGR, prolonged pregnancy*

Table 1.2 Relevance of History and Diagnosis (*cont.*)

First Trimester, up to 12 Weeks	Second Trimester, 13–28 Weeks	Third Trimester, up to 40 Weeks
Up to 5 rads is permissible	Loss of foetal movements—may be due to *IUD*	Loss of foetal movements—may be due to *IUD*
Burning and frequency of micturition indicates *UTI* UTI—has impact on pregnancy like threatened abortion, pre-term labour, IUGR	If pathological oedema is present, H/O blurring of vision, epigastric pain, vomiting, diminished urine output should be elicited *(symptoms of imminent eclampsia)* Breathlessness, fatigue, swelling of legs may indicate *anaemia complicating pregnancy* Breathlessness, swelling of legs, palpitation, recurrent respiratory infection, blood-stained sputum may indicate *heart disease complicating pregnancy*	If pathological oedema is present, similar history as in second trimester is to be elicited to rule out imminent eclampsia, anaemia and heart disease complicating pregnancy
H/O first trimesters scan done dating and NT	*H/O anomaly scan done* between 18 and 20 weeks	H/O growth scan done

FGR, Foetal growth restriction; IUD, intra-uterine death; NT, nuchal translucency; PPROM, pre-term premature rupture of membrane; PROM, premature rupture of membrane; UTI, urinary tract infection.

- Sometimes woman may conceive in the lactation period, in such cases LMP is not reliable.
- Woman may tell her LMP in the months according to regional Tamil months or express her LMP some days after or before an important day like Pongal or Diwali. One should know about this to calculate EDD.

Determination of gestational age when LMP is not known
- If patient can remember the date of single coitus, it is quite reliable to predict the expected date with accuracy.
- If conception occurred with induction of ovulation with drugs like clomiphene, HCG and follicular study was done, date of ovulation will be known.
- Date of quickening—probable date of delivery can be arrived by adding 20 weeks in primi, 22 weeks in multi from date of quickening.
- Per vaginal examination findings in first trimester.
- Height of uterus in second trimester.
- Palpation of foetal parts at the earliest by 20 weeks.
- Detection of foetal heart by hand Doppler by 10–12 weeks and auscultation of foetal heart at the earliest by 20 weeks by foetoscope.
- Previous available records like urine pregnancy test date.
- Dating scan by USG.

MARITAL HISTORY
- Duration of marriage
- Whether consanguineous marriage—find out degree of consanguinity
  - First degree—Siblings (Incest)
  - Second degree—Maternal uncle
  - Third degree—Cousins
- If there is history of planning—(postponement) enquire about contraception and it's type
- If history of infertility is present, investigations done and treatment taken should be elicited

PAST OBSTETRIC HISTORY
Previous obstetric events must be documented in chronological order.

Following relevant history about abortion is to be elicited:
- Gestational age at the time of abortion.
- Whether abortion was spontaneous/induced and certified by doctor.
- Whether USG was done and if so whether foetal death occurred after cardiac activity. If there was no cardiac activity, no foetal pole it means blighted ovum.
- Whether curettage was done or medical abortion done.
- Post-abortal period—H/O fever, H/O blood transfusion.
- History of any preceding events like fever, infection, trauma, drug intake or long travel.
- When did she establish periods after abortion?
- Sudden rupture of membrane with painless expulsion of foetus, which may indicate cervical incompetence.
- In Rh −ve woman whether anti-D was given—following abortion.
- H/O recurrent abortions.
- History of abnormal pregnancy like ectopic pregnancy, vesicular mole to be elicited.

Previous pregnancy, labour and delivery—following details are to be elicited:
- History regarding antenatal care, antenatal complications, intrapartum complications, post-partum and post-natal complications to be elicited
- Period of gestation at the time of delivery—pre-term, term or post-term
- One should know whether it is domiciliary delivery or hospital delivery conducted by dhai, midwife or doctor
- Spontaneous onset of labour pains or labour was induced [if labour was induced, whether cervical ripening agent—gel (PGE2) or augmentation with (oxytocin) drip was given]
- Duration of labour—prolonged labour may be due to CPD, malpresentation, malposition and might result in asphyxiated baby or IUD
- If episiotomy was given or any vaginal lacerations were present; if so whether they were sutured
- Whether natural vaginal delivery/forceps/vacuum/assisted vaginal breech delivery
- History of excessive bleeding after delivery (PPH)/manual removal of placenta/blood transfusion should be elicited
- Weight of the baby, whether cried immediately after birth, roomed with the mother or in NICU, how long breast fed and present condition of the baby

- If weight of the baby is >3.5 kg/stillbirth—rule out GDM in subsequent pregnancy
- If there was history of IUD—find out whether fresh/macerated or anomalous baby
- If there was history of neonatal death—find out regarding anomaly of the baby
- In Rh −ve woman, whether anti-D was given in the antenatal period or after delivery
- Example: Full-term normal vaginal delivery—male baby weighing 3.1 kg—3 years alive and healthy

In lower segment caesarean section, following details are to be noted:
- Whether it was elective or emergency LSCS
- Probable indication—recurrent (contracted pelvis) or non-recurrent (breech, placenta previa, malposition and presentation, abruption, failure to progress, eclampsia, big baby, foetal distress etc.)
- H/O blood transfusion, post-operative distension, repeated urinary tract infection (UTI), wound sepsis, resuturing, fever, duration of hospital stay
- Details regarding the newborn should be elicited as in vaginal delivery
- Interval between previous LSCS and the subsequent pregnancy (after 18 months, women can be allowed for vaginal birth after caesarean section—VBAC)

Example: Full term LSCS—indication breech presentation, female baby 3.5 kg—2 years alive and healthy. Post-operative period uneventful.

In previous history of pre-term delivery, following details are to be noted:
- History of precipitating factors like anaemia, fever, UTI, pre-eclampsia, IUGR, pre-term premature rupture of membrane (PPROM)
- Whether spontaneous or induced for obstetric reasons like severe pre-eclampsia, IUGR, oligohydramnios with Doppler changes
- Weight of the newborn
- Whether newborn was in NICU and for how long
- Milestones of the baby

Post-partum period—following details are to be elicited:
- History of PPH/H/O blood transfusion.
- Fever/pain/lochia—healthy or offensive (to rule out puerperal sepsis).
- Retention of urine, frequency of urine, fever (UTI).
- History suggestive of deep vein thrombosis (unilateral leg oedema with pain, redness).
- When she resumed her periods after delivery and regularity of menstrual cycle?

Lactation—following details are to be elicited:
- When did the woman start lactation, within half an hour or later or after some medications?
- History of sore nipple or retracted nipple or breast abscess.
- Complete failure of lactation.
- How long she was lactating?

Contraceptive history
H/O IUCD insertion/contraceptive pill use/barrier method following previous pregnancy.

PAST MEDICAL HISTORY

- This is very important because medical disorder has effect on pregnancy and pregnancy has effect on medical disorder.
- Drugs taken for certain medical diseases also have impact on the foetus.
- Medical condition can remain the same during pregnancy or worsen.
- Diabetes—insulin dependent or not and medications taken for the same.
- Heart disease—rheumatic heart disease or congenital.
- H/O cardiac surgery/valve prosthesis/pacemaker/taking cardiac drugs and anti-coagulants.
- Thyroid—hypo- or hyperthyroidism and medication taken.
- Epilepsy—duration and therapy—mono or triple drugs.
- Hypertension—duration and drug taken.
- History suggestive of systemic lupus erythematosus (SLE), anti-phospholipid antibody syndrome (APLA—skin lesion, thrombosis, recurrent pregnancy loss).
- Bronchial asthma—medication/corticosteroids usage.
- Tuberculosis—drug therapy.
- H/O allergy, blood transfusion.
- Drug taken for any other chronic illness.

PAST SURGICAL HISTORY

General surgical
Cholecystectomy/appendicectomy/laparotomy

Gynaecological surgery
- Laparoscopy/myomectomy/CPT repair/VVF repair
- Amputation of cervix, Fothergill's operation
- Any problems with anaesthesia in previous surgery

FAMILY HISTORY

- H/O diabetes, hypertension, history of twins
- Hereditary diseases like haemoglobinopathies, genetic disorders, congenital anomalies in siblings
- History of pre-eclampsia in mother and siblings

PERSONAL HISTORY

- History of drug abuse/smoking—may lead to FGR; alcohol—may lead to foetal alcohol syndrome
- History regarding bowel habits, micturition, sleep pattern, appetite should be taken

PHYSICAL EXAMINATION

Physical examination is to be done after taking permission politely to examine the woman.

Physical examination in obstetrics is unique in many aspects. The technique for physical examination involves skill and it is different from other specialties. When male doctor examines the pregnant woman, a female attendant should be available.

GENERAL EXAMINATION

This is of utmost importance because it gives an overview about the pregnant woman.

Stature
- Skeletal framework of a person can be noted as average/short stature/tall. Height of the woman is to be noted in centimetre.
- Short stature is 145 cm and less.

Nourishment
- Thin built/moderately built/obese

Weight
- Pre-pregnant weight has to be noted to calculate weight gain during pregnancy
- Calculation of BMI—weight in kilograms/height in square metres

<18.5	Underweight
18.5–25	Normal
25–29.9	Overweight
>30	Obesity

- *Underweight and obesity* can cause antenatal and perinatal complications
- *Total weight gain during pregnancy: 9–12 kg*

Total weight gain during first trimester: 1 kg; not much weight is gained due to vomiting and there may be loss of weight.

Second trimester: 3–4 kg
Third trimester: 4–6 kg

When weight gain is more than 1/2 kg/week, it may be early manifestation of pre-eclampsia—due to occult oedema.

Underweight women	should gain 12–14 kg
Average weight women	should gain 10–12 kg
Overweight women	should gain 8–10 kg
Obese women	should gain <8 kg

Causes of increased weight gain during pregnancy:

Multiple pregnancy, pre-eclampsia, polyhydramnios, gestational diabetes with macrosomia or obesity

CASE 1 OBSTETRIC HISTORY TAKING AND EXAMINATION

Causes of decreased weight gain during pregnancy:

FGR, anaemia, malnutrition, thin build

In prolonged pregnancy:
There may be drop in weight after crossing EDD due to oligohydramnios or increase in weight may be due to macrosomia after crossing EDD

Anaemia
- Site to look for pallor—lower palpebral conjunctiva, nail beds, tip of the tongue, soft palate, palms and soles (Fig. 1.1 A-D).

Cyanosis
- May be due to heart disease, cor pulmonale.
- Sites to look for peripheral cyanosis—hands, feet, fingers, toes and nail beds.
- Sites to look for central cyanosis—tongue, lips.
- Concomitant peripheral (Fig. 1.2A) and central cyanosis (Fig. 1.2B) may be present.

Jaundice
Sites to look for jaundice (Fig. 1.3) are upper bulbar, conjunctiva, under surface of tongue, soft palate, sole, palm and skin. Jaundice can be due to hepatitis, haemolysis, HELLP syndrome, cholestatic jaundice of pregnancy, sepsis.

Clubbing
Clubbing is associated with (Fig. 1.4) any disease featuring chronic hypoxia like congenital cyanotic heart disease/sub-acute bacterial endocarditis/atrial myxoma (benign tumour)/lung disease/gastrointestinal and hepatobiliary disease.

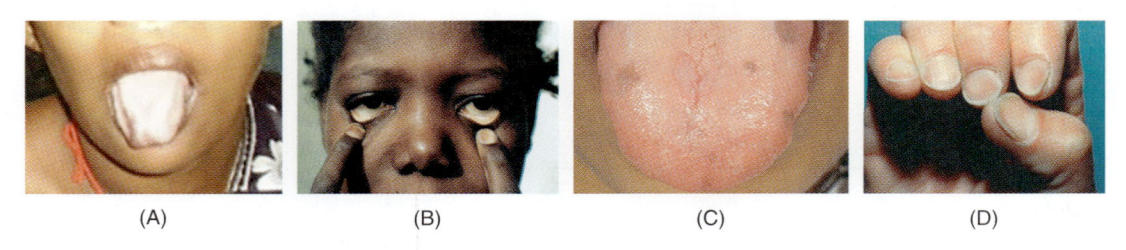

(A)   (B)   (C)   (D)

FIGURE 1.1

Site to look for pallor: (A) Pale Tongue (B) lower palpebral conjunctiva (C) Tip of the Tongue (D) Nail Beds

From Daftary, S.N., Manual of Obstetrics, fourth ed., p. 106, Fig 13.1A–C.

HISTORY   17

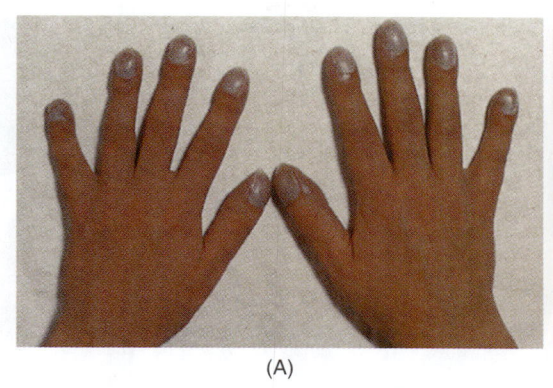

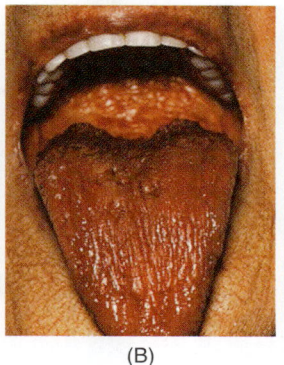

FIGURE 1.2

(A) Peripheral Cyanosis and (B) Central Cyanosis

Source: Part (A): Approach to the patient with possible cardiovascular disease. In: Goldman L., Schafe A.I. (Eds.), Goldman's Cecil Medicine, twenty fourth ed. Imprint Elsevier. pp. 246–255, Part (B): General patient examination and differential diagnosis. In: Glynn M., Drak W.M. (Eds.), Hutchison's Clinical Methods, twenty fourth ed. Imprint Elsevier.

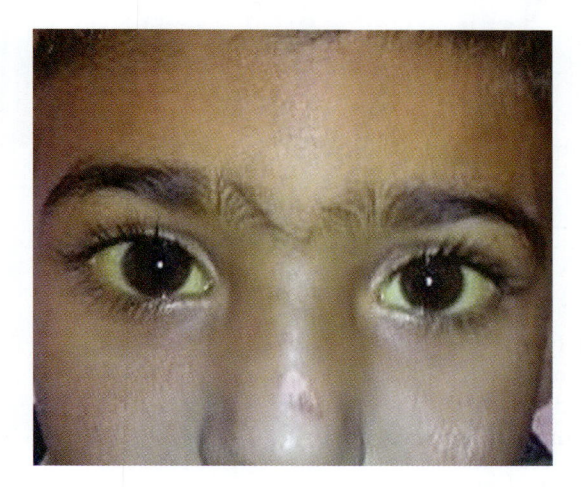

FIGURE 1.3   Jaundice

Others:
- Grave's disease (autoimmune hyperthyroidism)—in this case, it is known as thyroid acropachy.
- Familial and racial clubbing and 'pseudo-clubbing' (occurs often in people of African descent).
- Vascular anomalies of the affected arm, such as an axillary artery aneurysm (in unilateral clubbing).

Pedal oedema
- Pedal oedema may be bilateral or unilateral, pitting or non-pitting oedema
- Site to be examined for pedal oedema—pressure applied just above medial malleolus for at least 30 s; anterior surface of the lower third of shin; the dorsum of foot (Fig. 1.5A–C)
- Other sites—Puffiness of face, dorsum of hand, sacrum, abdominal wall (Fig. 1.5D), vulva (Fig. 1.5E)

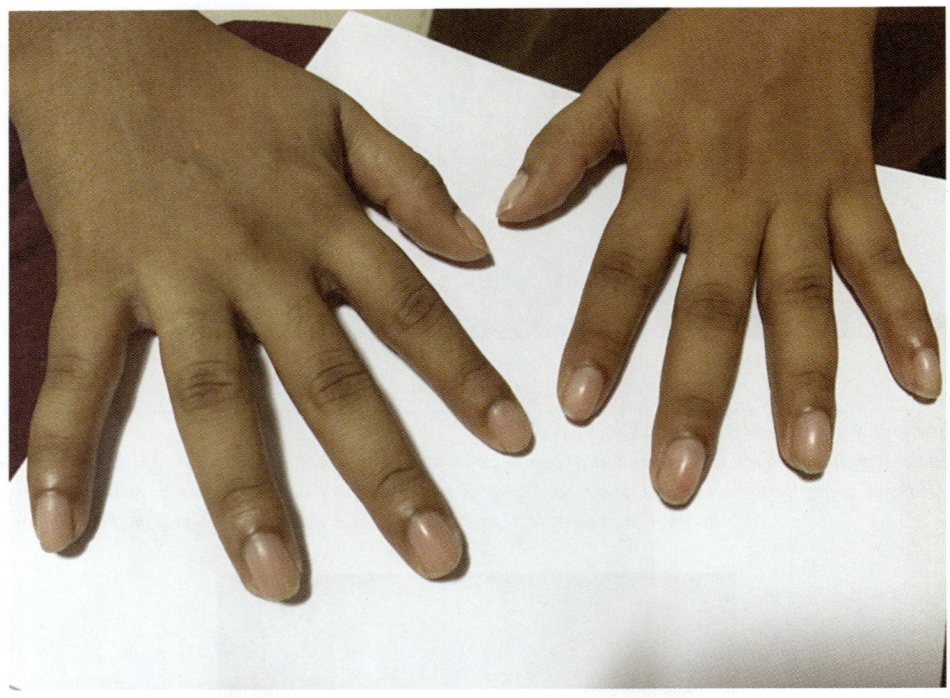

FIGURE 1.4 Clubbing

Physiological oedema
- Disappears after 12 h of rest
- Present only in the dependent parts like ankle and feet
- Mostly present in third trimester
- Not accompanied by diminished urine output

Reasons for physiological oedema
- Pressure on IVC by gravid uterus
- Vasodilatation—due to progesterone
- Change in colloid and hydrostatic pressure
- Na and H_2O retention due to oestrogen and progesterone
- Increase in aldosterone

Pathological oedema	May be due to anaemia, pre-eclampsia, heart disease, renal disease, hepatic disorders, hypoproteinaemia
Unilateral	Deep vein thrombosis, cellulitis, filariasis
Non-pitting	Myxoedema

FIGURE 1.5

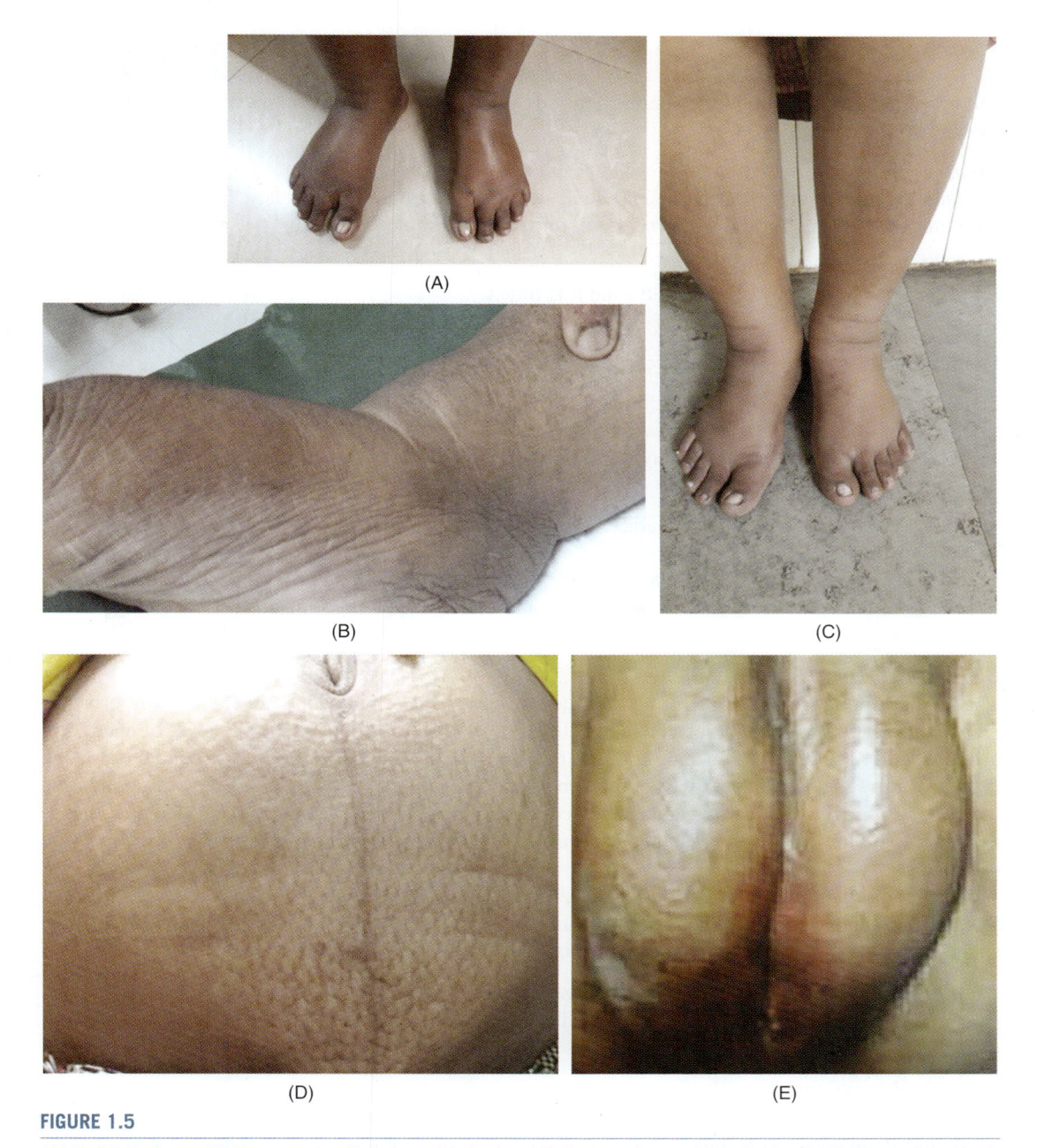

(A) Pedal Oedema, (B) Pressure Applied above Malleolus, (C) Oedema lower third of shin, (D) Oedema abdominal wall (E) Vulval Odema

Varicosities of legs
Varicose veins in the legs and vulva may appear for the first time or get aggravated during pregnancy and it is due to obstruction of the venous return by gravid uterus. Usually varicosities are seen in later months of pregnancy (Fig. 1.6).

Breast examination
In antenatal period, milky discharge may indicate either placental insufficiency, FGR or IUD. Breast lump may be detected for the first time. Look for retracted nipple.

Thyroid enlargement
Multi-nodular goitre may be noticed for the first time.

Tongue, teeth, gum
Examined for—glossitis, stomatitis, caries teeth, gingivitis.

Temperature
- Fever may be due to bacterial/viral infections.
- PROM with chorioamnionitis may result in rise in temperature.

Pulse
- Rate, rhythm, volume, special character, whether felt in all peripheral vessels and radio femoral delay to be noted.
- *Normally in pregnancy, pulse rate increases by about 10–15 beats/min.*
- Tachycardia indicates—heart disease, anaemia with CCF, hyperthyroidism, febrile conditions, infection.

Blood pressure measurement (Fig. 1.7):
This is an important measurement for pregnant women. This can be done either in sitting or semi-recumbent posture with slight left lateral tilt. In all positions, arm should be at the level of heart. Appropriate cuff should be chosen and should be tied firmly. Cuff should go 1.5 times around the arm and bladder width should be at least 40% of the arm circumference. By palpating radial pulse after inflating the cuff, systolic blood pressure can be assessed roughly. Bell or diaphragm can be placed over the inner aspect of elbow joint over brachial pulse; cuff is inflated 20–30 mmHg higher than systolic pressure obtained by palpation.

To record blood pressure: Pressure is released slowly so that mercury descends every 2 mm/beat. Systolic pressure is recorded when repetitive sounds are heard first. In pregnancy, disappearance of the sound—Korotkoff 5 (NICE 2008 guidelines) is taken as diastolic blood pressure.

Examination of cardiovascular and respiratory system
It is very essential; woman may come for medical care for the first time and conditions like asymptomatic heart disease can be diagnosed.

Abdominal examination
- Procedure to be explained to the patient. Pregnant woman is asked to empty the bladder. Examiner should stand on the right side of the pregnant woman to examine her. When male doctor examines the patient, one female attendant should be with him. Pregnant woman is examined in dorsal position, with semi-flexed thigh. Abdomen is fully exposed from xiphisternum to pubic symphysis with the other parts covered.

HISTORY 21

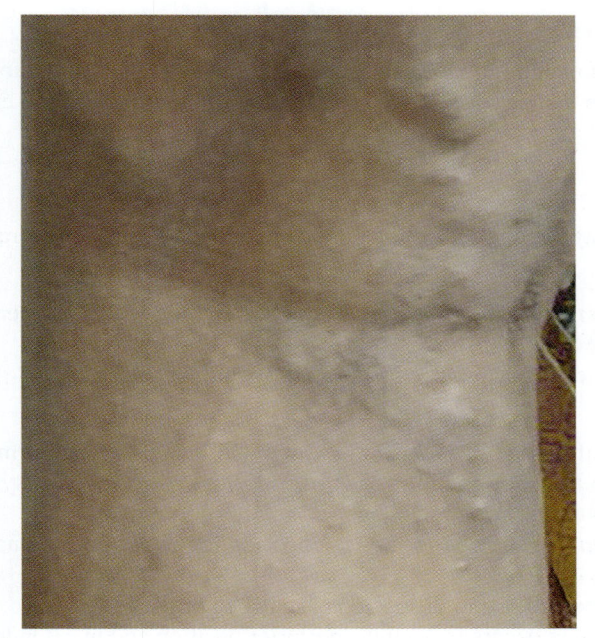

FIGURE 1.6 Varicose Veins

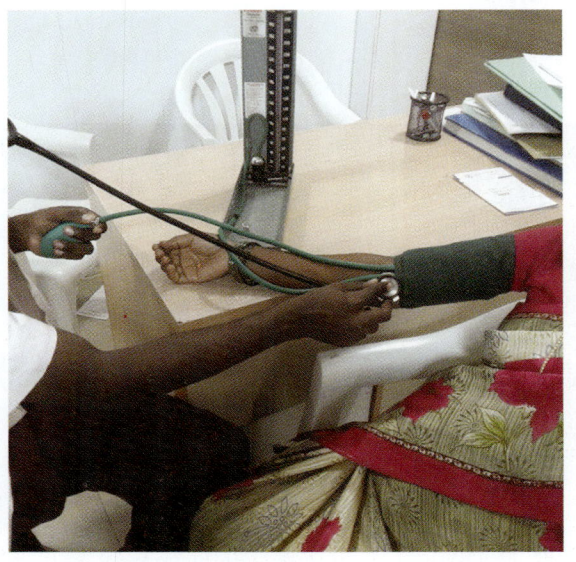

FIGURE 1.7 Method of Blood Pressure Measurement

OBSTETRIC EXAMINATION
The art of obstetric examination includes inspection, palpation and auscultation like other abdominal examination, but certain manoeuvres and techniques are different in obstetric examination.

INSPECTION
Uterine enlargement may be longitudinal (cephalic or breech) or transverse (transverse lie).

Striae gravidarum (Fig. 1.8)
- Linear marks due to rupture of elastic fibres due to stretching which is recent (seen in obesity, Cushing's syndrome also).
- *Striae albicans* is due to previous pregnancy and is white in colour.

Linea nigra (Fig. 1.9)
It is the cutaneous manifestation of pregnancy, which will be a dark line normally from umbilicus to pubic symphysis. It can also be sometimes seen from xiphisternum to pubic symphysis. It is probably due to melanocyte-stimulating hormone of anterior pituitary.

Abdominal wall oedema: can be due to pre-eclampsia, CCF either due to anaemia, heart disease or renal disease
- Umbilicus may be everted due to distension or may be normal
- Sub-umbilical flattening occurs in occipito-posterior position and in extended breech presentation

If scar is present, following points are noted:
- Scar—healthy or unhealthy
- Longitudinal or transverse or other
- Presence of incisional hernia

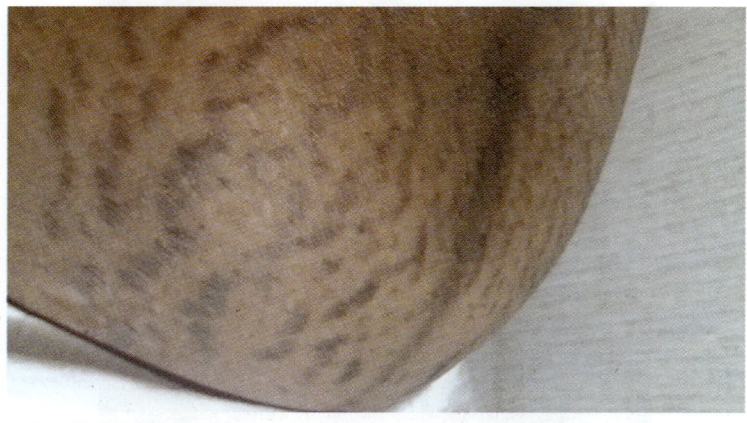

FIGURE 1.8 Striae Gravidarum

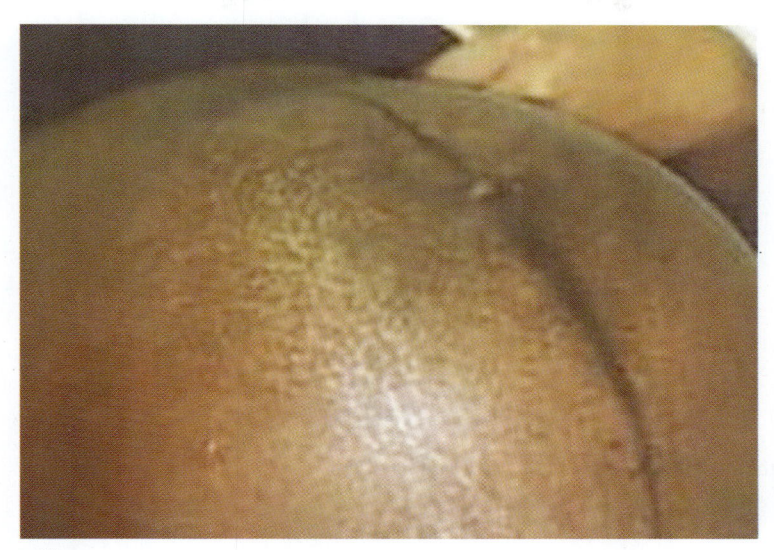

FIGURE 1.9 Linea Nigra

- Presence of keloid
- Pfannenstiel scar may be hidden by pubic hair line
- Infra-umbilical laparoscopic scar may not be clearly visualised

PALPATION

To find out the height of uterus in relation to lunar months, abdomen is arbitrarily divided as follows:
- *From pubic symphysis to umbilicus is divided into three equal parts*
    - Uterine enlargement will be within pelvis up to 12 weeks of pregnancy; uterus becomes palpable per abdomen after 12 weeks (Fig. 1.10)
    - First line of division corresponds to—16 weeks of pregnancy
    - Second line of division—corresponds to 20 weeks of pregnancy
    - At the level of umbilicus—corresponds to 24 weeks of pregnancy
- *From umbilicus to xiphisternum is divided into three equal parts*
    - First line of division above umbilicus corresponds to—28 weeks of pregnancy
    - Second line of division—corresponds to 32 weeks
    - Level of xiphisternum—corresponds to 36 weeks
    - At term the uterine size comes back to the level of 32 weeks but flanks will be full
- *Method:* Palpation will produce some discomfort for the pregnant woman and hence all palpation should be gentle

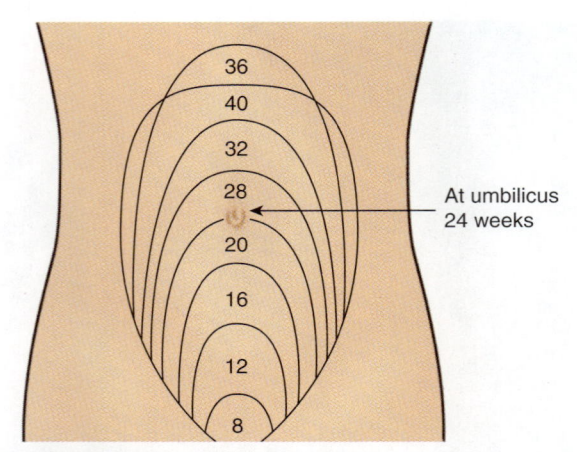

FIGURE 1.10 Arbitrary Lines Corresponding to Gestational Age

- Dextrorotation of the uterus (after 32 weeks) is corrected by pushing the uterus with right hand to the midline
- Dextrorotation is due to the presence of sigmoid colon on the left

Height of the fundus
Height of the fundus is felt with ulnar border of the left hand by moving the left hand downwards from xiphisternum to the upper most level of fundus. First resistance felt is the height of the fundus of the uterus (Fig. 1.11).

Conditions where height of the uterus is bigger than period of amenorrhoea:
- Wrong dates
- Full bladder
- Multiple pregnancy
- Polyhydramnios
- Big baby
- Pelvic tumours complicating pregnancy—ovarian/fibroid
- Vesicular mole

Conditions where height of uterus is lesser than period of amenorrhoea:
- Oligohydramnios
- Transverse lie
- IUD
- FGR
- Missed abortion
- Mistaken dates
- Delayed conception—in irregular periods

PALPATION 25

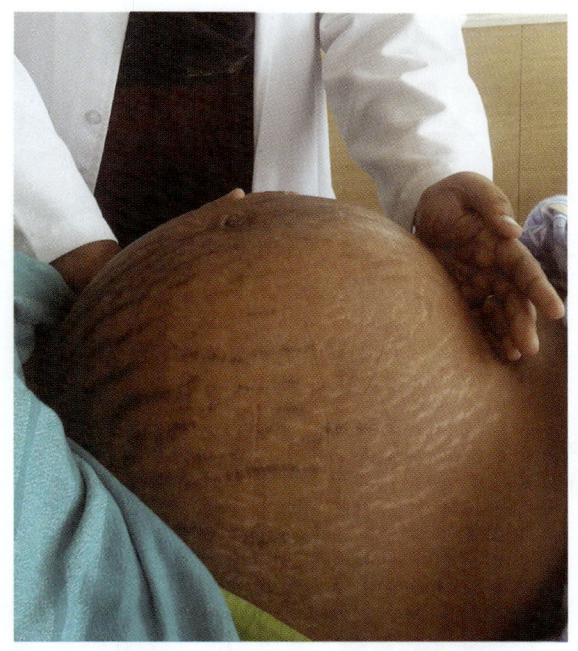

FIGURE 1.11 **Height of Fundus**

> Leopold's manoeuvres—obstetric four grips. First three grips are done by the examiner by facing the pregnant woman's face.

Fundal grip
Fundus is palpated with two hands to find out which part of the foetus is occupying the fundus of the uterus. If it is broad, soft, bulky, not independently ballotable foetal part, then it is breech occupying the fundus. When it is hard, round, independently ballotable foetal part, it is the head of the foetus occupying the fundus (Fig. 1.12).

Umbilical grip
One hand is placed on each side of the uterus and when smooth, curved and hard uniform resistance is felt, it is the back of the foetus and when multiple small nodules are felt, they are the limb buds (Fig. 1.13).

First pelvic grip
Pawlik's grip: Ulnar border of right hand is kept over the pubic symphysis and then with cupped right hand with thumb on one side and other fingers on opposite side, one can grip the foetal part, which occupies the

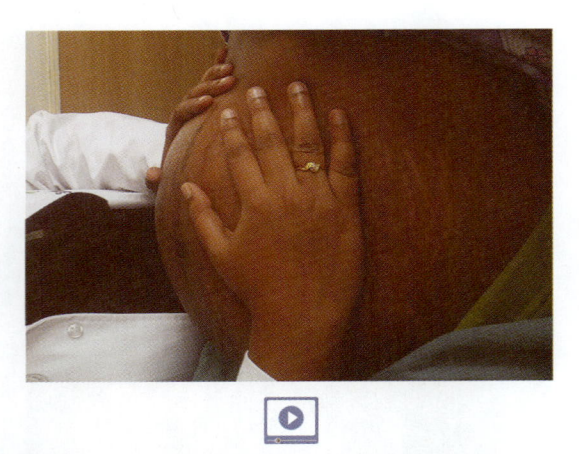

FIGURE 1.12 FUNDAL GRIP

Scan to play Antenatal examination

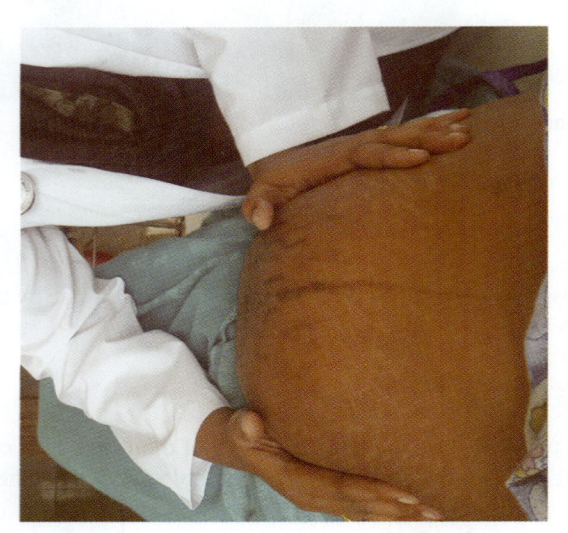

FIGURE 1.13 Umbilical Grip

lower pole of the uterus. If it is hard, round, independently ballotable foetal part it is head of the foetus. If it is broad, soft, irregular, not independently ballotable foetal part then it is the breech. If this grip feels empty it is due to transverse lie (one cannot feel any foetal part in lower pole of uterus) (Fig. 1.14).

Second pelvic grip
Examiner should face the pregnant woman's feet. The purpose is, four fingers of both hands are placed on either sides at the lower abdomen and deep palpation is made in the direction of the pelvic brim. The fingers of one hand will palpate the occiput and the other the sinciput (Fig. 1.15).

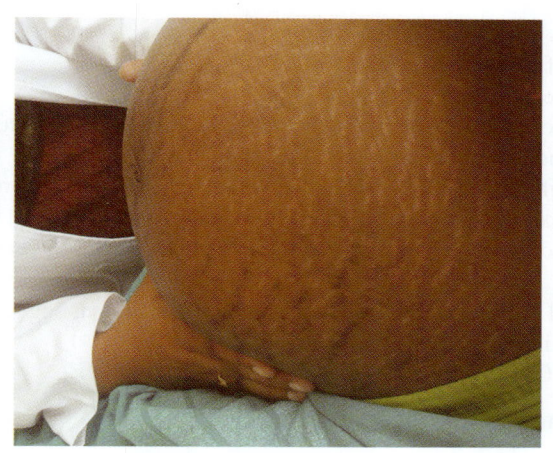

FIGURE 1.14 First Pelvic Grip

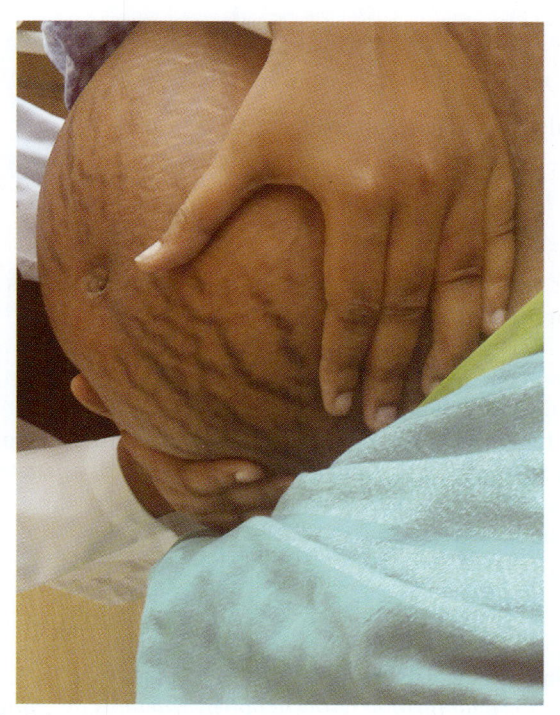

FIGURE 1.15 Second Pelvic Grip

28   CASE 1 OBSTETRIC HISTORY TAKING AND EXAMINATION

Second pelvic grip is done for the following reasons:
- To confirm findings of first pelvic grip
- To find out whether head is engaged or not
- To find out the attitude of head, whether well-flexed, deflexed or extended by noting the relative position of sinciput and occiput
   - If sinciput is at higher level than occiput—it is flexed head—vertex presentation
   - In deflexed head, both occiput and sinciput will be at the same level
   - In extended head, occiput will be at higher level and sinciput at lower level as in brow and face presentation
- If hands diverge, head is engaged and if hands converge, head is unengaged (in primi, head is engaged at 38 weeks, in multi, at the time of labour)
- To find out if there is CPD

Second pelvic grip is not done when head is floating.

Reasons for mobile head at term in primi:
- Wrong dates
- Prematurity
- Placenta previa
- Polyhydramnios
- Multiple pregnancy
- Contracted pelvis, CPD
- Cord around the neck
- Tumours in the lower uterine segment

Foetal cause for mobile head-hydrocephalus

AUSCULTATION

- In cephalic presentation, foetal heart will be heard below umbilicus
- In occipito-anterior or posterior positions, the foetal heart sound (FHS) is heard in the spinoumbilical line on the same side as the back
- In occipito-posterior, FHS is heard more towards the flanks
- In breech presentation, foetal heart will be heard above umbilicus
- In transverse lie, foetal heart will be heard at the level of umbilicus
- In multiple gestation, two foetal hearts will be heard with the difference of 10 beats/min and two observers should hear the foetal hearts in two different areas well separated from each other
- Foetal heart can be heard with bell or diaphragm of stethoscope or Pinard's foetoscope placed over back of foetus; hand Doppler can also be used

PERCUSSION

Generally, it is not used in obstetric examination.
   It is used only to check for fluid thrill in cases of polyhydramnios as follows:
When abdomen is overdistended due to polyhydramnios, skin is stretched and shiny. Patient or the attendant keeps the ulnar border of one hand over the abdomen in the midline. Examiner taps with one

hand on one side of the abdomen and with the other hand placed at the same level on the other side of the abdomen, feels the fluid thrill.

Other findings to be noted:
- *Shelving sign*—at term as the head gets engaged, there is falling forward of the uterus and when the mother sits, due to falling forward of the uterus, the examiner can keep (rest) the hand over the fundus of the uterus—called shelving sign
- *Uterus contracting or relaxing*
- *Amount of liquor*
- *Size of the baby*
- *Special points to be noted during examination*, for example:
    When woman complains of abdominal pain—palpate for uterine contraction and relaxation and it indicates true labour pains.
    When she complains of bleeding PV—palpate for uterine contractions and relaxation.
    When uterus is tense and tender, it indicates abruptio placenta and when uterus is tender and contour not made out, it indicates rupture uterus.
    When uterus is well relaxed with bleeding PV—diagnosis of placenta previa, vasa previa/local causes in cervix can be made.
    When along with uterine enlargement if there is a separate swelling with tenderness—it can be either ovarian mass, which has undergone torsion or red degeneration of the fibroid.
    When there is previous LSCS with suprapubic tenderness or bulge, it indicates scar dehiscence.
    When there is bulge on the skin over the abdominal scar without tenderness and it is reducible, it may be due to incisional hernia.

Measurements

Symphysiofundal height: This measurement is taken with an empty bladder and after correcting dextrorotation. It is the distance between the upper border of symphysis pubis to the upper or highest level of fundus. The highest point of uterine fundus is palpated and measurement is made from this point downwards with a tape to the highest point of pubic symphysis.
- From 20–36 weeks, SFH corresponds in centimetres to gestational age in weeks ±2 cm.
- When SFH is less by 4 cm to the normal—suspect FGR/oligohydramnios/wrong dates/IUD/transverse lie.
- When SFH is more—suspect polyhydramnios/multiple pregnancy/wrong dates/big baby/pregnancy with maternal ascites/tumour complicating pregnancy/foetal ascites (Fig. 1.16).

Gravidogram: Graphical representation of height of uterus (measured from fundus to pubic symphysis); it is a simple method to assess foetal growth measured during every visit.

After 20 weeks, SFH increases by 1 cm/week till 36 weeks.

Abdominal girth: Girth of the abdomen is measured at the level of umbilicus (Fig. 1.17). After 30 weeks, abdominal girth is to be measured. At term, it is 90–100 cm.

In average built person, *it is 30 in. or 75 cm at 30 weeks* and thereafter it increases by 1 in. or 2.5 cm/week—It is *100 cm or 40 in. by 40 weeks.*

Adequacy of liquor: If liquor is decreased, the uterus is found hugging the foetus, foetal parts may not be felt easily and abdominal girth may be less than period of gestation.

Foetal weight estimation: Johnson's formula (clinical method)
It is applicable only in cephalic presentation.

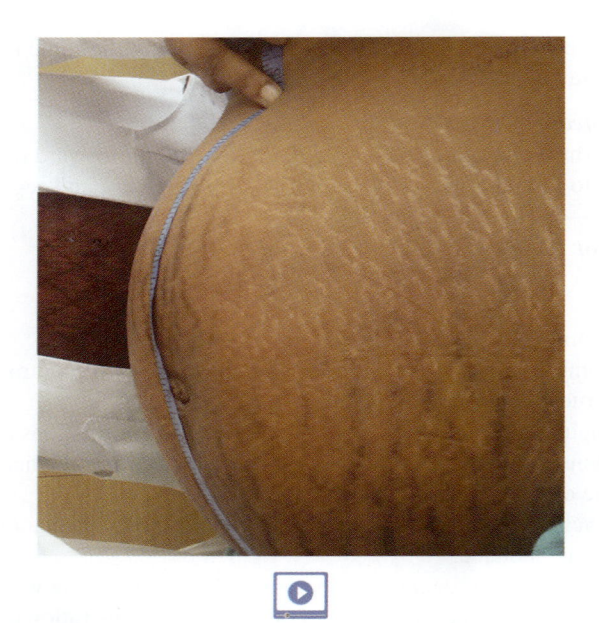

CASE 1 OBSTETRIC HISTORY TAKING AND EXAMINATION

FIGURE 1.16 SFH MEASUREMENT

Scan to play Antenatal examination

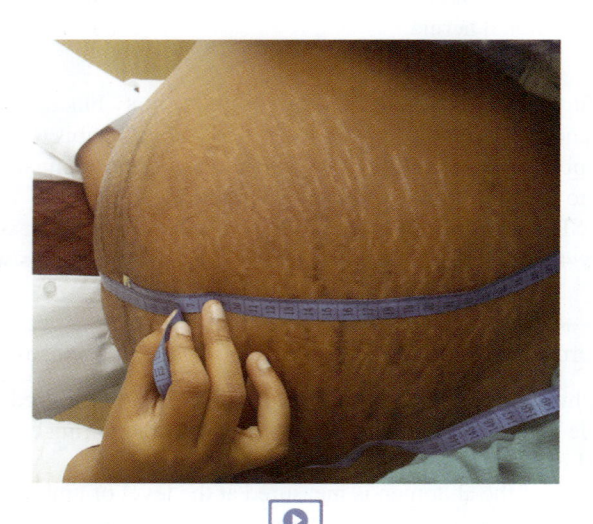

FIGURE 1.17 ABDOMINAL GIRTH

Scan to play Antenatal examination

In unengaged head, foetal weight = fundal height in centimetres − 12 × 155 g
In engaged head, foetal weight = fundal height in centimetres − 11 × 155 g

Foetal weight can be estimated by USG using BPD, AC, HC, FL biometry measurements.
McDonald's rule—To assess gestational age:

Height of fundus in centimetres × 2/7 = duration of pregnancy in lunar months
Height of fundus in centimetres × 8/7 = duration of pregnancy in weeks

PER VAGINAL EXAMINATION

Done in following circumstances:
- To confirm pregnancy
- When there is history of first trimester bleeding
- Routinely at 38 weeks in primi or nulliparous women to assess pelvis and CPD
- If pregnant woman comes with labour pains
- If there is history of PROM, S/E done prior to PV
- To assess length of cervix in women with H/O pre-term labour
- To assess Bishop's score if induction of labour is contemplated

P/V is done in cases of primi or nulliparous women to assess pelvis and CPD at 38 weeks (in indicated cases)
- Pelvic capacity can be estimated clinically by evaluating various measurements with the middle and index finger of right hand during bimanual examination

  To asses pelvis, index and middle fingers of right hand are introduced into vagina to find out the following:
    - Whether sacral promontory is reached or not
    - Bay of sacrum is well curved or not
    - Whether sacrosciatic notch admits two fingers or not
    - Pelvic side walls parallel or convergent
    - Whether ischial spines are prominent
    - Whether ischial spines are reached when fingers are spanned
    - Pubic arch well-curved or not, pubic angle is acute or obtuse
    - When clenched fist is kept between ischial tuberosities, whether it admits four knuckles or not
    - Coccyx is mobile or tipped

For features of adequacy of pelvis, refer CPD case 11.
Assessment of CPD
Munro Kerr Muller's method (this is done to assess for CPD and the degree): Index and middle fingers of the right hand are kept in the vagina at the level of ischial spines and right thumb over the pubic symphysis. With left hand, push the head into the pelvic brim downwards and backwards.
- If the head goes in—no CPD
- If head is flush with pubic symphysis—minor degree CPD
- If there is overriding—major degree CPD

  CPD is best assessed only at the onset of labour.

SUMMARY

Name... Occupation............................... Age…... Socioeconomic class...............
Gravida....................................... Para.. Booked..
Immunised, LMP/EDD....................... H/O amenorrhoea/period of gestation ....

Her complaints, significant and relevant present, past history, general examination findings, vitals and obstetric examination findings with relevant available investigations should be summarised.

DIAGNOSIS

- *Clear, concise and logic way of reporting should be done.*
- Primi …. Age …… EDD ….. term gestation/single live foetus with FH rate …… in cephalic presentation.

  Reporting: *Should form the basis for necessary investigations.*
  Differential diagnosis: May not be applicable to all obstetric cases except in multiple pregnancy, polyhydramnios, overdistended abdomen.

INVESTIGATIONS

Routine investigations done in antenatal care are given in Table 1.3.

Role of Dating scan:
- To find out if pregnancy is intra-uterine or extra-uterine
- Viable or not viable
- Number of sacs—single or multiple
- CRL: 7–12 weeks—dating (discrepancy 3–4 days). Accuracy of CRL decreases after 12 weeks
- To assess gestational age
- Normal or abnormal pregnancy—ectopic, vesicular mole
- Associated adnexal mass, uterine anomaly
- Nuchal translucency (NT) —more than 3 mm strong marker for chromosomal abnormalities like Down's syndrome

Anomaly scan is done at 18–20 weeks because of the following:
- Most of the major structural anomalies can be detected
- MTP is allowed till 20 weeks, if lethal anomaly is present
- Useful in assessing gestational age, when dating scan is not done
- For placental localisation
- Base line record of foetal biometry
- Useful in diagnosing multiple gestation, when USG is not done previously
- Amount of liquor

Table 1.3 Routine Investigations Done in Antenatal Care

Name of the Investigations	First Visit	When to Repeat	Importance
Urine routine examination	Booking	In all visits	When albumin is present—rule out pre-eclampsia. If pus cells >5, do culture and sensitivity. When sugar is present, rule out GDM
Hb, PCV	Booking	28 and 36 weeks, more frequently when anaemia is suspected or diagnosed	As per WHO Hb < 11 g.%: anaemia As per CDC Hb < 11 g.% in first trimester and third trimester and Hb < 10.5 g in second trimester: anaemia
Blood grouping and Rh typing	Booking	If not done in booking, it should be done in subsequent visit	If mother is Rh −ve, husband's blood group and Rh type to be done ICT to be done for the patient, if husband is positive
HIV after counselling HbsAg, VDRL	Booking	If not done in booking, it should be done in subsequent visit	Refer to ICTC when HIV +ve
Thyroid profile	Booking	Can be done	Can pick up thyroid dysfunction early and treat
Blood sugar	GCT GCT in high risk case	GCT—24–28 weeks in low risk In high risk, if GCT is negative in booking visit, repeat GCT done—28 and 32 weeks	Screening for gestational diabetes
USG	Booking—dating scan NT—11–13.6 weeks, can also pick up some anomalies like anencephaly	18–20 weeks—anomaly scan—(target scan) USG in third trimester—for foetal growth	
Screening tests	First trimester screening for chromosomal anomalies in high risk cases: 11–13.6 weeks, NT scan, PAPPA (pregnancy-associated plasma protein) βHCG	Triple screening test for chromosomal anomalies in high risk—15–18 weeks, AFP, unconjugated estriol, βHCG, and in quadruple test along with this inhibin A tested	Screening for chromosomal and neural tube defects in high-risk patients

AFP, Alpha-foetoprotein; GCT, glucose challenge test.

CASE 1 OBSTETRIC HISTORY TAKING AND EXAMINATION

KEY POINTS

Presentation The part of the foetus which lies in the lower pole of uterus and 96% are cephalic, 3% podalic and others 1%.
Presenting part Is the foetal part which overlies the internal os and when cervix dilates, it is felt by examining finger.
Attitude Relation of foetal parts to one another. Commonest is universal flexion.
Lie Relationship of the long axis of the foetus to long axis of uterus.
Position Relation of denominator to the different quadrants of the pelvis.
Denominator Is the fixed bony point, which comes in contact with various quadrants of pelvis (occiput in vertex, mentum in face, sacrum in breech, acromion in shoulder).
Largest transverse diameter of the skull Biparietal diameter—9.5 cm
Shortest transverse diameter of the skull Bitemporal diameter—8 cm
Engaging diameter in vertex presentation Sub-occipito-bregmatic diameter—9.5 cm
Engaging diameter in face presentation Sub-mento-bregmatic diameter—9.5 cm
Engaging diameter in brow presentation verticomental—13.5 cm
Engaging diameter in deflexed head as in occipito-posterior occipito-frontal—11 cm
Vertex Is the quadrangular or diamond-shaped area bounded anteriorly by bregma, posteriorly by posterior fontanelle and parietal eminence on either side.
Engagement The greatest engaging diameter of the presenting part has gone through the pelvic brim and presenting part will be at the level of ischial spines or below on per vaginal examination. In vertex, greatest transverse engaging diameter is biparietal diameter—9.5 cm.
Labour Is the process by which products of conception are expelled by the mother after period of viability either spontaneously or with external aid to complete it.
Normal or natural labour When a full-term foetus presenting by vertex is expelled by natural efforts unaided within a period of 24 h without maternal and foetal complications, it is called normal or natural labour.
Pre-term labour If labour sets in after 28 weeks before 37 weeks.
Term pregnancy 37–42 weeks.
Post-term pregnancy If pregnancy extends beyond 42 completed weeks.

FREQUENTLY ASKED QUESTIONS

1. Define gravida, para.
2. What is the importance of age, socioeconomic status?
3. What is booking and it's significance?
4. What will you do in antenatal care during first visit and subsequent visit?
5. How will you immunize antenatal mother?
6. How do you differentiate physiological pedal oedema and pathological oedema? And how is physiological pedal oedema caused?
7. What are the causes for pathological oedema?
8. What are the causes for uterus bigger or smaller than period of amenorrhoea?
9. What is lie, position, attitude, presentation and presenting part?

10. What is engagement?
11. What are the causes for mobile head at term in primi?
12. What information do you get when you do fundal grip, umbilical grip?
13. What information do you get in first and second pelvic grip?
14. How and when will you do pelvic assessment in primi?
15. What is dating scan? What is it's significance? What is NT and when will you do it and what is it's importance?
16. When will you do target scan or anomaly scan and why?
17. What is gravidogram?
18. What are the causes for hyperemesis gravidarum?
19. What are the routine investigations to be done in antenatal period?
20. What is denominator? And what are the denominators in different presentations?
21. Define normal labour.
22. What is quickening? When does it occur in primi and multi?
23. How will you calculate EDD? Whose rule is it? What percentage of women deliver on EDD?
24. What is Johnson's formula?
25. What is McDonald's rule?
26. Define elderly primi. What are the risks in elderly primi?
27. What are the problems of teenage pregnancy?
28. What information do you get in first trimester USG?

CASE 2

NORMAL PREGNANCY

PATIENT'S DETAILS
Name.. Age................. Address........................... Occupation..............
Socioeconomic Class.......................... Gravida, Para, Live, Abortion, (G......... P......... L......... A.........)
Booked/Unbooked........................ Immunisation....................... LMP............ EDD

H/O............months of amenorrhoea/period of gestation

PRESENT COMPLAINTS
Patient may present with period of amenorrhoea/gestational age as per LMP with following complaints:
- Lethargy
- Easy fatigability
- Swelling of the feet
- Palpitation
- Breathlessness

HISTORY
HISTORY OF PRESENT ILLNESS
- Elicit history in relation to onset, duration, severity.

MENSTRUAL HISTORY, MARITAL HISTORY, PAST OBSTETRIC HISTORY, PAST MEDICAL AND SURGICAL HISTORY, FAMILY HISTORY, PERSONAL HISTORY
- Refer Case 1.

EXAMINATION
GENERAL EXAMINATION AND OBSTETRIC EXAMINATION
- Refer Case 1.

CASE 2 NORMAL PREGNANCY

SUMMARY
- Name….. Age ….. booked….. immunised—— no significant complaints
- If positive findings are present in general examination—mention it
- Mention about obstetric examination findings
- Mention about available investigations

DIAGNOSIS
Mention about Gravida …… Para …. EDD …..…… Single foetus or Multiple ….Live… in ———-Presentation

INVESTIGATIONS
- Refer Case 1.

CASE DISCUSSION
- *Elderly primi*: when woman is pregnant at 35 years and above
- *Short primi*: height less than 145 cm
- *Grand multigravida*: is one who has been pregnant 5 times or more
- *Grand multipara*: is one who has already had five or more deliveries beyond period of viability
- *Ripening of cervix*: during which cervix becomes soft, cervical length shortens and dilatation of cervix occurs
- *Pre-labour*: This is the period, woman feels more frequent tightening of uterus and this occurs few days before onset of labour
- *Show*: Release of mucous plug from cervical canal with blood due to dilatation and effacement of cervix

MECHANISM OF LABOUR
It is a series of changes in position that the foetus undergoes during it's passage through the parturient canal with minimal difficulty.

Following are the cardinal movements of head in vertex presentation:
- *Engagement*: It is when the greatest diameter of the head has passed successfully through the inlet that is when the bi-parietal diameter has passed through the pelvic brim and lower most portion of vertex would be at the level of the ischial spines.
- *Descent*: It occurs secondary to uterine action in first and second stage of labour.
- *Flexion*: When the head descends to the pelvic floor and meets the resistance of pelvic side walls, flexion occurs.
- *Internal rotation*: The shape of the bony pelvis and direction of the pelvic floor muscles in addition to the well-flexed head will help the head to rotate into anterio posterior position.

In a well-flexed head the occiput will meet the pelvic floor and will guide the direction of the rotation
- *Extension*: The head is delivered by extension. First the bregma and then the face and chin appear in succession over the posterior vaginal opening and perineum.
- *Restitution*: As soon as the head escapes from the vulva, the head aligns itself with the shoulder by 45-degree rotation and thus neck is untwisted.
- *External rotation*: To deliver, the shoulders have to undergo internal rotation bringing bisacromial diameter into the anterior–posterior diameter of pelvis and external rotation of head occurs simultaneously.

  The obstetrician will rotate the head making the face of the foetus looking to medial aspect of the maternal thigh.
- *Delivery of the shoulders*: The anterior shoulder is under the symphysis pubis and delivers first and the posterior shoulder delivers subsequently.

Stages of Labour	
Stage	Events
First stage	From onset of true labour pains to full cervical dilatation
Second stage	From full dilatation to delivery of foetus or foetuses
Third stage	Delivery of the placenta
Fourth stage	2 h following placental delivery

CAUSES FOR FIRST TRIMESTER BLEEDING
- Threatened abortion
- Missed abortion
- Inevitable abortion
- Vesicular mole
- Ectopic pregnancy
- Local causes—cervical polyp, cancer cervix with pregnancy

AMTSL—active management of third stage of labour
- Administration of oxytocin 10 units IM within 1 min after birth of the baby making sure that there is no undiagnosed multiple gestation—*a critical component*.
- Wait for the cord pulsation to stop and then cord should be clamped.
- Controlled cord traction during uterine contraction. Left hand is kept just above the mother's pubic bone and pressure is applied over the uterus in a cephalad direction. At the same time with other hand the cord is pulled firmly, steadily in a downward direction during uterine contraction.
- Jerky and forcible pulling is avoided to prevent inversion of uterus.
- Uterine massage after placenta is delivered helps the uterus to contract and also to assess uterine contraction.
- **Indications for early cord clamping**: Rh isoimmunisation/foetal distress/HIV mother.

40 CASE 2 NORMAL PREGNANCY

EPISIOTOMY
Also known as perineotomy

- *Definition*: It is a surgical incision of the perineum and posterior vaginal wall done during second stage of labour to quickly enlarge the passage to expedite the delivery.
- *Timing of episiotomy*: It is given during crowning of the head at the vulva and head should not recede into the vagina in between contractions.
    In case of breech, episiotomy is given when the breech is climbing the perineum.
- *Types of episiotomy*:
    - Mediolateral
    - Median
    - Lateral
- *Commonly used episiotomy*: Mediolateral after giving local infiltration with 1% xylocaine and given at midpoint of vulvar rim at 15–20 degree either right or left directed towards ischial tuberosity, to avoid anal sphincter.
- *Episiotomy repair*: Lithotomy position, clean the area with antiseptic. Repaired in three layers with local infiltration given before giving episiotomy (Fig. 2.1).
    - *First layer*—Vaginal mucosa—take suture with 1–0 chromic catgut beyond apex of cut wound and start suturing with continuous interlocking stitch.

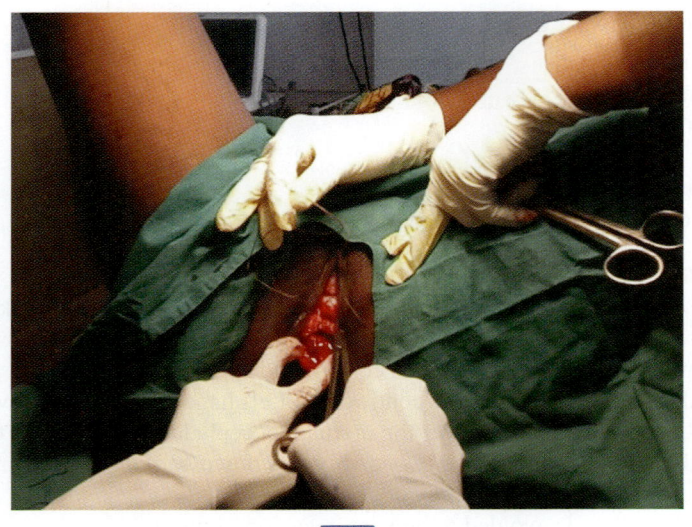

FIGURE 2.1 Suturing of Vaginal Mucosa

Scan to play Episiotomy suturing

- *Second layer*—Muscles are opposed and dead space obliterated to prevent vulval haematoma.
- *Third layer*—Skin and subcutaneous tissue—sutured by interrupted mattress suture or subcuticular stitches.
- *Indications*: Not used as a routine; used in following conditions:
  - Rigid perineum
  - When perineal tear is anticipated like big baby, breech delivery, face to pubis delivery, shoulder dystocia and instrumental delivery
- *Advantages of mediolateral episiotomy over other types*:
  - Reduces the trauma to perineum
  - Reduces the maternal pushing effort; incision can be extended, if necessary
  - If extension occurs, rectum is not affected
- *Complications of episiotomy*:
  - Immediate: Extension to rectum and anal sphincter, vulval haematoma
  - Delayed: Infection, wound gaping
  - Remote: Dyspareunia

LACERATED PERINEUM

First degree	Laceration of the vaginal mucosa and perineal skin
Second degree	Lacerations of perineal muscles and perineal body
Third degree	Lacerations of the perineum including anal sphincter
Fourth degree	Involvement of anal sphincter, anal and rectal mucosa

Differentiating Points Between True Labour Pains and False Labour Pains	
True Labour Pains	**False Labour Pains**
Occurs at regular intervals, with increasing frequency, duration and intensity	Does not occur at regular intervals; frequency, duration and intensity does not increase
Radiates to back and thigh	Does not radiate
Accompanied by show	Not accompanied by show
Associated with progressive dilatation and effacement of cervix	Not associated with progressive dilatation and effacement of cervix
Not relieved by enema or analgesia	Relieved by enema or analgesia

Differential Diagnosis of Pain Abdomen at Term	
Causes	**Conditions**
Pregnancy related	False labour pain, true labour pain, abruptio placenta
Pregnancy with	Fibroid undergoing red degeneration
Pregnancy with other causes	UTI, gastritis, appendicitis, ureteric colic, gastroenteritis

KEY POINTS

- Cardinal movements that are taking place during mechanism of labour are engagement, desent, flexion, internal rotation, extension, restitution and external rotation.
- Timing of episiotomy: In vertex, it is given during crowning of the head at the vulva and head should not recede into the vagina in between contractions. In case of breech, episiotomy is given when the breech is climbing the perineum.
- Commonly used episiotomy is mediolateral so as to avoid injury to the anal sphincter.
- Components of AMTSL—Administration of Oxytocin 10 units IM within 1 min after birth of the baby, pressure over the uterus in a cephalad direction and controlled cord traction during uterine contraction and uterine massage.
- There are four different degrees of perineal lacerations. In first degree vaginal mucosa and perineal skin are involved, in second degree perineal muscles and perineal body are torn, in third degree lacerations include perineum including anal sphincter, in fourth degree anal sphincter, anal and rectal mucosa are involved.

FREQUENTLY ASKED QUESTIONS

1. What do you mean by false labour pains and true labour pains?
2. What are the stages of labour? What is show?
3. What information do you get in first trimester USG?
4. How will you conduct labour?
5. When will you give episiotomy?
6. What are the signs of separation of placenta?
7. What are the causes for first trimester bleeding?
8. What is AMTSL—active management of third stage of labour?

A CASE OF ANAEMIA COMPLICATING PREGNANCY

CASE 3

PATIENT'S DETAILS

Name.. Age.................. Address.......................... Occupation.............
Socioeconomic Class......................... Gravida, Para, Live, Abortion, (G......... P......... L......... A ....)
Booked/Unbooked........................ Immunisation....................... LMP............ EDD

H/O............ months of amenorrhoea/period of gestation

PRESENT COMPLAINTS

Patient may present with period of amenorrhoea with following complaints:
- Lethargy
- Easy fatigability
- Swelling of face, arms, abdominal wall and feet
- Palpitation
- Breathlessness
- Chest pain

HISTORY
PRESENT HISTORY

- History elicited in relation to onset, duration, severity and treatment with parenteral iron/blood transfusion.

MENSTRUAL HISTORY

- Previous history of excessive menstrual flow to be elicited as it may result in pre-conceptional anaemia and during pregnancy

MARITAL HISTORY AND OBSTETRIC HISTORY

- Refer Case 1.

To view the lecture notes log in to your account on www.MedEnact.com

CASE 3 A CASE OF ANAEMIA COMPLICATING PREGNANCY

Past obstetric history
Following history has to be elicited:
- History of anaemia in previous pregnancy/blood transfusion/APH/PPH/iron, folic acid intake/history suggestive of puerperal sepsis, failure of lactation and deep vein thrombosis (could be due to anaemia in previous pregnancy)
- Number of children, spacing (if pregnancy occurs within 2 years, more iron is required to replenish the iron stores)
- History of low birth weight (LBW) babies, duration of lactation

Past history
Following history has to be elicited:
- Melena, haematemesis, bleeding piles, epistaxis, dysentery
- Bleeding tendency or prolonged bleeding after injury
- Worm infestation, walking barefoot
- Malnutrition, chronic diarrhoea or excessive vomiting
- Malaria, chronic illness
- Epilepsy (anti-epileptic drugs result in folic acid deficiency)
- Anti-coagulant, any other prolonged drug therapy
- Recurrent urinary tract infection
- History suggestive of haemolytic anaemia
- Irregular antenatal check-up and intake of folic acid and iron

PAST SURGICAL HISTORY

If woman gives history of gastrojejunostomy, that may be the cause for anaemia.

PAST MEDICAL HISTORY

- H/O malaria, chronic illness like tuberculosis, rheumatoid arthritis, chronic drug intake, Intolerance to iron, H/O gastrointestineal disorders, H/O parenteral iron and blood transfusion to be elicited.

FAMILY HISTORY

- Sickle cell anaemia
- Thalassaemia

PERSONAL HISTORY

- Food habits—vegetarian/non vegetarian
- Beetle nut chewing

EXAMINATION
GENERAL EXAMINATION

- Refer Case 1.

Specific points to be noted in anaemia:
- *Nutritional status*: Build and stature—patient may be under nourished. Patient may have lack lustre hair
  - Mouth—bald tongue, glossitis, stomatitis may be present
- *Pedal oedema*: May be due to cardiac failure or due to associated hypoproteinaemia
- *Jaundice*: Suggestive of haemolytic anaemia
- *Weight*: Poor weight gain may be present
- *Pulse*: Tachycardia (indicates cardiac failure)
- *Blood pressure*: To be carefully checked since anaemia can be associated with pre-eclampsia
- *JVP*: JVP may be raised in CCF
- *CVS*: Tachycardia, systolic murmur less than grade 3 (haemic murmur) and sometimes cardiomegaly
- *R.S*: Increased respiratory rate/basal rales may be present when there is congestive cardiac failure
- *Abdomen*: Hepatosplenomegaly suggestive of haemolytic anaemia

- Hepatomegaly may be present when there is congestive cardiac failure

OBSTETRIC EXAMINATION

Examination is done like any other case (refer Case 1).
- If multiple pregnancy is made out on examination, anaemia may be associated.
- Height of the uterus to be carefully palpated, SFH and abdominal girth to be measured carefully because foetus may develop FGR/oligohydramnios and uterine size may be lesser than the period of amenorrhoea.

SUMMARY
- Mrs………Age……..Socioeconomic Class…..Gravida, Para, Booked/Immunised, LMP…..EDD……admitted for……H/O Months of amenorrhoea…../period of gestation
- With complaints of swelling of legs/breathlessness/or any other symptoms and taking iron/has taken treatment or transfusion
- *On general examination*: mention about anaemia, pedal oedema/dyspnoea. If JVP is raised mention about it and about hepatomegaly if present
- *On obstetric examination*: mention about height of the uterus ….lie… presentation/single/multiple……head engaged or not…..FHR....
- *Investigation* reports if available, mention about it

DIAGNOSIS
- Mrs………. Age………. Gravida………. Para at …………… weeks of pregnancy……single or multiple……….live foetus……….with mild/moderate/severe anaemia (if report available, mention it) in cardiac failure or not, baby FGR or not.

46 CASE 3 A CASE OF ANAEMIA COMPLICATING PREGNANCY

INVESTIGATIONS
- **Hb, RBC, PCV**
- *Normal values of MCV/MCH/MCHC and colour Index*
  Normal values
  - Mean corpuscular volume: 75–95 μm^3; mean corpuscular haemoglobin: 26–31 pg
  - Mean corpuscular haemoglobin concentration: 34%
  - Colour index: 1; when <1: hypochromic; >1: hyperchromic
- *Peripheral smear can indicate the following*:
  - Type of anaemia: Hypochromic, microcytic, anisocytosis, poikilocytosis—iron deficiency anaemia (Fig. 3.1)

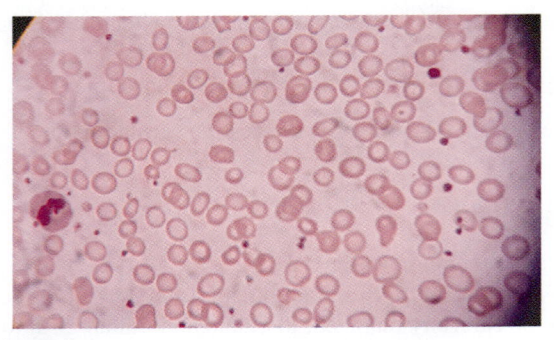

FIGURE 3.1 Iron Deficiency Anaemia

- Hyperchromic, macrocytic, hypersegmentation of neutrophils, presence of megaloblasts/Howell–Jolly bodies—megaloblastic anaemia (Fig. 3.2)

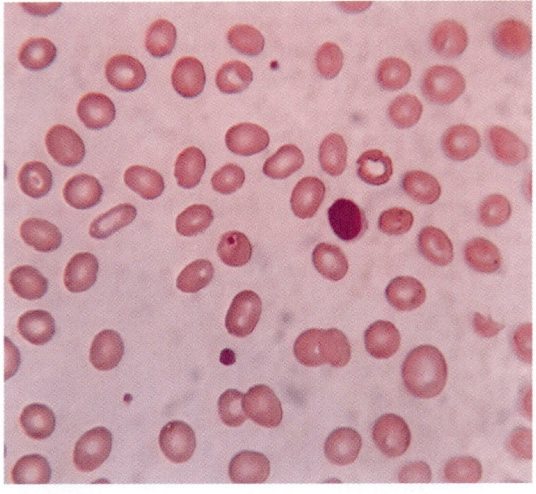

FIGURE 3.2 Megaloblastic Anaemia

- Red cell morphology (sphero/eliptocytes, sickle cells) (Fig. 3.3)

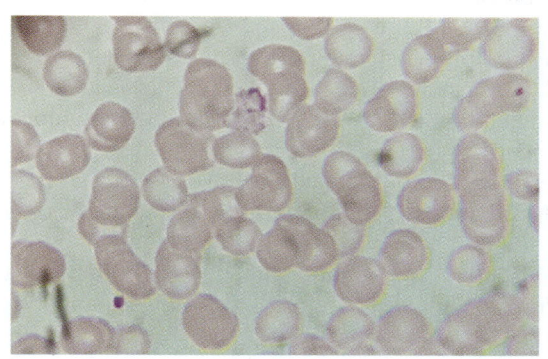

FIGURE 3.3 Malarial Parasite

- Malarial parasites, inclusion bodies may be present
- Presence of eosinophils may be due to hookworm infestation
- Abnormal cells may be due to leukaemia
- ***Platelet count***: Normal value, 1.5–4 lakhs/mm^3
  Platelet—*deficient in idiopathic thrombocytopenic purpura (ITP)*
- ***Reticulocyte count***: Presence of reticulocytes during treatment denotes response
- ***Blood group, Rh type***
- ***Bleeding time, clotting time***
- ***Buffy coat***: Blood is centrifuged at 3000 rpm/30 min, which will result in three layers.
  - Plasma
  - Buffy coat
  - RBC

  Buffy coat will contain hypersegmented neutrophils and platelets.
- ***Stool examination for***: ova cyst, occult blood (in hookworm infestation, 0.03–0.05 mL of blood/day/worm is lost)
- ***Urine***: protein, sugar, pus cells and culture sensitivity
  Recurrent UTI can lead to anaemia. Pre-eclampsia may be present along with anaemia
- ***Serum protein***: to rule out hypoproteinaemia
- ***In iron deficiency anaemia***: following investigations are to be done:
  - Serum iron, total iron binding capacity (TIBC), serum ferritin
  - Normal values: total serum iron—65–120 µg/dL, TIBC—300–400 µg/dL, serum ferritin—15–200 µg/L

Specific to iron deficiency:

- Hb < 10 g.%, RBC < 3.2 million/mm^3, PCV < 30%, MCV < 75 µm^3, MCH < 25 pg, MCHC < 30%, serum iron <30 µg/dL, TIBC > 400 µg/dL, serum ferritin <12 µg/L, high red cell distribution width (RDW)

- Peripheral smear: Hypochromic microcytic picture with anisocytosis and poikilocytosis
- *Recent investigative procedures for iron deficiency anaemia*: Serum transferrin receptor/free erythrocyte protoporphyrin
- *In megaloblastic anaemia*: following investigations are to be done:
  - Serum folate, RBC folate, serum B12, methylmalonic acid and homocysteine
  - Normal values: Serum folate, 3–8 ng/mL, RBC folate >150 µg/mL, serum vitamin B12, 150–900 pg/mL

  Specific for megaloblastic anaemia: Hb less than 10 g.%,
  - Peripheral smear: Macrocytic hyperchromic, hypersegmentation of neutrophils, Howell–Jolly bodies
  - MCV > 100 µm^3, MCH > 33 pg, serum folate <3 ng/mL, RBC folate <80 µg/mL, serum B12 level <90 pg/mL
  - Serum iron: normal
- *Specific investigation for haemoglobinopathies*: Haemoglobin electrophoresis, acid elution test, serum bilirubin, osmotic fragility test
- *Bone marrow study*: Usually deferred during pregnancy. It is done when patient is not responding to therapy
- *For foetal assessment*: Daily foetal movement count, maternal weight gain, SFH, abdominal girth measurement at every visit and if FGR is suspected serial USG and Doppler

CASE DISCUSSION

1. Commonest form of anaemia in pregnancy in India: dimorphic due to nutritional deficiency of iron, folic acid and B12.
2. Definition of anaemia: Decrease in oxygen carrying capacity of blood due to quantitative and/or qualitative decrease in RBC and Hb concentration of blood
3. Degrees of anaemia: According to Centers for Disease Control and Prevention, Anaemia in pregnancy is defined as: Hb < 11 g/dL in the first trimester and third trimester and < 10.5 g/dL in the second trimester.
4. ICMR classification of anaemia in pregnancy

Mild	10–10.9 g/dL
Moderate	7–10 g/dL
Severe	4–7 g/dL
Very severe (decompensated)	<4 g/dL

5. FOGSI classification of anaemia in pregnancy

Mild	8–10 g/dL
Moderate	6.5–8 g/dL
Severe	<6.5 g/dL

CASE DISCUSSION

6. According to WHO: Hb < 11 g/dL is considered as anaemia in pregnancy
7. According to FOGSI: Hb < 10 g/dL is considered as anaemia in pregnancy
8. Causes for increased iron requirement during pregnancy:
   a. Foetus, placenta—300 mg
   b. Maternal Hb mass expansion—500 mg; loss by excretion—200 mg
   c. Parturition, lactation—300 mg
   d. Conservation of iron due to amenorrhoea—300 mg; net total requirement—1000 mg
9. Physiological anaemia occurs in pregnancy because increase in plasma volume during pregnancy is 40%–50% and increase in RBC mass is only 20%–30%. Hence there is haemodilution, which results in decrease in Hb concentration
10. Criteria for physiological anaemia (Fig. 3.4):

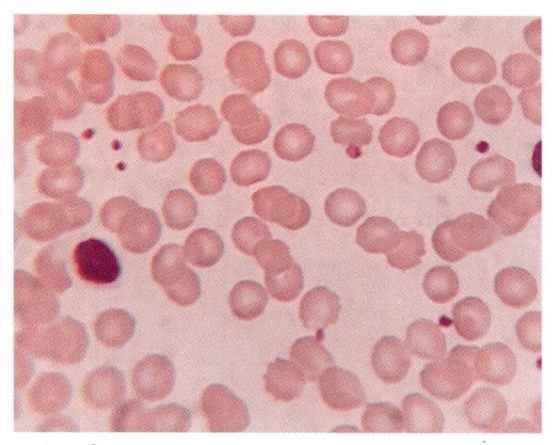

FIGURE 3.4 Normocytic Normochromic

   a. Lower limit of Hb—10 g/dL
   b. RBC—3.2 millions/mL
   c. PCV—30%
   d. Normal morphology in peripheral smear
11. National Anaemia Prophylaxis Programme:
   a. All pregnant and lactating mothers should receive 100 mg of elemental iron and 0.5 mg of folic acid and children aged 1–5 years should receive 20 mg of elemental iron and 0.1 mg of folic acid daily for at least 100 days.
   b. *The 12 by 12 initiative*: Aim is to achieve Hb of 12 g/dL by the age of 12 years by 2012.
12. Calculation for iron requirement:
   a. 2.4 × weight in kilograms × Hb deficiency in grams + 1000 mg (to replenish the stores) = total milligrams required
   or 0.3 × wt. in pounds × deficiency of HB in per cent +500 mg

13. Iron deficiency occurs in three stages:

First stage	Depletion of iron stores decrease in ferritin
Second stage	Decrease in serum iron and increase in TIBC
Third stage	Iron deficiency anaemia

14. The effects of anaemia on mother and foetus:
    a. Maternal: Pre-eclampsia, abruptio, pre-term delivery, precipitate labour, congestive cardiac failure
    b. Foetal: LBW babies—IUGR, pre-term, IUD
15. Choice of therapy depends on: Severity of anaemia, type of anaemia, duration of pregnancy, associated complications
    a. *Mild anaemia*—Oral iron in therapeutic dose is given.
       – Diet rich in iron and folic acid is advised.
       – Deworming is done (Albendazole 400 mg stat).
    b. *In severe anaemia in any trimester and moderate anaemia in late third trimester*—Packed cell transfusion is given (Table 3.1).

Table 3.1 Three Different Modality of Antenatal Anaemia Treatment

Oral Iron	Parenteral Iron	Packed Red Cell Transfusion
<30 Weeks—moderate anaemia	Pregnancy 30–36 weeks with moderate anaemia	>36 Weeks and severe anaemia in any trimester
When oral iron contraindicated—parenteral iron	IM or IV	

16. Indications for parenteral iron therapy: Intolerance to oral iron, non-compliance of the woman, unpredictable absorption, moderate anaemia
17. Different parenteral iron preparations:
    a. Iron dextran complex, iron sorbitol citric acid complex and iron sucrose
    b. Iron sucrose—Advantage is that there is no need for test dose
    c. Dose 100 mg in 100 mL of normal saline intra-venous in 15 min/day (to be given in 15 min to prevent free radicals)
    d. Maximum 200 mg/day, 600 mg/week
    e. *Rate of improvement after iron therapy*: 0.7 g/100 mL/week
       Time taken for improvement after oral and parenteral iron therapy: 21 days but within a week reticulocytes appear
18. *Daily requirement of iron*: Non-pregnant 2–3 mg/day
    In pregnancy, 6–7 mg/day. Only 10% of iron taken orally is absorbed
19. Factors influencing iron absorption—Phytates, tannins, phosphates and calcium—**Decrease iron absorption**
    Vitamin C, amino acids, citric acid—**Increase iron absorption**

20. *Each ferrous sulphate tablet*: Contains 333 mg, which contains 100 mg of elemental iron (previously 200 mg tablet has 60 mg of elemental iron) Prophylatic oral iron therapy—tablet $FeSO_4$ once daily; therapeutic iron therapy—tablet $FeSO_4$ thrice daily
21. *Daily requirement of folic acid*: 500 μg/day
22. Role of blood transfusion: Packed cell—is to be given to reduce overload
    a. Packed cell is given in severe anaemia in any trimester and moderate anaemia in advanced pregnancy, in emergency operative procedure, acute blood loss and in haemoglobinopathies
    b. *One unit of packed cell increases Hb by 1 g/100 mL and effect is seen after 24–48 h*
23. Management of anaemia complicating pregnancy during labour:
    a. Wide bore IV line—maintenance
    b. Propped up position
    c. Reserve blood—packed cell transfusion is given, if indicated
    d. Prophylactic antibiotics
    e. Cut short second stage of labour
    f. Active management of third stage of labour
    g. If women comes in CCF—O_2, diuretics, digoxin, antibiotics, partial exchange transfusion to be given; vitals and intake and output to be monitored
24. Intrapartum, post-partum and post-natal complications of anaemia in pregnancy: Subinvolution of uterus, cortical vein thrombosis, deep vein thrombosis, high maternal morbidity, mortality
25. Indications for recombinant human erythropoietin: Refractory iron deficiency anaemia and in patients with chronic renal disease. Dose of 150 IU/kg is given subcutaneously thrice a week
26. Partial exchange transfusion—*Not used nowadays*; packed cell transfused through one cubital vein with simultaneous withdrawal of blood from other cubital vein; volume withdrawn should be less than that is transfused.

KEY POINTS

- Anaemia in pregnancy is a major public health problem in India since it is direct cause for 20% of maternal death and indirect cause for 20% of maternal death.
- According to WHO: Hb < 11 g/dL is considered as anaemia in pregnancy; according to FOGSI: Hb < 10 g/dL is considered as anaemia in pregnancy and according to CDC: Hb < 11 g/dL in the first trimester and third trimester and <10.5 g/dL in the second trimester.
- Commonest anaemia during pregnancy is iron deficiency and it can be dual, both iron and folic acid deficiency.
- There is increased iron requirement during pregnancy for foetus, placenta, for RBC expansion, blood loss during pregnancy. Net requirement during pregnancy is 1000 mg.
- Due to physiological changes in pregnancy there is increase in plasma volume to 50% and RBC cell mass increases only to 20%, there is fall in haemoglobin concentration and haematocrit resulting in haemodilution termed as physiological anaemia of pregnancy.
- Symptoms may be easy fatigue, breathlessness, palpitations, pedal oedema and signs are pallor, glossitis, tachycardia, haemic murmur and may result in CCF.
- Effect of anaemia during pregnancy on mother are pre-eclampsia, abruptio, pre-term labour and on foetus are IUGR, IUD, prematurity, LBW.

CASE 3 A CASE OF ANAEMIA COMPLICATING PREGNANCY

- Three modalities of antenatal management are oral iron, parenteral iron and blood transfusion.
- In mild anaemia, oral therapy is given. When there is intolerance to oral iron, non-compliance, malabsorption, parenteral iron is given. In severe anaemia in any trimester and moderate anaemia in late trimester, packed cell transfusion is given.
- Management during labour are oxygen, propped up position, packed cell transfusion if indicated, prophylactic antibiotics, cut short second stage of labour, active management of third stage of labour and if CCF occurs treat CCF.

FREQUENTLY ASKED QUESTIONS

1. What is physiological anaemia and criteria for diagnosing it?
2. Why is there increased iron requirement during pregnancy?
3. What is the dose of oral prophylactic and therapeutic iron in pregnancy?
4. What are the effects of anaemia on mother and foetus?
5. What are the causes for iron deficiency anaemia?
6. What are the stages of iron deficiency?
7. How will you diagnose iron deficiency anaemia?
8. What is buffy coat?
9. How will you calculate iron requirement?
10. What are the factors determining the management of anaemia?
11. What are the different types of iron therapy, it's advantage and disadvantages? How long will it take to increase the Hb?
12. What are the other types of anaemia? What are the clinical features of megaloblastic anaemia, it's investigations and management?
13. What is the antenatal management of anaemia during pregnancy?
14. How will you manage anaemia complicating pregnancy during labour?
15. What are the intrapartum, post-partum and post-natal complications of anaemia in pregnancy?

CASE 4

A CASE OF HYPERTENSION IN PREGNANCY

PATIENT'S DETAILS

Name... Age.................. Address........................... Occupation.............
Socioeconomic Class......................... Gravida, Para, Live, Abortion, (G......... P......... L......... A.........)
Booked/Unbooked........................ Immunisation...................... LMP............ EDD

H/O............ months of amenorrhoea/period of gestation

(*AGE*—Teen age and elderly primi are more prone for pre-eclampsia, *Parity*—primi—more prone for pre-eclampsia)

PRESENT COMPLAINTS

Patient may present with period of amenorrhoea with following complaints:
All complaints must be in chronological order.
- C/O undue weight gain
- History of high blood pressure prior to pregnancy and taking treatment for the same
- C/O swelling—oedema
  - *Site*—dependent parts: ankle, feet, below knee and lower limbs; non-dependent parts: hands, abdominal wall, face, pre-sacral region, vulva
  - *Duration*
  - *Whether disappears with rest*
    If oedema is present, rule out other causes like anaemia, heart disease, liver disease, renal disease, deep vein thrombosis, and chronic hypertension with CCF.
- H/O diminished urine output/diminished foetal movements/painful bleeding PV—due to abruptio placenta
- Ask for imminent symptoms like H/O headache, visual disturbances, giddiness, epigastric pain (due to stretching of liver capsule), vomiting, diminished urine output—*indicates severe pre-eclampsia, imminent eclampsia*

HISTORY
MENSTRUAL HISTORY
- Refer Case 1.

To view the lecture notes log in to your account on www.MedEnact.com

MARITAL HISTORY
- Refer Case 1.

OBSTETRIC HISTORY
Past obstetric history
- In previous pregnancy, H/O pre-eclampsia to be elicited (following details namely gestational age at which it was diagnosed, severity, induction of labour, mode of delivery/weight of the baby, alive or dead to be elicited)
- H/O GDM—its onset and type of treatment

PAST MEDICAL HISTORY
- Other predisposing factors like diabetes, recurrent UTI, renal disease, hypertension to be ruled out (if woman is taking medication dose and type of anti-hypertensive drug, it is to be elicited)

PAST SURGICAL HISTORY
- Refer Case 1.

FAMILY HISTORY
- H/O pre-eclampsia in mother/siblings (autosomal trait)/hypertension/diabetes

PERSONAL HISTORY
- Smoking

EXAMINATION
GENERAL EXAMINATION
- Refer Case 1.
  Specific points to be noted in pre-eclampsia:

- *Build*—obese/moderate/thin
- *Weight*—pre-pregnant weight should be asked for and present weight is to be taken to assess excessive weight gain
  - Daily weight measurement is to be done
  - Weight gain more than ½ kg/week gives evidence of occult oedema

EXAMINATION

- *Oedema*—importance to be given to the site of oedema apart from pedal oedema
  - Oedema seen in the morning as soon as patient gets up from bed is always pathological.
  - *In pre-eclampsia, non-dependent oedema may be seen in the following sites*:
    - Face, dorsum of hand and abdominal wall along with dependent area like lower limbs (Figs 4.1–4.3), vulva (Fig. 4.4) and pre-sacral area
  - For causes and differentiating points for physiological and pathological oedema—refer Case 1

Grading of Oedema	
Grade 1	Mild—both feet/ankles
Grade 2	Moderate—both feet plus lower limbs, hands and arms
Grade 3	Severe—generalised, bilateral pitting oedema, including both feet, legs, arms, abdominal wall, face
Grade 4	Anasarca

- *Anaemia* can co-exist, which may be due to haemolysis due to HELLP syndrome
- *Jaundice* (HELLP syndrome)
- *Deep tendon reflexes*
- *Blood pressure measurement*: This should be measured in semi-recumbent position—45-degree tilt or in sitting posture with arm at the level of heart with proper size cuff, properly tied. When

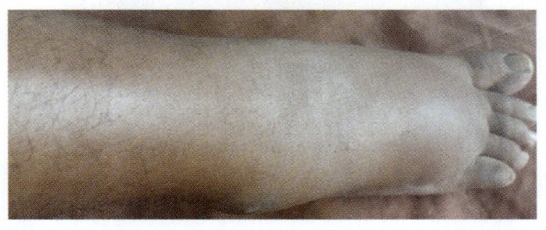

FIGURE 4.1 Bilateral Pedal Oedema

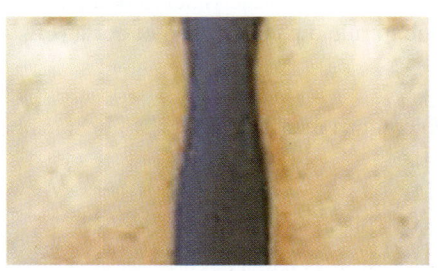

FIGURE 4.2 Oedema Below Knee

56 CASE 4 A CASE OF HYPERTENSION IN PREGNANCY

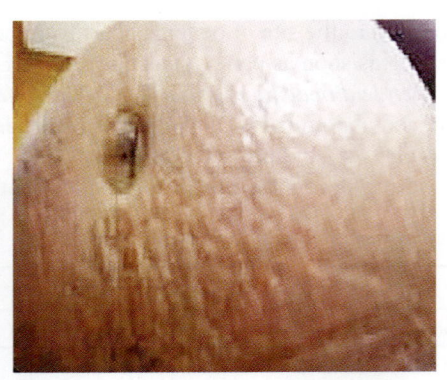

FIGURE 4.3 Oedema of Abdominal Wall

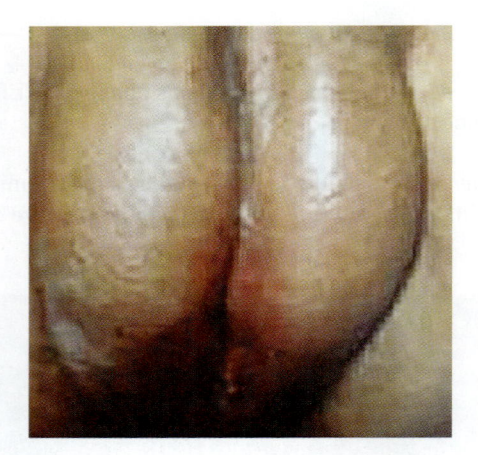

FIGURE 4.4 Vulval Oedema

small size cuff is used for bigger arm circumference women, it will show false high blood pressure. The disappearance of sound (Korotkoff V) is considered for diastolic BP since in pregnancy the peripheral vascular resistance is less. When blood pressure is high in upper arm, one should check in the lower limb to rule out coarctation of aorta (Fig. 4.5).

If BP is high, repeat after 4–6 h to confirm measurements.

OBSTETRIC EXAMINATION
Examination is done as in any other case (refer Case 1).

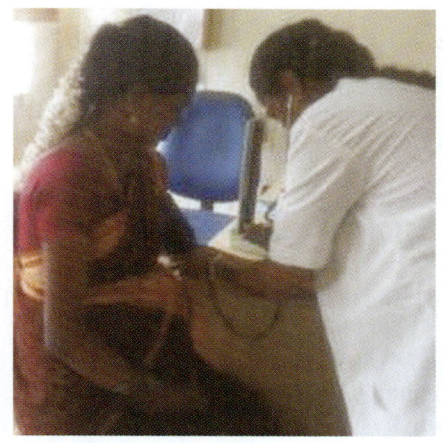

FIGURE 4.5 **Blood Pressure Measurement**

Following examination findings may be present:
- Oedema of abdominal wall
- Height of the uterus—may correspond to period of gestation
- In oligohydramnios/FGR—height will be less
- In multiple gestation—height of uterus will be bigger (multiple pregnancy may be a predisposing factor for pre-eclampsia)

SUMMARY
- Mrs……………………………… Age…….. Socioeconomic Class…….. Gravida, Para, Booked/immunised, LMP…….....…….. EDD ………..…… admitted with H/O………..…… months of amenorrhoea/gestational age/with c/o pedal oedema/diminished foetal movements/bleeding PV/diminished urine output/blurring of vision/headache/vomiting/draining PV
- General examination findings—oedema, anaemia, blood pressure.
  CVS/RS -findings
- Obstetric examination findings—height of the uterus (corresponding or not), uterus acting or not, tense or tender, lie of the foetus, size of the baby, foetal heart rate

DIAGNOSIS
Gravida………… Para………… period of gestation………… EDD with mild/severe pre-eclampsia (if urine protein result is available) or gestational hypertension with viable foetus single or multiple …… in…… presentation.

INVESTIGATIONS

Laboratory investigations for pre-eclampsia:
- *Urine*—Albumin by dipstick method
    Urine albumin trace = 0.1 g/L
    1+ = 0.3–1 g/L
    2+ = 1–3 g/L
    3+ = 3–10 g/L
    4+ = 10 g/L
  - Proteinuria—presence of more than 0.3 g/L in 24 h urine or 1 g/L in random specimen on two occasions
  - Urine—deposits—pus cells, casts—hyaline, epithelial, granular, RBC casts (underlying renal disease). Hyaline casts, epithelial cells and few RBC may be present in pre-eclampsia
  - Urine—culture and sensitivity
  - Urine for 24 h protein
  - Urine—sugar
- *Blood*
  - Haemoglobin, PCV (PCV may be increased due to haemoconcentration)

For haemolysis	Peripheral smear—schistocytes in peripheral smear/LDH
Platelet count	Grading of thrombocytopenia
Grade 1	$>1,00,000$ mm^{-3}
Grade 2	$50,000–1,00,000$ mm^{-3}
Grade 3	$<50,000$ mm^{-3}

  - Blood group, Rh type
  - Bleeding time, clotting time
  - Blood sugar
  - Renal function test: blood urea, serum creatinine
  - Serum uric acid—more than 4 mg/dL (has prognostic value)
  - Coagulation profile: serum fibrinogen
    – Prothrombin time—PT
    – Activated prothrombin time—APTT
  - Liver function test: serum bilirubin, AST/ALT

Optic fundus examination:

Fundal changes: Grade 0	Normal
Grade 1	Constriction of arterioles
Grade 2	Arteriolar spasm, alteration in ratio of vein: arteriole 3:2 to 3:1
Grade 3	Oedema, haemorrhage, exudates
Grade 4	Papilloedema

INVESTIGATIONS

Table 4.1 Hypertensive Disorders in Pregnancy

Hypertensive Disorders in Pregnancy	Diagnostic Features
Gestational hypertension	BP 140/90 mmHg or more occurring for the first time after 20 weeks of pregnancy in a previously normotensive woman without proteinuria. Blood pressure will come to normal within 12 weeks of delivery. Final diagnosis is possible only after post-natal period.
Pre-eclampsia	Blood pressure of 140/90 mmHg or more measured on two occasions 4–6 h apart, accompanied by proteinuria (greater than 0.3 g/L in 24 h urine or greater than 1 g/L in random sample) occurring after 20 weeks of pregnancy in a previously normotensive woman.
Mild pre-eclampsia	Blood pressure—140/90 mmHg but <160/110 with proteinuria—1+
Severe pre-eclampsia	Blood pressure of 160/110 mmHg and above/symptoms like occipital head ache, vomiting, visual disturbances, persistent epigastric pain Proteinuria of >3 g/L in 24 h/(>2+) Oliguria <400 mL/24 h/platelet count < 100,000/mL/HELLP syndrome Serum creatinine >1.1 mg/dL Fundus changes—Grade 3 and 4/pulmonary oedema/FGR Now the terminology used is pre-eclampsia with or without severe features
Eclampsia	Occurrence of convulsions in a patient with pre-eclampsia with no coincidental neurological disease
Chronic hypertension	Persistent blood pressure values over 140/90 mmHg in either pre-pregnancy or prior to 20 weeks and persist 12 weeks post-partum
Superimposed pre-eclampsia on chronic hypertension	New onset proteinuria after 20 weeks gestation, sudden increase in BP or proteinuria in woman with hypertension before 20 weeks

Significance—shows severity of disease. Grade 3 and 4 fundal changes are indications for termination of pregnancy irrespective of gestational age

Assessment of foetal wellbeing
- Daily foetal movement—kick chart
- Serial USG—to rule out IUGR and oligohydramnios
- Modified biophysical profile (NST + AFI)
- Doppler of the foetal vessels—umbilical artery, middle cerebral artery, ductus venosus

HYPERTENSIVE DISORDERS IN PREGNANCY
Case discussion
Hypertensive disorders in pregnancy are explained in Table 4.1.

BASIC PATHOLOGY OF PRE-ECLAMPSIA IN SHORT
- Vasospasm (imbalance between vasodilators—PGI_2, NO and vasoconstrictors—angiotensin 11, thromboxane A2, endothelin 1)

- Endothelial dysfunction and damage (due to oxidative stress and inflammatory mediators like cytokines and interleukins). These changes can affect almost all vessels especially those of uterus, kidney, brain and liver
- Pathophysiology is inadequate secondary invasion of cytotrophoblast into spiral arteries leading to ineffective vascular remodelling resulting in insufficient placental perfusion.

> Pre-eclampsia is not a preventable disease but severity and complications can be anticipated and treated.

HIGH RISK FACTORS FOR DEVELOPING PRE-ECLAMPSIA
- Primi gravida
- Maternal age more than 35 years
- Obesity
- Multiple pregnancy
- Vesicular mole
- APLA syndrome
- H/O previous PE, family H/O PE in mother, sister
- Thrombophilias—Protein S, Protein C deficiency, Factor V Leiden mutation
- Existing diabetes mellitus, chronic hypertension, renal disease

PREDICTORS OF PRE-ECLAMPSIA
- *Mean arterial pressure (MAP)* = $\dfrac{\text{systolic} + (\text{diastolic} \times 2)}{3}$
  More than 90 mmHg in second trimester predicts pre-eclampsia; more than 105 mmHg may be diagnostic for pre-eclampsia
- *Absence of mid-trimester fall of BP*
- *Gants's roll over test*—done at 28–30 weeks. Increase in diastolic BP by >20 mmHg when patient lies in supine position from left lateral position
- *Persistent uterine artery diastolic notch* in Doppler at 24 weeks
- *Angiotensin sensitivity test*
- *Foetal–placental unit endocrine dysfunction*: HCG, AFP, PAPP A, Inhibin A, placental protein 13
- *Renal dysfunction*: serum uric acid, microalbuminuria, urinary calcium, fibronectin, thromboxane
- *Placental growth factor*—PIGF, vascular endothelial growth factor (VEGF), endoglin
- *Others*: cell-free foetal DNA
- *Endothelial dysfunction*: platelet count

PREVENTION OF PRE-ECLAMPSIA

- Regular antenatal check-up
- Low—dose aspirin, 75 mg in prevention of early onset PE; in high risk women, APLA syndrome, previous history of pre-eclampsia.
- Calcium supplementation
- Anti-oxidants like vitamin C, vitamin E, fish oil

Differentiating Features Between Mild and Severe Pre-Eclampsia	
Pre-Eclampsia	**Clinical Features**
Mild	BP > 140/90 mmHg but <160/110 mmHg persist even after 4 h with proteinuria—1+
Severe	BP > 160/110 mmHg Head ache, visual disturbances, vomiting Proteinuria >3 g/24 h Oliguria <400 mL in 24 h Platelet count < 100,000/mL HELLP syndrome Serum creatinine >1.1 mg/dL Fundus changes—Grade 3 and 4 Pulmonary oedema FGR

Anti-Hypertensive Drugs Used in Pregnancy				
Drugs Used	**Dose**	**Maintenance and Maximum**	**Mode of Action**	**Contraindication**
Labetalol	100–200 mg	b.i.d. or t.i.d.	Alpha and beta blockers	Asthma and CCF
Nifedipine	10–20 mg	b.i.d. or t.i.d.	Calcium channel blockers	Unstable angina pectoris, LVF
Alpha-methyldopa	250–500 mg	t.i.d. or q.i.d.—max—2 g	Central	Depression, Parkinson symptoms, angina, chronic heart failure
Hypertensive crisis				
Labetalol	10–20 mg IV every 10 min	Maintenance—40 mg/h, max—300 mg	Alpha and beta blockers	Cardiac failure bronchospasm
Hydralazine	5 mg/30 min	Maintenance 10 mg/h, max—30 mg IV	Peripheral vasodilators	Recent heart attack, disease of the arteries of the heart, stroke

ACE inhibitors absolutely contraindicated.

MANAGEMENT
GENERAL MANAGEMENT OF PRE-ECLAMPSIA

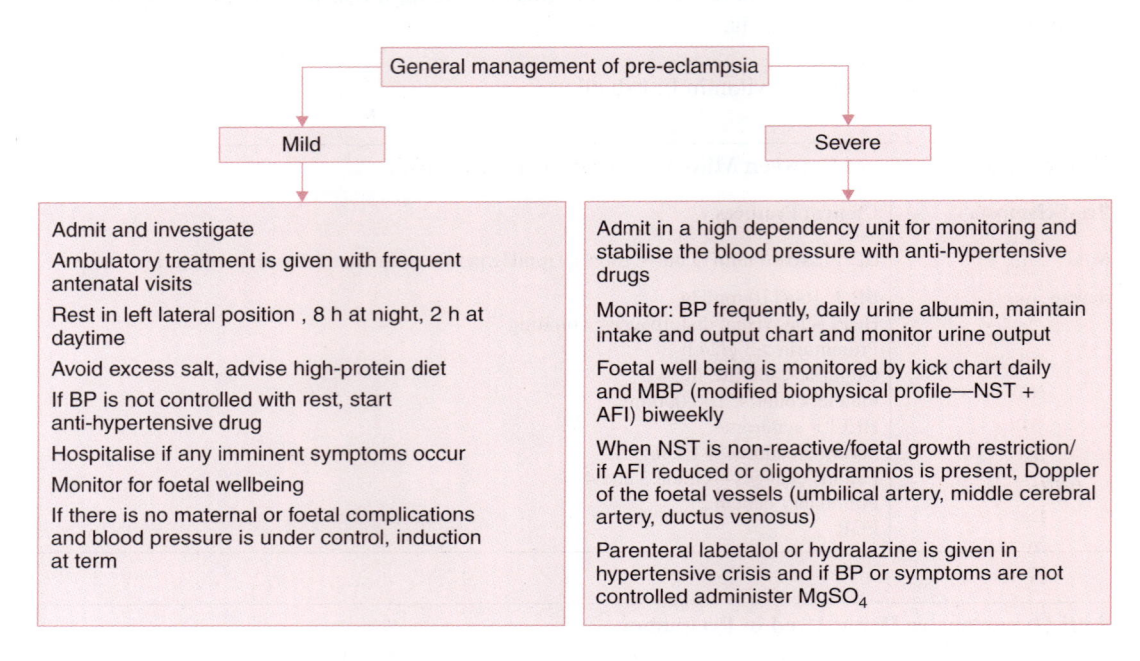

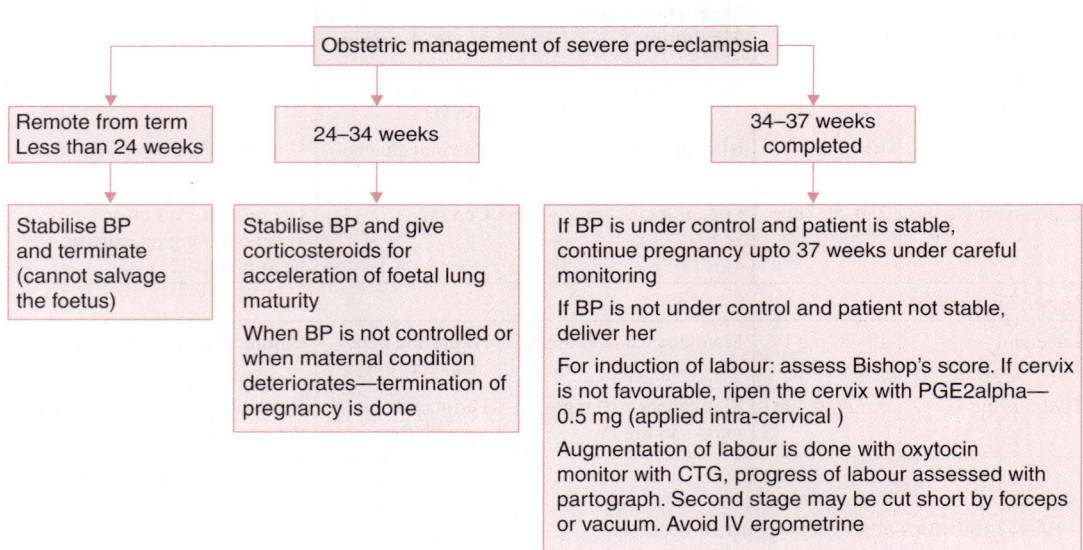

General management of pre-eclampsia

Mild
- Admit and investigate
- Ambulatory treatment is given with frequent antenatal visits
- Rest in left lateral position, 8 h at night, 2 h at daytime
- Avoid excess salt, advise high-protein diet
- If BP is not controlled with rest, start anti-hypertensive drug
- Hospitalise if any imminent symptoms occur
- Monitor for foetal wellbeing
- If there is no maternal or foetal complications and blood pressure is under control, induction at term

Severe
- Admit in a high dependency unit for monitoring and stabilise the blood pressure with anti-hypertensive drugs
- Monitor: BP frequently, daily urine albumin, maintain intake and output chart and monitor urine output
- Foetal well being is monitored by kick chart daily and MBP (modified biophysical profile—NST + AFI) biweekly
- When NST is non-reactive/foetal growth restriction/ if AFI reduced or oligohydramnios is present, Doppler of the foetal vessels (umbilical artery, middle cerebral artery, ductus venosus)
- Parenteral labetalol or hydralazine is given in hypertensive crisis and if BP or symptoms are not controlled administer $MgSO_4$

Obstetric management of severe pre-eclampsia

Remote from term Less than 24 weeks
- Stabilise BP and terminate (cannot salvage the foetus)

24–34 weeks
- Stabilise BP and give corticosteroids for acceleration of foetal lung maturity
- When BP is not controlled or when maternal condition deteriorates—termination of pregnancy is done

34–37 weeks completed
- If BP is under control and patient is stable, continue pregnancy upto 37 weeks under careful monitoring
- If BP is not under control and patient not stable, deliver her
- For induction of labour: assess Bishop's score. If cervix is not favourable, ripen the cervix with PGE2alpha— 0.5 mg (applied intra-cervical)
- Augmentation of labour is done with oxytocin monitor with CTG, progress of labour assessed with partograph. Second stage may be cut short by forceps or vacuum. Avoid IV ergometrine

INDICATIONS FOR CAESAREAN SECTION
- *Emergency caesarean section*: if there is no progress in labour/abnormal CTG or partogram in labour
- *Elective caesarean section*: in cases of foetal compromise—FGR, oligohydramnios
- Other risk factors like malpresentation, CPD, elderly primi, BOH

MANAGEMENT OF ECLAMPSIA
- *General management*
  - Admit in HDU
  - Railed cot
  - O_2
  - Clear air way
  - Insert mouth gag
  - Continuous bladder drainage
  - Intake output chart
  - Intravenous line with wide bore needle
  - Antibiotics
  - Monitor—pulse, BP, RS, urine output
- *Anti-hypertensives management*
  - Labetalol: IV bolus of 20, 40 and 80 mg every 10 min to total of 300 mg followed by 2 mg/min infusion
  - Hydralazine: 5–10 mg IV bolus every 20 min till BP is controlled. Infusion—0.5–10 mg/h. If no success with 20 mg IV or 30 mg IM, consider another drug
- *Anti-convulsant management*—Pritchard's regime—$MgSO_4$

Inj. magnesium sulphate:
- Mode of action: at motor end plate, it suppresses the acetylcholine release and sensitivity
- Acts by competitive inhibition of calcium ion at motor end plate
- Uses of magnesium sulphate:
  - In pre-term labour, it can be used as tocolytic agent
  - In severe pre-eclampsia, it is given as prophylaxis against eclampsia
  - In eclampsia, it reduces intra-cerebral oedema and has specific anti-convulsant action on cerebral cortex
  - Pritchard's regime: each ampoule contains 2 mL of 50% solution equivalent to 1 g of $MgSO_4$
- Loading dose—4 g of 20% $MgSO_4$, given slowly IV over a period of 3–5 min (4 ampoule—8 mL contains 4 g $MgSO_4$, mix it with 12 mL of water which makes it 20 cc (4 g) of 20% of $MgSO_4$)
- Followed by 5 g of $MgSO_4$ (10 mL—5 ampoule of 50%) in each buttock IM
- Subsequently—5 g of $MgSO_4$ IM (10 mL—5 ampoule of 50%) administered on alternate buttock every 4 h depending upon the blood pressure, clinical and biochemical parameters
- Continue till 24 h after the last fit or delivery whichever is later
- Monitor the following: knee jerk should be present, respiratory rate >16 min^{-1}, urine output >30 mL/h. Therapeutic level of serum magnesium—4–7 mEq./L
- Antidote: calcium gluconate—10 mL of 10% IV

Zuspan regime: 4 g $MgSO_4$ IV as bolus over 10 min followed by 1 g IV as infusion till 24 h after last fit

- *Obstetric management*
  - Stabilise and deliver immediately
  - If fits are controlled, if cervix favourable, and good progress in labour or if labour is imminent—allow vaginal delivery
  - Uncontrolled fits/if cervix is unfavourable—LSCS
- *Management of complications*: treatment based on the complication

COMPLICATIONS OF PRE-ECLAMPSIA
- *Maternal*:
  - Eclampsia
  - Pre-term labour
  - Abruptio placenta
  - Oliguria and anuria—renal failure
  - Papilloedema, cortical blindness, retinal detachment
  - HELLP syndrome
  - Pulmonary oedema
  - Cerebral haemorrhage
  - Post-partum collapse
  - Disseminated intra-vascular coagulation (DIVC)
  - CCF

HELLP syndrome: feature of haemolysis, elevated liver enzymes, low platelet count—warrants immediate delivery.

- *Foetal complication*: Foetal growth restriction, IUD, prematurity, intrapartum asphxia, perinatal mortality

Role of diuretics in pre-eclampsia—used only in pulmonary oedema and CCF.

Hypertensive disorder is the most frequent condition associated with abruption.

ABRUPTIO PLACENTA
- *Definition of APH*: bleeding from genital tract after 28 weeks of pregnancy before delivery of foetus
- *Causes of APH*:
  - Abruptio—Premature separation of a normally situated placenta
  - Placenta previa
  - Circumvallate placenta
  - Vasa previa

- Rupture of marginal sinus
- Unclassified
- Coincidental local factors—Cx polyp, erosion, cancer cervix
- *Page classification of abruptio placenta*:

Grade 0	Retroplacental clots seen after delivery
Grade I	External bleeding only
	Mild uterine tetany
	No foetal or maternal distress
Grade II	Possibly external bleeding
	Uterine tetany and tenderness
	Foetal distress or death
	No maternal distress or shock
Grade III	Uterine tetany
	IUD
	Maternal shock or coagulation defects

- *Complications of abruptio placenta*:

Maternal	PPH, shock, DIVC, renal failure, maternal death
Foetal	IUD, prematurity

- *Management of abruptio placenta*:
  - In abruptio placenta—patient may present, after period of viability, with concealed or revealed bleeding PV with pain in abdomen and with history of amenorrhoea
    On examination, uterus may be tense, tender with or absent foetal heart
  - If foetus is dead—it denotes severity (>1/3rd placental separation) and warrants early delivery
  - When foetus is alive and mature—deliver early by caesarean section, if vaginal delivery is not imminent
- *General management*

In all cases after initial examination and assessing the severity of blood loss, patient should be sedated.

- Bladder catheterised for hourly monitoring of urine output
- In cases of severe blood loss, compatible blood to be transfused to treat the shock
- Blood for coagulation profile to be done
- Monitor vitals and coagulation profile

- *Obstetric management*
  - Mild cases—ARM and augmentation of labour (ARM will help to control bleeding and hasten labour)
- *Principal line of management of severe cases*
  - Combat shock and replace blood loss
  - Relieve uterine distension by ARM
  - Hasten labour by oxytocin augmentation
  - Watch for coagulation and renal failure
- *Indications for LSCS*
  - If labour is not well established
  - If progress of labour is slow
  - If the patient deteriorates
- *Couvelaire uterus*: in abruptio placenta, blood may extravasate into the uterine musculature called as utero placental apoplexy with dark ecchymotic changes over serosa, called as Couvelaire uterus

Abruptio placenta—management of each case is individualised.

KEY POINTS

- Pre-eclampsia is not preventable but severity and complications can be anticipated and if treated promptly eclampsia can be prevented.
- Basic pathology in pre-eclampsia is vasospasm caused by imbalance between prostacyclin PGI2, PGE2 prostaglandin and thromboxane and endothelial dysfunction caused by oxidative stress.
- Predictive tests are not much valuable.
- Pre-eclampsia can be with or without severity but both can cause maternal and foetal complications.
- Pre-eclampsia should be differentiated from other hypertensive disorders in pregnancy.
- Best treatment for pre-eclampsia is to stabilise blood pressure, vigilant monitoring for maternal and foetal wellbeing, anticipate complications, treat it and appropriate timing and mode of delivery.
- For uncontrolled severe pre-eclampsia and imminent eclampsia prophylactic anti-convulsant MgSO$_4$ therapy to be started.
- Basic principle in management of eclampsia are general management, anti-hypertensive and anti-convulsant therapy, management of complications and expedite delivery.

FREQUENTLY ASKED QUESTIONS

1. Define pre-eclampsia.
2. Classify hypertensive disorders in pregnancy.
3. What is the etiopathogenesis of pre-eclampsia?

FREQUENTLY ASKED QUESTIONS

4. What is the pathophysiology of pre-eclampsia?
5. What are the risk factors for pre-eclampsia?
6. What are the clinical and diagnostic criteria for severe pre-eclampsia?
7. What is proteinuria and how much does 1+ to 4+ proteinuria in urine indicate?
8. What are the investigations for a case of pre-eclampsia?
9. What are the fundal changes and its significance?
10. What is HELLP syndrome and management?
11. What is the importance of serum uric acid?
12. What is $MgSO_4$ regimen? How will you monitor?
13. What is the antenatal foetal surveillance in pre-eclampsia?
14. Prediction and prevention of pre-eclampsia?

CASE 5

A CASE OF PROLONGED (POST-TERM) PREGNANCY

PATIENT'S DETAILS

Name.. Age................. Address.......................... Occupation.............
Socioeconomic Class.......................... Gravida, Para, Live, Abortion, (G......... P......... L......... A..........)
Booked/Unbooked......................... Immunisation....................... LMP............ EDD

H/O............ months of amenorrhoea /period of gestation

PRESENT COMPLAINTS

Patient may present with period of amenorrhoea with following complaints:

Following history is elicited:
- By how many days she has crossed her EDD?
- Is she sure of her LMP?
- Regularity of her menstrual cycle
- Conceived spontaneously or after induction of ovulation?
- History of taking oral contraceptive pill and did she have regular periods after stopping the pill?
- Sedentary lifestyle
- Date of urine pregnancy test done
- Details of dating scan, target scan, growth scan—if USG reports are available, it helps to assess gestational age
- Pelvic and abdominal examination records in early pregnancy, if available
- Date of quickening
- H/O of taking prostaglandin inhibitors—NSAID, aspirin
- Whether she is feeling foetal movements well/diminished foetal movements or loss of foetal movements

HISTORY

MENSTRUAL HISTORY, MARITAL HISTORY, PAST HISTORY, SURGICAL HISTORY, FAMILY HISTORY, PERSONAL HISTORY
- Refer Case 1.

To view the lecture notes log in to your account on www.MedEnact.com

CASE 5 A CASE OF PROLONGED (POST-TERM) PREGNANCY

OBSTETRIC HISTORY
- **In multi**—previous history of post-datism and in placental sulphatase deficiency—prolonged pregnancy can recur
- Age of the first child
- When did she establish her periods after child birth and whether the cycles were regular or she conceived during lactation amenorrhoea
- Whether she conceived soon after abortion?
- H/O spontaneous conception/whether conceived after induction of ovulation

FAMILY HISTORY
- Prolonged pregnancy can occur due to placental sulphatase deficiency

EXAMINATION
GENERAL EXAMINATION
- Refer Case 1.

OBSTETRIC EXAMINATION
- Fundal height of the uterus
- Whether flanks are full
- Shelving sign present or not
- Amount of liquor clinically—diminished or not
- Feel of the head—hard or not
- Presenting part—mobile/unengaged/engaged
- Girth of abdomen—when liquor is less, girth reduces
- Assessment of foetal weight

PER VAGINAL EXAMINATION
- Pelvic assessment/Bishop scoring/CPD assessment by Munro Kerr Muller method
- Hard head may be felt through fornix

SUMMARY
- Mrs………Age………Gravida…..Para……admitted with……
- …H/O... months amenorrhoea with crossing her dates/with regular cycles/conceived spontaneously/by induction of ovulation/good foetal movements/diminished foetal movements/bleeding PV/draining PV
- Include positive general examination findings/about CVS/RS
- Obstetric examination findings—whether uterus is term and flanks are full, shelving sign, clinically about liquor, size of the foetus, lie of the foetus, feel of the head, mobile or unengaged, foetal heart rate

DIAGNOSIS

Mrs………Age………Gravida……Para……period of gestation by dates………she has crossed her dates by………days that is post-dated by………days

INVESTIGATIONS

- Routine (basic) investigations
- Clinically—assess pelvis, Bishop score and assess CPD
- *USG*: For gestational age by BPD, FL, AC, HC, foetal weight, amount of liquor, placental localisation
- **Modified biophysical profile (NST + AFI)**
- **Doppler**: umbilical artery, middle cerebral artery, ductus venosus

CASE DISCUSSION

Reliability of the EDD:

- *Excellent dates*
  - Sure of LMP, previous three consecutive cycles are regular
  - No recent OC pill use
  - Uterine size correlates with dates + USG between 16 and 24 weeks
  - Inadequate clinical information but two USGs between 16 and 24 weeks and linear growth correlates with EDD
- *Good dates*
  - Adequate clinical information + one USG at 24 weeks
- *Poor dates*
  Any clinical situation different from following:
  - If LMP is not known
  - Conceived during lactational amenorrhoea
  - Conceived soon after stopping oral pill
  - When LMP is uncertain or woman has not had three regular cycles
- *When LMP is not known, EDD is calculated in the following ways*:
  - Early PV examination findings
  - Date of positive urine pregnancy test
  - Early dating scan
  - Date of quickening (20 weeks in primi, 16–18 weeks in multi)
  - Induction of ovulation with follicular study (266 days are added to date of ovulation to arrive at EDD)
  - SFH measurements after 20 weeks
- *Term pregnancy* is pregnancy after 37 completed weeks to 42 weeks
- *Post-term or prolonged pregnancy* is one that has lasted 294 days or 42 weeks or more from 1st day of LMP

Table 5.1 Bishop Score

Score	Dilatation	Effacement	Station	Cervical Consistency	Cervical Position
0	Closed	0–30	−3	Firm	Posterior
1	1–2	40–50	−2	Medium	Mid-position
2	3–4	60–70	−1	Soft	Anterior
3	+>5	+>80	+1, +2	Soft	Anterior

- *Post-mature syndrome*—described by Clifford is foetus born of prolonged pregnancy. Neonate will have wrinkled, peeling skin coated with meconium, overgrown nails, well-developed palm and sole creases, reduced subcutaneous fat and wizened old man appearance
- *Modified biophysical profile*—AFI + NST
- *Bishop score*: based on effacement, dilatation, position, consistency of cervix, station of the head (Table 5.1)
  If Bishop score is high, it is favourable for induction.
  If <6: Ripen the cervix with intra-cervical gel—Dinoprostone 0.5 mg

MANAGEMENT
MANAGEMENT OF PROLONGED PREGNANCY

- *Wait up to 41 weeks* when modified biophysical profile is normal and Bishop score is unfavourable.
- *Induce at 40 weeks*
- If there are obstetric complications
- If Bishop's score is favourable
- If NST is non-reactive
- If there is oligohydramnios
- In the presence of macrosomia

> Pregnancy with complications like GDM Rh −ve pregnancy, pre-eclampsia, RPL, FGR, elderly primi—**should not be allowed to go beyond 40 weeks**

METHODS OF FOETAL SURVEILLANCE BEYOND DATES

- *Daily foetal movement count* (DFMC)—Kick chart, normal is 3 kicks/1 h
- *Foetal alarm signal*—less than 10 movements/12 h indicates foetal compromise and needs further evaluation
- Less than four in 12 h can result in IUD

- Cardiff count to 10:
  - After a meal patient is given a piece of thread and asked to put knot whenever she perceives a foetal movement till 10 movements are perceived. Starting time and ending time are noted
  - If <10 foetal movements are perceived in 12 h—foetal compromise. Practical difficulty in this method, woman has to notice foetal movement from 9 a.m. to 9 p.m.
  - Hence she is advised to put foetal kick chart (FKC) for 1 h in the morning, 1 h in the afternoon and 1 h in the evening

MANNING'S BIOPHYSICAL PROFILE

It includes NST and monitoring the following points in USG:

- Foetal breathing movements
- Foetal gross body movements
- Foetal tone
- AFI
- Each component is given a score of 2
- Since it takes minimum of 30 min to finish the test as the foetal breathing, foetal movement may not be present for 30 min during sleep cycle, and may need stimulation, nowadays it is not used

MODIFIED BIOPHYSICAL PROFILE (NST + AFI) BIWEEKLY

- NST—Basis—Autonomic influences mediated by sympathetic and parasympathetic impulses has impact that affect the foetal heart rate which results in beat-to-beat variability
- With foetal movements, there is acceleration of foetal heart rate when foetus is not hypoxic

Interpretations
NST reactive:
- Baseline rate 110–160 beats/min
- Normal beat-to-beat variability, 5–15 beats/min
- Two or more accelerations of 15 beats/min lasting for 15 s, in response to a foetal movement over a period of 20 min
- Absence of late or variable decelerations

NST non-reactive: Anything which does not meet the previously mentioned criteria
- In foetal sleep cycle—absence of foetal heart rate accelerations may be there. So extend the duration of NST for further period of 20 min or stimulate the foetus by using the vibroacoustic stimulation test (VAST)

AMNIOTIC FLUID INDEX

It is a measurement done with USG (Fig. 5.1).
- It is the sum of the largest vertical pockets of amniotic fluid measured in four quadrants of the uterus (free of cord or foetal structures)
- AFI: 8–20 is normal

CASE 5 A CASE OF PROLONGED (POST-TERM) PREGNANCY

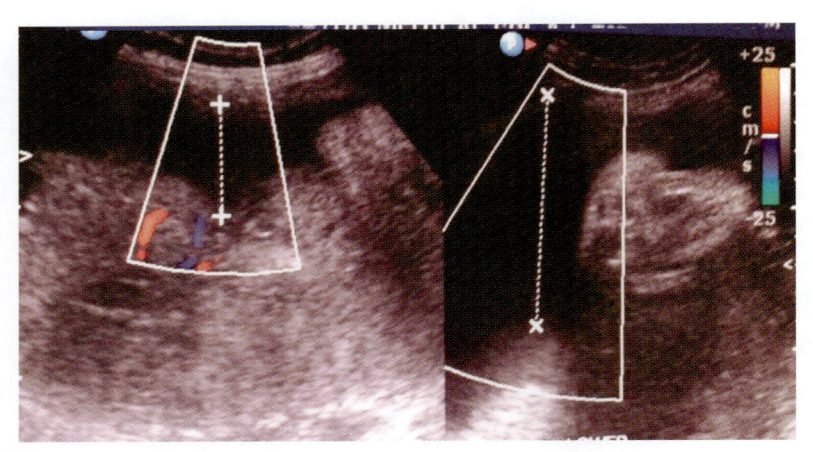

FIGURE 5.1 AFI Measurements

- Oligohydramnios: AFI, 5 cm or single pocket less than 2 cm; polyhydramnios: AFI, 25 cm or single pocket more than 8 cm

DOPPLER VELOCIMETRY

Whenever foetus is at risk of hypoxia, Doppler will show sequential changes in foetal blood vessels.
- Doppler study is done in the umbilical artery, middle cerebral artery and ductus venosus
- When all three vessels show normal S/D ratio—*no foetal hypoxia*
- When umbilical artery shows reduced diastolic flow or absent or reversed flow—*foetus is hypoxic*. Reversed flow is an *ominous sign*
- Middle cerebral artery shows changes due to preferential cerebral flow (brain sparing effect) *to compensate for hypoxia*
- Ductus venosus show changes when foetus goes for cardiac failure and *death is imminent*

INDUCTION OF LABOUR IN PROLONGED PREGNANCY

- Induction is done at 41 weeks because she may get in to spontaneous labour after 40 weeks
- Induction is done, when there is no foetal compromise and no maternal complications at 41 weeks and earlier if there is evidence of foetal compromise and maternal complications
- After 41 weeks, there is increased incidence of meconium aspiration syndrome and perinatal morbidity due to placental insufficiency

Pre-requisites for induction of labour
- Rule out CPD, Bishop score to be assessed
- If cervix is favourable, score more than 6/13—induction with ARM and Syntocinon can be done
- If cervix is unfavourable, score less than 6/13—intra-cervical PGE$_2$ gel is applied for ripening the cervix. Three doses of PGE$_2$ (Dinoprostone) can be repeated at 6th hourly interval
- Progress of labour monitored by partogram
- ARM is done in active labour

MANAGEMENT

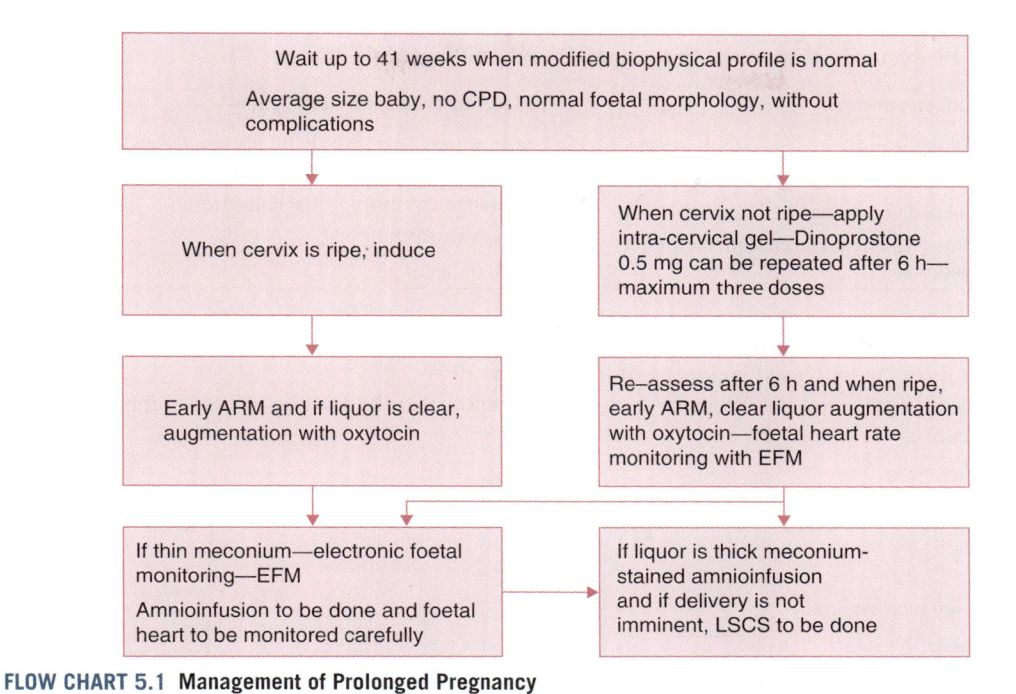

```
┌─────────────────────────────────────────────────────────┐
│ Wait up to 41 weeks when modified biophysical profile   │
│ is normal                                                │
│ Average size baby, no CPD, normal foetal morphology,    │
│ without complications                                    │
└─────────────────────────────────────────────────────────┘
```

FLOW CHART 5.1 Management of Prolonged Pregnancy

- If liquor is clear or thin meconium stained augmentation of labour with oxytocin can be done
- If liquor is meconium-stained moderately, amnioinfusion to be done and foetal heart to be monitored carefully during the progress of labour and augmentation of labour with oxytocin can be done
- If liquor is thick meconium-stained—amnioinfusion and LSCS to be done, if delivery is not imminent

Indications for LSCS:
- Macrosomia with CPD
- Complicated prolonged pregnancy
- Severe oligohydramnios
- Reversed or absent end diastolic flow in umbilical artery
- Non-reactive NST/oligohydramnios
- Thick meconium-stained liquor
- Failed induction
- Non-reassuring CTG in labour (Flow chart 5.1)

COMPLICATIONS OF PROLONGED PREGNANCY

Maternal (Table 5.2)
- When there is no placental insufficiency—macrosomia

Table 5.2 Problems in Prolonged Pregnancy Based on Placental Changes

Placenta With Insufficiency	Placenta Without Insufficiency
Lead to oligohydramnios	Macrosomia, and hard skull bone results leading to dystocia, prolonged labour, shoulder dystocia
Cord compression due to oligohydramnios	Operative and instrumental deliveries
Meconium stained liquor due to GI maturity	Traumatic PPH
Oligohydramnios and hypoxia leads to meconium aspiration syndrome	Birth trauma

- Macrosomia can lead to prolonged labour/increased operative deliveries/instrumental deliveries/shoulder dystocia/increased incidence of birth trauma PPH
- When there is placental insufficiency—oligohydramnios, thereby leading to cord compression and foetal distress

Foetal

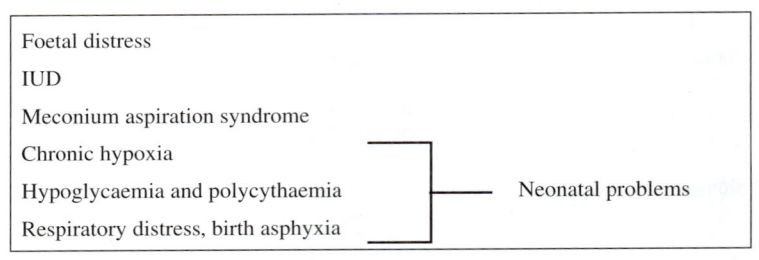

Foetal distress
IUD
Meconium aspiration syndrome
Chronic hypoxia
Hypoglycaemia and polycythaemia ⎤
Respiratory distress, birth asphyxia ⎦ — Neonatal problems

Post-term pregnancy can lead to oligohydramnios

OLIGOHYDRAMNIOS

Other causes for oligohydramnios:
- Pre-eclampsia
- PROM
- FGR
- Intra-uterine infection
- Renal agenesis in foetus
- Obstruction of urinary tract
- Posterior urethral valve
- Chromosomal anomaly
- *Problems of early onset oligohydramnios*:
  - Pulmonary hypoplasia
  - Limb deformities like talipes
  - Amniotic adhesions or bands can lead to deformity
- *Problems of late onset oligohydramnios*:
  - Cord compression

Table 5.3 Management of Oligohydramnios

Antepartum	Intrapartum
No specific treatment	If Doppler normal and NST reactive—ARM to be done
Rest in left lateral position	If liquor—moderate meconium—amnioinfusion, careful monitoring of foetal heart rate and augmentation of labour with oxytocin
Monitor with antenatal foetal surveillance	
Search for renal malformation and when lethal anomaly is diagnosed, termination is offered	If liquor is thick meconium—if delivery is not imminent—LSCS

- Increased operative deliveries
- Meconium aspiration syndrome (MAS) chronic hypoxia
- Foetal distress
- *Diagnosis of oligohydramnios*:
  - Height of uterus smaller than period of amenorrhoea; uterus hugs the foetus
  - USG: AFI < 5 cm (Table 5.3)
- *Indications for LSCS*:
  - Thick meconium—if labour is not imminent
  - If NST—non-reactive
  - Doppler shows absent or reversed end diastolic flow
  - For obstetric indications

KEY POINTS

- Post-term pregnancy is pregnancy continuing beyond 42 weeks.
- Factors leading to post-term pregnancy are prior prolonged pregnancy, sedentary habit, elderly primi, obesity, occurs in family, placental sulphatase deficiency, undiagnosed anencephaly due to abnormal hypothalamic adrenal axis.
- Early assessment of gestational age by dating scan can reduce the incidence of post-term pregnancy.
- In post-term pregnancy, physiological changes occur in the placenta, liquor and foetus.
- When there is placental insufficiency, it causes oligohydramnios; when there is no placental insufficiency, it will result in macrosomia.
- In post-term, induction is done at 41st week. Till then antepartum surveillance is done.
- Induction done at 41 weeks, if there is no maternal complication, normal liquor, average size bay, no CPD and normal morphology.
- When cervix is favourable, early ARM and augmentation of labour is done with oxytocin and if cervix is not ripe, it can be done by applying intra-cervical Dinoprostone 0.5 mg (PGE_2 gel) and re-evaluation done after 6 h.
- When ARM is done, if liquor is clear, augment with oxytocin. If liquor is thick meconium-stained, if labour is not imminent, do LSCS.
- Maternal risk is increased due to labour dystocia, shoulder dystocia, increased incidence of instrumental delivery, operative delivery and PPH.
- Perinatal morbidity and mortality is increased from 0.4% at 37 weeks to 11.5 per 1000 at 43 weeks.

CASE 5 A CASE OF PROLONGED (POST-TERM) PREGNANCY

FREQUENTLY ASKED QUESTIONS

1. What is term pregnancy? What is prolonged/post-term pregnancy? What is post-maturity?
2. How will you establish gestational age when LMP is not known?
3. How will you calculate EDD when menstrual cycle is irregular?
4. What are the biometries in USG that will give you gestational age?
5. When do you induce labour in prolonged pregnancy?
6. Why you want to wait till 41 weeks?
7. How will you monitor foetal wellbeing till 41 weeks?
8. What are the causes for oligohydramnios?
9. What is the management of oligohydramnios?
10. What is biophysical profile?
11. What is modified biophysical profile?
12. What is the role of Doppler in post-datism?
13. What is Bishop score?
14. What are the methods of induction?
15. How will you monitor the progress of labour?
16. What are the maternal and foetal complications of prolonged pregnancy?
17. What are the neonatal complications? What are the complications of macrosomia?
18. What are the indications for caesarean in prolonged/post-term pregnancy?

CASE 6

A CASE OF PREGNANCY FOLLOWING CAESAREAN SECTION

PATIENT'S DETAILS

Name................................... Age................ Address......................... Occupation..............
Socioeconomic Class........................ Gravida, Para, Live, Abortion, (G......... P......... L.......... A.........)
Booked/Unbooked........................ Immunisation...................... LMP............ EDD

H/O............ months of amenorrhoea/period of gestation

PRESENT COMPLAINTS

Patient may present with period of amenorrhoea with following complaints:
 Admitted for safe confinement or history of pain—duration/site of pain/draining or bleeding PV/painful micturition is elicited. Enquire about foetal movements.

HISTORY

MENSTRUAL HISTORY, MARITAL HISTORY, PAST MEDICAL SURGICAL HISTORY, OBSTETRIC HISTORY, FAMILY HISTORY

- Refer Case 1.

Past obstetric history in detail
- In previous vaginal delivery, weight of the baby/alive or not/NICU admission/history of difficult forceps delivery

Regarding previous LSCS delivery, elicit the following:
- When was LSCS done in relation to EDD—term or pre-term?
- What is the indication for caesarean? (Whether it is recurrent or non-recurrent?)
- Whether emergency or elective LSCS?
- In discharge summary, check about whether resuturing done, whether there is mention about inverted T incision or extension of uterine angles.

To view the lecture notes log in to your account on www.MedEnact.com

In emergency LSCS, following history is to be elicited:
- How long was she in labour?
- When did membranes rupture?
- Was there any induction or acceleration of labour done?
- H/O prolonged labour or failed forceps, done after trial of labour.
- LSCS for H/O painless bleeding PV or painful bleeding PV or malpresentation.
- H/O blood transfusion.

If elective LSCS done:
- Find out indication (whether due to malpresentation, CPD, FGR, bad obstetric history)

Enquire about the following post-operative problems:

Distension of abdomen	
Wound infection	All these indicate infection, which can weaken the scar and lessen uterine scar integrity
Urinary tract infection	
Fever in puerperium	
Foul smelling lochia	

Resuturing:
- Duration of hospital stay (prolonged stay in the hospital indicates wound sepsis or other complications)

Regarding baby:
- Whether baby cried immediately, weight of the baby, whether baby was with the mother or admitted in NICU; condition of the baby at present

EXAMINATION
GENERAL EXAMINATION
- Refer Case 1.

Presence of maternal tachycardia may be due to scar dehiscence.

OBSTETRIC EXAMINATION
Apart from routine examination, describe the following:
- Nature of abdominal scar—vertical—mid-line or paramedian or Pfannenstiel
- Presence of puckering, keloid, incisional hernia over the scar
- Palpation done for suprapubic tenderness or bulge, from right to left to elicit uterine scar tenderness (Fig. 6.1)

EXAMINATION   81

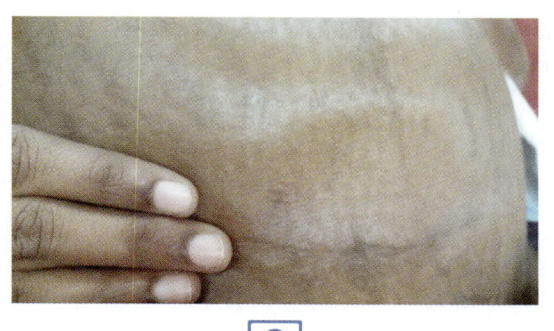

FIGURE 6.1   Palpation in the Suprapubic Area

▶ Scan to play How to elicit Scar tenderness in previous LSCS Pregnancy

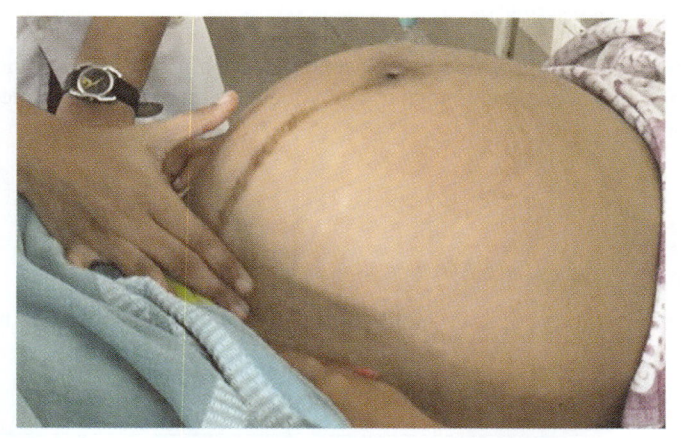

FIGURE 6.2   Palpation Done in the Suprapubic Area in Vertical Abdominal Scar

- In vertical abdominal scar also, palpation is done in the suprapubic area to elicit lower segment caesarean scar tenderness (Fig. 6.2).
- Palpation is done to find out foetal lie, position and presentation—whether head is engaged or not and size of the foetus to decide about vaginal birth after caesarean section (VBAC).

SUMMARY
- Mrs………..Gravida…..Para……admitted with……….
- H/O months amenorrhoea/period of gestation with previous H/O caesarean done for recurrent/non-recurrent indication/no complaints but for safe confinement/labour pains

- Include positive general examination findings/pulse/CVS/RS.
- Obstetric examination findings—gestational age/lie/presentation/if vertex, whether engaged/foetal heart rate/no suprapubic tenderness.

DIAGNOSIS
Gravida……Para……period of gestation, with previous caesarean section single/live foetus in vertex/breech presentation.

INVESTIGATIONS
- Routine investigations
- Haemoglobin
- Blood group, Rh type, cross-matching
- Blood urea, sugar
- *USG*: To confirm foetal position, viability, placental location if anterior over the scar or low lying (probability of placenta accreta, increta, percreta to be thought of and to be ruled out by Doppler), amount of liquor

CASE DISCUSSION
DEFINITION OF CAESAREAN DELIVERY
Delivery of the foetus after the period of viability through an incision on the abdominal wall and intact uterus.

Indications for Caesarean Section		
Absolute	**Relative**	**Recurrent**
1. Malpresentation (brow, transverse lie, persistent mento-posterior, footling, knee presentation) 2. Previous CS with obstetric complications 3. Prior full thickness myomectomy 4. Previous hysterotomy 5. CPD (major degree) contracted pelvis 6. Vaginal septum 7. Placenta previa (Type 3, 4, Type 2 posterior) 8. HIV infection 9. Coarctation of aorta with cerebral aneurysm 10. Cord presentation 11. First of twin non-vertex presentation 12. Cervical or fibroid in lower uterine segment 13. Pregnancy with cancer cervix	1. Severe pre-eclampsia and eclampsia when delivery is not imminent 2. FGR 3. GDM with macrosomia 4. Abnormal foetal Doppler 5. BOH 6. Abruptio placenta when delivery is not imminent 7. HSV infection with active lesion	1. Contracted pelvis 2. Vaginal septum

TYPES OF CAESAREAN SECTION
Lower segment caesarean section (only done nowadays) and classical section.

SCAR DEHISCENCE (INCOMPLETE SCAR RUPTURE—PERITONEUM INTACT)
It may be asymptomatic or there may be tenderness in the suprapubic area, tenesmus and tachycardia.

SYMPTOMS AND SIGNS OF RUPTURE UTERUS
Symptoms are sudden cessation of labour pains and feeling of something giving way.

It usually occurs in labour and is accompanied by maternal tachycardia, hypotension, shock, haematuria.

Uterine contour is lost.

Suprapubic bulge
Foetal parts are felt superficially, foetal heart will be absent.
Receding of the presenting part will be made out on pelvic examination.

Fresh bleeding PV
FH changes like loss of variability/bradycardia and late decelerations are the first signs of rupture uterus.

MANAGEMENT OF RUPTURE UTERUS
- Simultaneous resuscitation and laparotomy should be done
- Foetus and placenta are removed from abdominal cavity
- If rent is regular rent, repair and sterilisation done (if the woman has previous live baby)
- If there is no previous live baby defer sterilisation and in next pregnancy care is taken to deliver earlier by elective LSCS
- If rent is irregular and could not be repaired, caesarean hysterectomy has to be done

Identification of lower uterine segment: It is just below the reflection of the loose uterovesical fold of peritoneum.

Scar integrity:
- Scar may be weak when previous caesarean was done as an emergency for placenta previa or following prolonged labour (due to sepsis)
- *During present pregnancy, following conditions may cause weakness of scar*—pregnancy with polyhydramnios/multiple pregnancy/placenta previa delivery
- *If USG done between 36–38 weeks depicts lower uterine scar thickness of 3.5 mm or more, it indicates good scar integrity and woman can be allowed for VBAC*
- *In non-pregnant period when HSG shows more than 5 mm wedge, it indicates weak scar*

THE PRE-REQUISITES FOR ALLOWING PATIENT FOR TRIAL OF LABOUR AFTER CAESAREAN/VAGINAL BIRTH AFTER CAESAREAN
- Conducted in institution with facilities for immediate caesarean, blood bank facilities
- Counselling and informed consent

- Non-recurrent indication for previous LSCS
- Previous one LSCS
- Previous post-operative period uneventful
- H/O previous vaginal delivery, good indicator for successful vaginal delivery
- Interval between pregnancy must be more than 18 months
- In the present pregnancy: No other obstetric or medical complications, no CPD—should be average size baby with vertex presentation
- Spontaneous onset of labour is ideal
- No place for induction of labour in VBAC

MONITORING DURING VBAC

- IV fluids to be started with wide bore needle
- Solid diet should be avoided (to prevent aspiration)
- Blood to be cross-matched and kept ready
- Admission CTG and continuous electronic monitoring should be done
- Look for suprapubic tenderness or bulge, blood-stained urine

First stage:
- Monitor maternal pulse every 30 min, FHR every 15 min
- Monitor progress of labour by partogram
- ARM is done in active labour
- Pain relief measures are to be taken (epidural analgesia can be offered)

Second stage: Cut short by outlet forceps

Third stage: Active line of management
- After delivery, monitor for bleeding PV and pulse rate. If tachycardia and profuse bleeding PV is present, suspect rupture uterus.
- When you suspect rupture uterus, PV should be done to palpate lower uterine segment to check for scar integrity or rupture. (Routinely lower uterine segment is not palpated.)
- If rupture uterus is suspected, laparotomy should be done (there may be scar rupture, broad ligament haematoma, or bladder rent) (Table 6.1).

ADVANTAGES OF LSCS OVER CLASSICAL SECTION

- Scar dehiscence and rupture is less in LSCS—0.4%–1.5% (incidence of rupture uterus in classical CS—4%–9%)
- In lower segment, scar healing is good because lower segment is thin and approximation is good and less chance for haematoma formation
- Lower segment is quiescent in post-operative period
- During subsequent pregnancy, the stretch is parallel to the scar
- Chance of weakening of the scar by the placenta is unlikely
- Rupture may occur only during labour in LSCS scar (Table 6.2)

Table 6.1 Advantages and Disadvantages of VBAC

Advantages of Successful VBAC	Disadvantage of VBAC
1. Major surgery is avoided 2. Reduced risk of infection, haemorrhage and blood transfusion 3. Less costly	1. Woman will be anxious about outcome 2. Emergency LSCS in failed trial of labour 3. Risk of scar rupture which is 1%–2% has higher maternal morbidity/foetal morbidity and mortality

Table 6.2 Complications of Caesarean Section

During Surgery	Post-Operative	Remote
1. Anaesthesia complications 2. Difficulty in entering into the abdomen due to adhesions 3. Difficulty in delivering the head of the foetus due to high mobile head and in deeply engaged head in late labour 4. Haemorrhage due to atonicity, broad ligament haematoma due to extension of the incision laterally 5. Injury to bladder, ureter, bowel	1. Vomiting 2. Abdominal distension 3. Paralytic ileus 4. Intestinal adhesion can lead to intestinal obstruction 5. Fever 6. Wound infection 7. Urinary tract infection 8. Thromboembolism	1. Adhesions 2. Incisional hernia 3. Scar rupture during subsequent pregnancy 4. Scar endometriosis

INDICATIONS FOR CLASSICAL CAESAREAN IN MODERN OBSTETRICS

- Cancer cervix
- Fibroid in the lower uterine segment
- Dense adhesion in the lower uterine segment due to previous surgeries
- Conjoined twins
- Large vessels in lower uterine segment due to placenta previa
- Inability to approach lower segment due to kyphoscoliosis
- Neglected cases of shoulder presentation
- Extreme prematurity
- Post-mortem

Steps of LSCS: Refer Case 16.

INDICATIONS FOR CAESAREAN HYSTERECTOMY

Atonic PPH not responding to other management
Adherent placenta
Multiple fibroids complicating pregnancy
Intrapartum sepsis
Early-stage cancer cervix—radical hysterectomy

CASE 6 A CASE OF PREGNANCY FOLLOWING CAESAREAN SECTION

KEY POINTS
- With proper selection of women, they will be eligible to undergo trial of vaginal delivery following previous caesarean section.
- Successful VBAC results in vaginal delivery of a live foetus without scar rupture.
- VBAC should be conducted in hospital where facilities for emergency caesarean, blood bank and neonatologist are available.
- In scar dehiscence, there will be incomplete uterine scar separation and peritoneum is intact but in uterine rupture, there will be complete disruption of the uterine scar including visceral peritoneum.
- Earliest sign of scar dehiscence is foetal heart variability and for rupture uterus, simultaneous resuscitation and laparotomy should be done.

FREQUENTLY ASKED QUESTIONS
1. Define caesarean section.
2. What are the absolute and relative indications for LSCS?
3. What are the recurrent causes for LSCS?
4. What are the steps of LSCS? Refer Case 16.
5. What are the advantages of LSCS over classical section?
6. What are the complications of LSCS?
7. What are the indications for classical caesarean?
8. How do you determine scar integrity?
9. What are the pre-requisites for allowing patient for trial of scar/VBAC?
10. How will you conduct VBAC?
11. What are the signs and symptoms of scar rupture?
12. What are the advantages and disadvantages of VBAC?
13. What is the incidence of scar rupture in LSCS and classical caesarean section?
14. What are the signs and symptoms of rupture uterus and management?
15. What are the indications for caesarean hysterectomy?

CASE 7

A CASE OF HEART DISEASE COMPLICATING PREGNANCY

PATIENT'S DETAILS

Name.. Age.................. Address........................... Occupation..............
Socioeconomic Class......................... Gravida, Para, Live, Abortion, (G......... P......... L......... A.........)
Booked/Unbooked........................ Immunisation...................... LMP............ EDD

H/O............ months of amenorrhoea/period of gestation

PRESENT COMPLAINTS

Patient may present with period of amenorrhoea with following complaints or woman can be admitted for safe confinement in view of her heart disease (or) woman can be admitted for evaluation, investigations and management of heart disease.

Elicit the following history:
- Breathlessness on exertion, breathlessness while doing day-to-day activity, breathlessness at night (paroxysmal nocturnal dyspnoea), breathlessness at rest
- Palpitation, chest pain, syncope
- Swelling of legs (persists even after 12 h of rest)
- Cough with expectoration, haemoptysis
- Diminished urine output
- Details regarding care taken by obstetrician and cardiologist or drugs taken for cardiac failure/anti-coagulant
- History of foetal movements—normal or diminished (IUGR may be associated in heart disease)

HISTORY
MENSTRUAL HISTORY

Refer Case 1.

MARITAL HISTORY

Refer Case 1.

To view the lecture notes log in to your account on www.MedEnact.com

OBSTETRIC HISTORY
Refer Case 1.

Past obstetric history
- History of cardiac failure during previous pregnancy, grade of failure in that pregnancy (from history, grade to be found out)
- Mode of delivery
- Baby—Weight, Apgar score/any cardiac anomaly/alive healthy or dead
- In puerperium—H/O CCF/fever/thromboembolism/lactation failure
- Contraception—Nature of contraception practiced in between pregnancy

PAST SURGICAL HISTORY
- Refer Case 1.
- Cardiac corrective surgery (whether open or closed heart surgery)

PAST MEDICAL HISTORY
- H/O rheumatic fever (major and minor criteria), age at which it was diagnosed and treatment given
- H/O congestive cardiac failure
- History suggestive of thyrotoxicosis—like palpitation, loss of weight, tremors, diarrhoea
- Repeated respiratory infection
- History of drugs taken: current medications—digoxin, diuretics, penicillin, anti-coagulants, other antibiotics

FAMILY HISTORY
- H/O congenital heart disease in the family may lead to congenital heart lesion in the offspring

EXAMINATION
GENERAL EXAMINATION
- Patient comfortable at rest or dyspnoeic
- Cyanosis
- Clubbing
- Pallor—anaemia worsens failure
- Pedal oedema, oedema in other sites—could be due to CCF or pre-eclampsia, which can precipitate or worsen cardiac failure
- JVP—raised in cardiac failure
- Pulse rate—rhythm, volume, tension, character, whether felt in all peripheral vessels
- Blood pressure—associated pre-eclampsia can precipitate or worsen cardiac failure
- Respiratory rate

- Temperature—any febrile illness can precipitate cardiac failure; it could be due to infective endocarditis also
- Thyroid enlargement (thyrotoxicosis can precipitate CCF)

CARDIOVASCULAR SYSTEM
Should be examined in detail

- Palpation, percussion, auscultation to be done in detail in mitral, pulmonary, aortic and tricuspid area
- *Palpate*—site and type of apical impulse, palpable thrill
- *Auscultation*—heart rate
- First sound, second sound in all areas
- Presence of third sound
- Loud P2
- Arrhythmia
- Atrial fibrillation   — Indicates heart disease
- Murmur—systolic grade 3
- Diastolic murmur
- Thrill

RESPIRATORY SYSTEM
- Auscultate for basal crepitations and any evidence of infection

ABDOMINAL EXAMINATION
- Hepatomegaly with tenderness—indicates cardiac failure
  Splenomegaly—may indicate infective endocarditis

OBSTETRIC EXAMINATION
- It is done as usual. Special attention should be taken to find out intra-uterine growth restriction. Assess uterine and foetal size.

SUMMARY
- Mrs……Age……..Gravida…..Para……EDD admitted with…
- H/O…..months of amenorrhoea/period of gestation, with breathlessness/pedal oedema/diminished urine output/H/O paroxysmal nocturnal dyspnoea/mention about previous positive history like rheumatic fever/mention about her medication/surgery, if any
- Include her general examination/respiratory and cardiovascular system examination findings

CASE 7 A CASE OF HEART DISEASE COMPLICATING PREGNANCY

DIAGNOSIS

- Gravida……Para…… Age…period of gestation, EDD with, mention the type of heart lesion (mitral stenosis)…..class …according to [New York Heart Association (NYHA) classification] in sinus rhythm with single live foetus ……presentation

INVESTIGATIONS

- Routine basic investigations
- Haemoglobin
- Urine routine and culture and sensitivity
- Electrocardiogram
- Echocardiogram—to assess cardiac status, functional capacity, structural abnormality
- Blood urea and electrolytes—diuretics can cause electrolyte disturbance, which can precipitate cardiac failure
- X-ray chest only if absolutely necessary, after shielding the abdomen

CASE DISCUSSION
CARDIOVASCULAR CHANGES DURING PREGNANCY

- Blood volume increases by 40%, starts increasing from 5 weeks and reaches maximum at 32 weeks
- Cardiac output increases by 40% at 24–30 weeks, 50% in labour and soon after delivery, by 80% of pre-labour volume
- Pulse rate increases by 10 beats/min

Symptoms and Signs Due to Physiological Changes During Pregnancy That Mimic Heart Disease	
Symptoms That Mimic Heart Disease	Signs That Mimic Heart Disease
Breathlessness	Pulse rate increases by 10 beats/min
Dizziness	Shift of apical impulse to 4th left inter-costal space in the mid-clavicular line
Fatigue	
Swelling of the feet	Systolic murmur—grade 2 due to hyper-dynamic circulation
Palpitation	Mammary Soufflé

CONDITIONS WHICH CAN PRECIPITATE CARDIAC FAILURE

- Anaemia
- Thyrotoxicosis
- Infections (dental, respiratory, urinary tract)
- Obesity
- Tachycardia

- Atrial fibrillation
- Infective endocarditis
- Pre-eclampsia
- Multiple pregnancy
- Polyhydramnios
- Drugs like beta mimetics

NYHA classification: Depends upon the cardiac response to physical activity

Class 1	Uncompromised. Patients with cardiac disease but no limitation of physical activity.
Class 2	Slightly compromised. Patients with cardiac disease with slight limitation of physical activity. Patients will have discomfort with ordinary physical activity.
Class 3	Markedly compromised. Patients with cardiac disease with marked limitation of physical activity. Patients will have discomfort with less than ordinary physical activity.
Class 4	Severely compromised. Patients with cardiac disease with discomfort even at rest.

DRAWBACK OF NYHA CLASSIFICATION
Classification depends on symptoms and not on degree of structural abnormalities. The class may change at any time based on clinical features.

THE CRITERIA TO DIAGNOSE HEART DISEASE IN PREGNANCY
- Severe dyspnoea
- Orthopnoea and chest pain
- Haemoptysis
- Clubbing
- Cyanosis
- Systolic murmur more than grade 3
- Diastolic murmurs
- Arrhythmias
- Palpable thrill
- Cardiomegaly
- Echocardiogram showing structural and functional abnormality

Effect of Pregnancy on Heart Disease and Effect of Heart Disease on Pregnancy

Effect of Pregnancy on Heart Disease	Effect of Heart Disease on Pregnancy
CCF, pulmonary oedema, embolic manifestation, arrhythmias	In well-compensated rheumatic heart disease—outcome is usually good
Adverse effects seen between 28 and 32 weeks of gestation and after delivery	In cyanotic disease—spontaneous abortion, IUGR, prematurity can occur
	If mother has congenital cardiac lesion, 5%–10% foetus will have cardiac lesion and 50% will have same defect

TIME OF HOSPITALISATION IN CARDIAC DISEASE COMPLICATING PREGNANCY

Class 1 and 2—Admit, evaluate and then can be treated as out-patient
    Admit at 34 weeks or whenever complications arise
    Class 3 and 4—Admit throughout pregnancy

CONDUCT OF LABOUR IN A HEART DISEASE COMPLICATING PREGNANCY

First stage: No induction of labour
- 1st, 2nd and 3rd stage of labour—semi-recumbent position with backrest to avoid haemodynamic problems
- O_2 by re-breathing mask
- Wide IV line kept for emergency drugs
- Monitor pulse, BP
- Oxygen saturation monitored with pulse oximeter
- Urine output to be monitored

Infective endocarditis prophylaxis:
- Ampicillin (2 g) + 1.5 mg/kg Gentamycin (not to exceed 80 mg) to be given at the onset of labour and to be repeated 8th hourly. In case of allergy to ampicillin, vancomycin to be given
- Adequate analgesia to be given (when not contraindicated—epidural analgesia)
- Digoxin and diuretics—in case of CCF
- Avoid repeated PV examination

Second stage: Cut short 2nd stage with outlet forceps
- Avoid ergometrine

Third stage: Oxytocin IM can be given
- Monitor for CCF

COMPLICATIONS DURING ANTENATAL PERIOD, LABOUR AND IN PUERPERIUM

- Cardiac failure, infective bacterial endocarditis, pulmonary embolism, postpartum collapse
- In coarctation of aorta—dissection of aorta, rupture of co-existing berry aneurysm and intra-cranial haemorrhage can occur
- In Marfan's—dissection of aortic aneurysm can occur

INDICATIONS WHERE PREGNANCY IS TO BE AVOIDED

- In women with primary pulmonary hypertension
- Eisenmenger's syndrome
- In Grade 3 and 4 heart disease, pregnancy is avoided
- In above conditions, consider MTP in early pregnancy—first trimester after treating failure
- Woman is advised to become pregnant after corrective cardiac surgery, when indicated

INDICATIONS FOR CARDIAC SURGERY DURING PREGNANCY

- Recurrent CCF, failure to respond to medical management, tight mitral stenosis, pulmonary oedema
- Cardiac surgery is performed between 16 and 18 weeks

PLACE OF CAESAREAN SECTION IN HEART DISEASE COMPLICATING PREGNANCY
- Obstetric indications
- In coarctation of aorta, to prevent dissection of aorta and rupture of berry aneurysm

CONTRACEPTION IN HEART DISEASE COMPLICATING PREGNANCY
- Temporary—barrier method, mini pill or Inj. Depot medroxyprogesterone acetate are advised
- Oestrogen-containing pills may increase the risk of thrombosis and IUCD may be a source of infection which may lead to infective endocarditis and hence not recommended
- Permanent—tubectomy can be done after 2 weeks following delivery, if she is fit for surgery
- If husband is willing, vasectomy can be done

MATERNAL OUTCOME
Group I
- Low risk; mortality <1%
- ASD, VSD, corrected TOF, mitral stenosis class 1 and 2

Group II
- Moderate risk; mortality 5%–15%
- Mitral stenosis class 3 and 4, MS with AF, uncorrected TOF, uncomplicated coarctation of aorta, Marfan's with normal aorta

Group III
- High risk; mortality 25%–50%
- Primary pulmonary hypertension, Eisenmenger's syndrome, coarctation of aorta with valvular involvement, Marfan's syndrome with aortic involvement

Basic Principal in the Treatment of CCF	
Drug	Action
Bed rest and diuretics (IV frusemide 40–80 mg)	Reduces pre-load
Digoxin (0.5 mg IM followed by 0.25 mg tab)	Improves contractility
Vasodilators—hydralazine, IV nitroglycerin	Reduces afterload

RULE OF FIVE
- Haemodynamic changes starts from 5th week onwards
- It reaches maximum by 5 weeks before term
- Complications—CCF occur
- 5 min after delivery
- 5 h after delivery
- 5 days after delivery

ANTI-COAGULATION GUIDELINES

- If patient is on warfarin, substitute heparin during peak teratogenic period (6th to 12th week) and then change to warfarin up to 36 weeks
- INR should be maintained between 2.5 and 3
- Switch over to heparin 2 weeks before labour
- Stop heparin 6 h before delivery
- Restart heparin 6 h after vaginal delivery and 12 h after LSCS
- Start warfarin after 3 days and withdraw heparin
- Warfarin is safe during lactation

KEY POINTS

- Physiological changes start from 5th week onwards and reaches peak between 28 and 32 weeks and maintained till term.
- All patient with cardiac disease complicating pregnancy should deliver in hospital and should be admitted by 34 weeks or whenever complications arise in class 1 and 2 and in class 3 and 4 should be in the hospital throughout pregnancy.
- Women with cardiac disease should have proper pre-pregnancy counselling.
- Adequate analgesia should be provided during labour.
- Mostly these women deliver vaginally but caesarean is done for obstetric indications and in coarctation of aorta, to prevent dissection of aorta and rupture of berry aneurysm.
- Methylergometrin is contraindicated.
- Monitoring of the woman should be continued throughout puerperium.
- When medical termination is necessary, it should be done before 8 weeks.
- Surgical correction for cardiac lesion can be performed during second trimester but best done before pregnancy.
- Ideal time for tubectomy is beyond puerperal period but can be done after 14 days, if she is fit for surgery.

FREQUENTLY ASKED QUESTIONS

1. What are the cardiovascular changes during pregnancy?
2. What are the signs and symptoms that mimic heart disease in pregnancy?
3. What are the criteria to diagnose heart disease in pregnancy?
4. What are the signs and symptoms of cardiac failure?
5. How will you classify cardiac disease according to NYHA and what are its drawbacks?
6. What are the effects of pregnancy on cardiac lesion?
7. What are the effects of cardiac disease on pregnancy?
8. When will you admit patient with cardiac disease?
9. What are the factors which might worsen failure in pregnancy?
10. How will you manage labour in heart disease complicating pregnancy?

11. What are the complications to anticipate during antenatal period, labour and in puerperium?
12. What contraception will you advice?
13. What are the contraindications to pregnancy in heart disease?
14. What are the indications for cardiac surgery during pregnancy?
15. What are the factors determining the prognosis?
16. Place of caesarean section in heart disease complicating pregnancy?
17. How will you group the heart disease according to risk and maternal mortality?

A CASE OF MALPRESENTATION

CASE 8

PATIENT'S DETAILS
Name... Age.................. Address.......................... Occupation.............
Socioeconomic Class.......................... Gravida, Para, Live, Abortion, (G......... P......... L......... A ....)
Booked/Unbooked........................ Immunisation....................... LMP............ EDD

H/O............ months of amenorrhoea/period of gestation

PRESENT COMPLAINTS
Patient may present with period of amenorrhoea with following complaints:

- Admitted for safe confinement or H/O labour pains or draining PV
- Ask about foetal movements

SPECIAL HISTORY
History of epigastric or hypochondrial pain in breech due to the pressure of foetal head.

MENSTRUAL HISTORY
- Refer Case 1.

MARITAL HISTORY
- Refer Case 1.

OBSTETRIC HISTORY
- Refer Case 1.

Past obstetric history
- H/O previous malpresentation—may indicate uterine anomaly
- H/O mode of delivery/outcome/foetal malformation

To view the lecture notes log in to your account on www.MedEnact.com

CASE 8 A CASE OF MALPRESENTATION

Conditions which predispose to malpresentation
Relevant history for the following conditions to be asked for: multiple pregnancy, polyhydramnios, placenta previa, multiple pregnancy, mass in the lower pole of the uterus, contracted pelvis, multi-parity, anomaly of uterus, foetal anomaly like hydrocephalus, anencephaly.

FAMILY HISTORY, PERSONAL HISTORY
- Refer Case 1.

PAST SURGICAL HISTORY
- Refer Case 1.

EXAMINATION
GENERAL EXAMINATION
- Refer Case 1.

OBSTETRIC EXAMINATION
Breech presentation
- *Inspection*: sub-umbilical flattening may be there in extended breech.
- *Palpation*:
  - *Fundal grip* will reveal hard, round, independently ballotable foetal part, which indicates head. When not much ballotable—it is extended breech due to splinting action of the legs (Figs 8.1 and 8.2).
    In extended breech, head may be in the midline due to splinting by extended legs.
  - *Umbilical grip* smooth, curved hard, uniform resistance denotes back.
    Multiple small nodules felt on the other side denotes—limb buds.
  - *1st Pelvic grip* will reveal broad, soft, not independently ballotable foetal part which indicates breech in lower pole.
  - *2nd Pelvic grip* will assess whether breech is engaged or not.
- *Auscultation*: foetal heart is heard above the umbilicus on the same side as the back.

Transverse lie
- Uterus will be transversely enlarged.
- Height of the uterus will be smaller than period of amenorrhoea.
- Fundal and pelvic grip will be empty.
- Head will be in one or the other iliac fossa/lumbar region and breech will be in the opposite side.
- Foetal heart—heard at the level of umbilicus.
- Foetal heart will be heard easily in dorsoanterior position and indistinct in dorsoposterior position.

Face presentation
Since head is extended and it is longitudinal lie, sinciput will be at lower level than the occiput and occiput is in contact with the back and a depression will be felt between the foetal spine and head due to

EXAMINATION   99

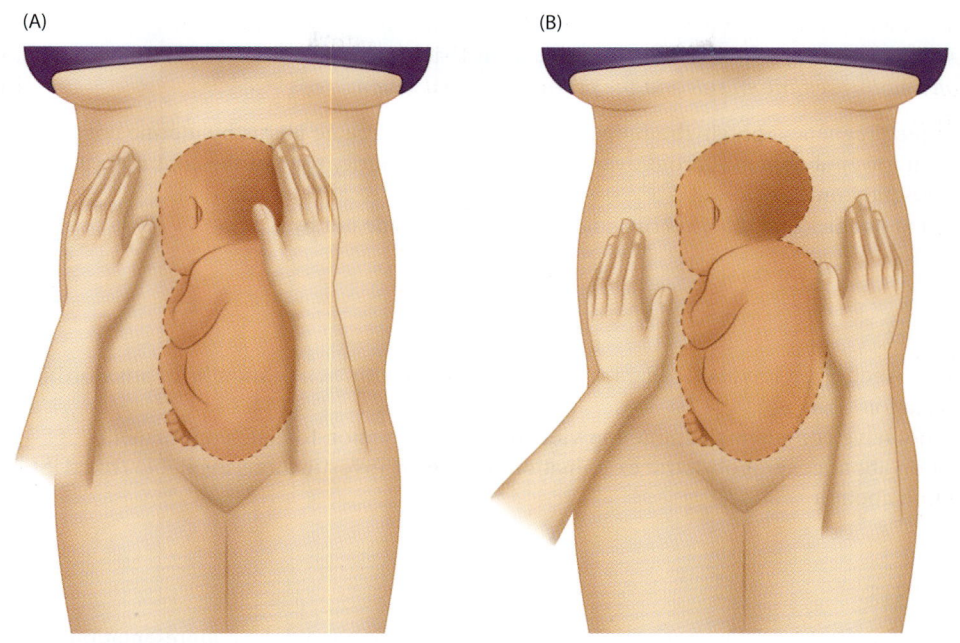

FIGURE 8.1   Various Grips in Breech
(A) Fundal grip and (B) umbilical grip.

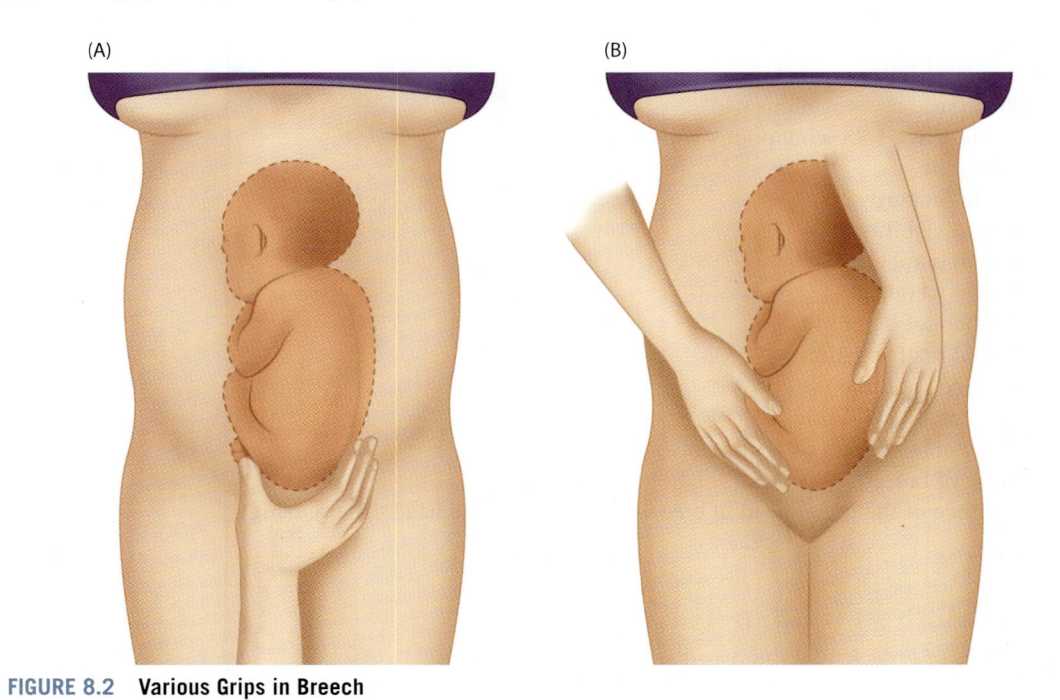

FIGURE 8.2   Various Grips in Breech
(A) 1st pelvic grip and (B) 2nd pelvic grip.

CASE 8 A CASE OF MALPRESENTATION

the extension of the head. When palpated from above, downwards in 2nd pelvic grip, cephalic prominence will be the occiput, felt at the same side as the back.

In any malpresentation, rule out the following by palpation:

- Multiple pregnancy, polyhydramnios, uterine anomaly (arcuate uterus by uterine contour), mass in lower abdomen (fibroid/ovarian tumour), prematurity (one of the common causes for malpresentation)
- Foetal anomalies and other uterine anomalies can be made out by USG

SUMMARY

- Mrs … Age……..Gravida …..Para……EDD admitted with……….months of amenorrhoea/period of gestation
- May not have complaints/admitted in view of malpresentation for safe confinement
- Mention about general/obstetric examination findings/if investigations available (like USG), mention about it

DIAGNOSIS

Age...Gravida...Para... EDD... period of gestation with mention about the malpresentation like breech/transverse lie.

INVESTIGATIONS

- Routine basic investigations
- By doing USG, following points will be made out:
    - Foetal lie
    - Foetal maturity
    - Foetal viability
    - Foetal number
    - Foetal weight
    - Amount of amniotic fluid
    - Foetal malformation
    - Uterine anomaly
    - Placental localisation
    - Mass in lower part of abdomen
    - Type of breech
    - Attitude of the foetal head in breech (extension of the head—star gazing)

CASE DISCUSSION-BREECH PRESENTATION

- *Incidence of breech*: at term: 3%–4% and 16% at 32 week

CASE DISCUSSION-BREECH PRESENTATION

Aetiology for Malpresentation		
Maternal Cause	**Foetal Cause**	**Placenta, Liquor, Cord**
CPD, obliquity of uterus, anomaly of uterus, multi-parity, tumour in the lower pole of uterus	Prematurity, foetal anomalies like hydrocephalus, anencephaly, multiple pregnancy	Cornual implantation of placenta, short cord, very long cord, placenta previa, polyhydramnios, oligohydramnios

- *Types of breech*:
    - Complete—universal flexion maintained
    - Incomplete—extended breech (frank breech); knee presentation; footling presentation

Three Stages in Labour and Three Methods of Vaginal Breech Delivery	
Three Stages in Mechanism of Labour in Breech	**Three Methods of Vaginal Breech Delivery**
1. Delivery of breech	1. Spontaneous breech delivery—without any assistance occurs in extreme pre-term baby
2. Delivery of shoulders	2. Assisted breech delivery with assistance by the obstetrician
3. Delivery of head	3. Breech extraction under GA delivered by the obstetrician fully

MECHANISM OF LABOUR

Engaging diameter—bitrochanteric.

- *Delivery of breech*:
    - Engagement: in left sacroanterior (LSA), breech engages in left oblique diameter
    - Descent with compaction
    - Internal rotation—anterior buttock rotates by 1/8 of the circle and hitches against the pubic symphysis
    - Lateral flexion—by a process of lateral flexion, breech is able to pass through the cavity and distends the perineum and is born
- *Delivery of shoulder*:
    - Engaging diameter—bisacromial diameter and shoulder engages in the same oblique diameter as breech
    - Internal rotation—anterior shoulder rotates by 1/8 of the circle and hitches against pubic symphysis; posterior shoulder is born first by lateral flexion followed by anterior shoulder
- *Delivery of the head*:
    - Engaging diameter—sub-occipito-bregmatic diameter: 9.4 cm. Head engages in opposite oblique diameter to that of buttocks
    - Descent with increasing flexion
    - Internal rotation—occiput rotates anteriorly and hitches against the pubic symphysis
    - Birth by flexion—nape of the neck pivots under the symphysis; chin, mouth, forehead and occiput are born by a movement of flexion

ASSISTED BREECH DELIVERY

Foetus is allowed to deliver up to the umbilicus and then assistance is given to the delivery of remaining parts of the foetus.

- *Basic principles*:
    - Never pull from below
    - Hands off till foetus is born till umbilicus
    - The feet may be hooked out, if required
    - Gentle suprapubic push by assistant
    - Back of the foetus is kept always facing the obstetrician
    - Cover the baby to prevent premature respiration
- *Conduction of assisted breech delivery*:
    - Once breech distends the perineum (climbing of perineum), woman must be advised to bear down with contractions
    - Episiotomy should be given
    - No touch policy must be adopted until the buttocks and lower back till the level of umbilicus is delivered
    - Baby must be wrapped in a clean cloth
    - Back of the foetus should always be anterior
    - Loop of umbilical cord is kept to one side to avoid compression
    - After spontaneous delivery of the first arm, buttocks must be lifted toward the mother's abdomen to enable the second arm to deliver spontaneously
    - Once the shoulders are delivered, the baby's body with the face down must be supported by obstetrician's forearm. If there is difficulty in delivering shoulders, Lovset's manoeuvre is done (posterior shoulder which is at a lower position is rotated, brought anterior and delivered first)
    - For delivery of the after-coming head, the foetus is allowed to hang unsupported from the maternal vulva, till the nape of foetal neck appears. Efforts are made to deliver the foetal head by grasping the ankles and sweeping it towards mother's abdomen (Marshall Burn's technique)
    - Other methods to deliver the head—Mauriceau–Smellie–Veit manoeuvre or by using Piper's forceps or axis traction forceps

BREECH EXTRACTION

- Entire body of foetus is delivered by obstetrician; done under GA—all steps of breech delivery are done actively by the obstetrician

TECHNIQUES TO DELIVER THE HEAD IN BREECH

- *Marshall Burn's technique*
    - When occiput is seen under the symphysis, steady traction is given on the feet and the baby is swung in an arc towards the mother's abdomen with simultaneous suprapubic pressure by the assistant and head is born by flexion.
- *Mauriceau–Smellie–Veit manoeuvre*
    - Foetal body rests upon the palm and forearm of the left hand and index and middle fingers of the same hand are applied over the malar bone to promote flexion of the foetal head.

- Two fingers of the right hand are hooked over the foetal neck and downward traction is applied, grasping the shoulders till the sub-occipital region or nape of neck appears under the pubic symphysis.
    Simultaneous gentle suprapubic pressure is given by assistant.
- The direction is changed and foetus is swung up over the mother's abdomen and head is born.
• *Forceps for the after-coming head*
    - By Piper's forceps or axis traction forceps.
    - Advantage of the forceps delivery is that it obviates the traction to the foetal spine, neck and jaw.
    - Controlled traction is applied over the foetal skull.

COMPLICATED BREECH
- When associated with maternal complications like APH, PE, previous CS etc., it is called complicated breech.

COMPLICATIONS OF BREECH DELIVERY *(INHERENT FOR BREECH DELIVERY)*
- PROM, cord prolapse, difficulty in delivering legs, arms and head
- Nuchal position of arms, incomplete cervical dilatation, impacted breech, birth asphyxia, birth trauma

EXTERNAL CEPHALIC VERSION (ECV) (Fig. 8.3A–B)
- No anaesthesia is required

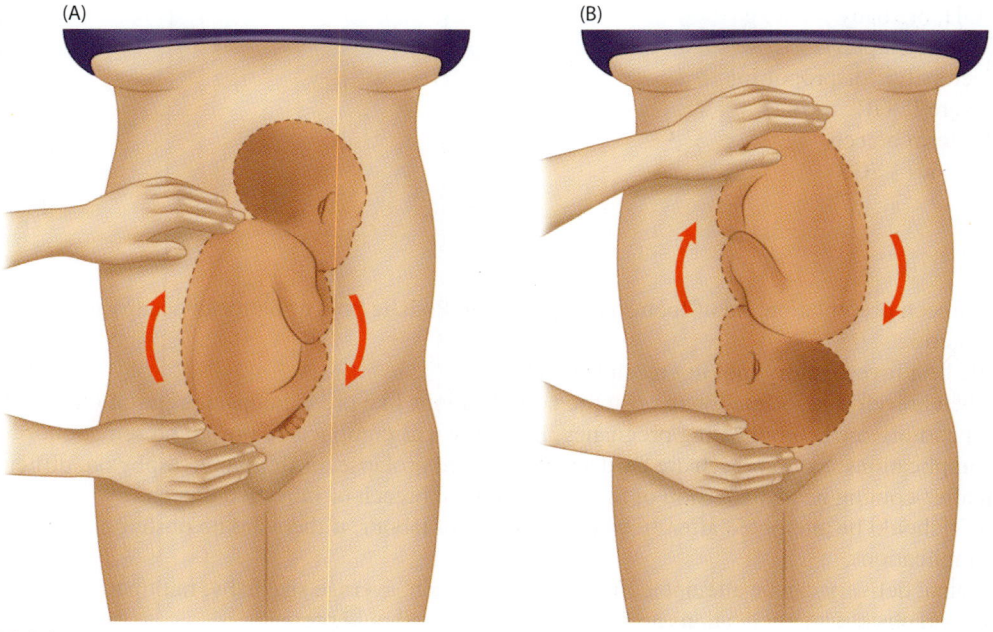

FIGURE 8.3

(A–B) External version to turn breech.

- Done at 36–37 weeks till onset of labour
- Map out the position of the baby
- With gentle stroking movements, bring the head down, keeping the flexion attitude of foetus
- Monitor FHR before, during and after the procedure
- *Indications for ECV*
  - Breech with no maternal complications
  - Aim is to increase the chance of vaginal delivery
- *Contraindications for ECV*
  - Multiple pregnancy, APH, IUGR, oligohydramnios, polyhydramnios, contracted pelvis, foetal anomaly, known congenital anomalies of uterus like septate, bicornuate uterus, previous CS, previous myomectomy/hysterotomy scar/obesity
- *Complications*
  - Abruptio placenta, pre-term labour, premature rupture of membranes, foetal distress
  - If ECV is done in Rh −ve woman, chance of Rh-isoimmunisation is present. Hence Anti-D is to be given

INDICATIONS FOR CAESAREAN IN BREECH PRESENTATION

- Primi with breech
- Footling presentation
- Knee presentation
- Breech with hyper-extended head—'star gazing' attitude
- Complicated breech—with maternal complications
- BOH, big baby >3.5 kg
- Contracted pelvis
- Foetopelvic disproportion
- Severe IUGR
- Pre-term breech
- Previous LSCS

KEY POINTS

- In breech presentation, lie of foetus is longitudinal. Podalic pole or buttocks occupy the lower pole of uterus.
- The best investigatory tool in breech is USG.
- When breech is associated with obstetric complications like pre-eclampsia or gestational diabetes or heart diseases complicating pregnancy, it is known as complicated breech presentation.
- Complications due to breech are cord accidents, cord prolapse, birth trauma, asphyxia, difficulty in after-coming head, extension of the arms, arrest of breech or impacted breech.
- ECV should be attempted after 36 weeks till onset of labour, if there are no obstetric complications.
- Vaginal delivery can be attempted, if it is a frank breech, average size baby, multiparous women with no obstetric complications and skilled obstetrician should present.
- Perinatal morbidity and mortality is increased in breech.

FREQUENTLY ASKED QUESTIONS

1. What is the aetiology for breech?
2. What are the types of breech and it's incidence?
3. What is the denominator in breech and what is the engaging diameter?
4. What is star gazing attitude in breech?
5. What is the mechanism of labour in breech delivery?
6. What are the techniques used for the delivery of the head in breech presentation?
7. What is Lovset's manoeuvre?
8. What is complicated breech?
9. What are the complications of breech delivery?
10. How do you conduct assisted breech delivery?
11. What is ECV, its indications and contraindications?
12. What are the indications for caesarean section in breech delivery?

CASE 9

A CASE OF MULTIPLE PREGNANCY

PATIENT'S DETAILS

Name.. Age.................. Address........................... Occupation..............
Socioeconomic Class......................... Gravida, Para, Live, Abortion, (G......... P......... L......... A ....)
Booked/Unbooked......................... Immunisation....................... LMP and EDD............

H/O............ months of amenorrhoea/period of gestation

PRESENT COMPLAINTS

Patient may present with period of amenorrhoea with following complaints.

The following history is to be elicited:
- Excessive distension of uterus
- Excessive vomiting in early months of pregnancy
- Excessive foetal movements
- Conception with ovulation induction drugs, assisted reproductive technique (ART)
- Pressure symptoms—haemorrhoids, swelling of legs, varicose veins
- Respiratory embarrassment—shortness of breath
- History suggestive of PE/anaemia
- Excessive weight gain

HISTORY
MENSTRUAL HISTORY
- Refer Case 1.

MARITAL HISTORY
- Refer Case 1.

OBSTETRIC HISTORY
Past obstetric history
- Refer Case 1.

To view the lecture notes log in to your account on www.MedEnact.com

CASE 9 A CASE OF MULTIPLE PREGNANCY

Present obstetric history
- H/O induction of ovulation
- ART
- Conception within 1 month of stopping OCP
- Patient may report with USG diagnosis of multiple pregnancy
- May give H/O bleeding PV (if there is placenta previa)

PAST MEDICAL AND SURGICAL HISTORY
- Refer Case 1.

PERSONAL HISTORY
- Refer Case 1.

FAMILY HISTORY
- H/O multiple pregnancy should be elicited.

EXAMINATION
GENERAL EXAMINATION

Special attention to be paid for the following details:
- Pallor
- Pedal oedema
- Hypertension
- Pressure symptoms
- Varicosity in lower limbs and vulva

OBSTETRIC EXAMINATION
- Uterus will be bigger than period of amenorrhoea from early pregnancy (other conditions like wrong dates, hydatidiform mole, polyhydramnios, macrosomia, fibroid or ovarian mass with pregnancy to be ruled out) (Fig. 9.1)
- Fundal height and abdominal girth will be greater than period of amenorrhoea
- Two foetal heads or three foetal poles should be made out distinctly by palpation to diagnose multiple pregnancy; multiple foetal parts will be felt
- Two foetal heart sounds should be heard by two different persons at two separate points significantly apart from each other with a difference of 10 beats/min to diagnose twin gestation
- Malpresentation is common
- Presentation of the first twin, that is the twin which occupies the lowest part of uterus should be noted
- Note whether the presenting part is engaged or not
- If polyhydramnios is present—confirm by fluid thrill

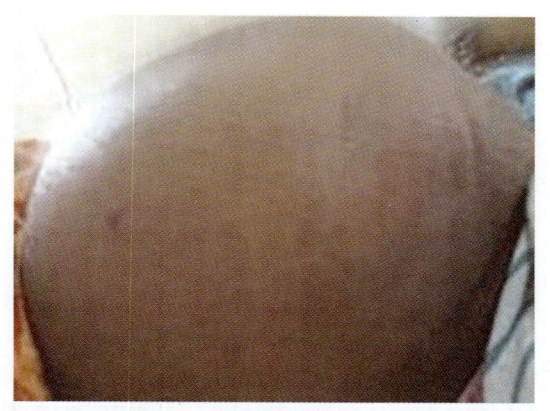

FIGURE 9.1 Over-Distended Uterus

SUMMARY

- Mrs …Age……..Gravida …..Para……EDD admitted with……….months amenorrhoea/period of gestation with over-distended uterus/pressure symptoms/respiratory symptoms with family history of twins or H/O taking drugs for induction of ovulation
- Mention about general examination/obstetric examination findings

DIAGNOSIS

- Age…Gravida…Para…EDD…period of gestation, twins. If anaemia/pre-eclampsia present, mention about it.

INVESTIGATIONS

- Haemoglobin
- Blood group, Rh type
- If anaemia is present—investigations for anaemia
- If pre-eclampsia is present—investigations for pre-eclampsia (fourfold increase in incidence of pre-eclampsia)
- *USG*:
  - *First trimester*—number of gestational sacs, chorionicity—lambda or twin peak sign in dichorionic twins, T-sign in monochorionic diamniotic twins (Figs 9.2 and 9.3)
  - 11–13.6 weeks—measurement of nuchal translucency
  - *Vanishing twin*—if earlier USG showed two sacs or two cardiac activity, but subsequent USG shows one sac or only one heart beat, then diagnosis of vanishing twin is made

110 CASE 9 A CASE OF MULTIPLE PREGNANCY

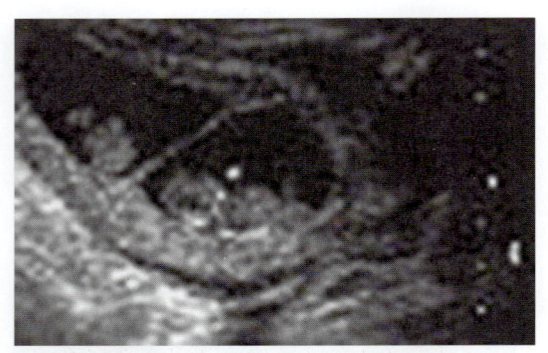

FIGURE 9.2 Monochorionic Diamniotic Twin

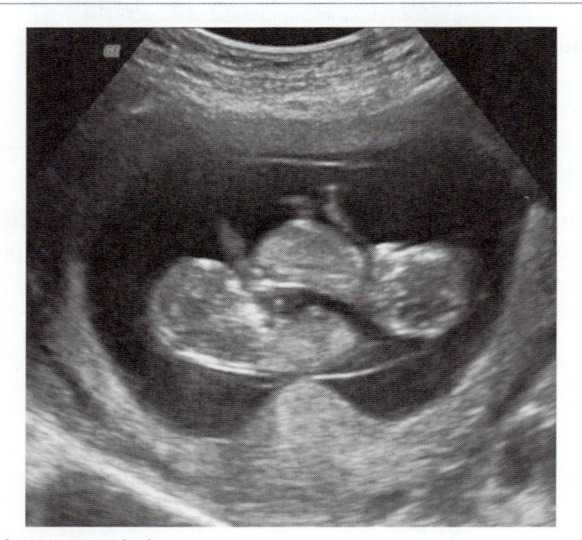

FIGURE 9.3 Monochorionic Monoamniotic

From J. Copel, Monochorionic monoamniotic twin gestations, Obstetric Imaging, Expert Radiology Series, 1st edition, Saunders: 2012, pp. 710–714.

- *Second trimester*—number of foetuses, position, localisation of placenta, number of placenta, foetal anomalies, discordant twin
- *Third trimester*—foetal growth, position, lie, presentation, weight of both the twins, localisation of placenta, amount of liquor
- *Discordant twins:*
  - Difference in BPD, 5 mm
  - Difference in abdominal circumference, 20 mm
  - 5% difference in HC
  - Difference of 15%–25% in estimated foetal weight
- *Twin-to-twin transfusion*:
  - This occurs in monochorionic placentation due to arteriovenous anastomosis with resultant net flow in one direction

QUINTERO'S CLASSIFICATION OF SEVERITY OF TWIN-TO-TWIN TRANSFUSION

Polyhydramnios in one sac and oligohydramnios in another:
- Stage 1: Discordant amniotic fluid volume
- Stage 2: Plus absent urine in donor bladder
- Stage 3: Plus abnormal Doppler of umbilical artery, ductus venosus
- Stage 4: Ascites or frank polyhydramnios in either twin
- Stage 5: Demise of either foetus

CASE DISCUSSION

- Incidence of monozygotic twin is constant, 1 in 250
- Binovular twins incidence is influenced by heredity, race, age, parity

PROGNOSIS OR OUTCOME IS INFLUENCED BY THE CHORIONICITY RATHER THAN THE ZYGOSITY

- Determination of chorionicity can be performed by USG. Different sex, two separate placenta, thick inter-twin membrane, presence of 'twin peak' sign or 'lambda sign' denotes dichorionicity.
- By USG, thick inter-twin membrane at 6–9 weeks aided at 11–14 weeks by 'lambda' sign is diagnostic of dichorionicity.
- Monochorionicity is associated with thin inter-twin septum and 'T' sign.

Determination of Zygosity

Differentiating Points	Monozygotic Twin	Dizygotic Twin
Placenta	Single	2 or may be fused
Membrane	Intervening membrane—two amnions (when division occurs after 8 days)	4 (2 chorion and 2 amnions)
Vascular communications	Present	Absent
Sex	Same	Same or different
Blood group	Same	Same or different
DNA and finger prints	Same	Different
Skin graft	Accept	Reject
Identical	Usually identical	Not identical

ANTENATAL MANAGEMENT OF MULTIPLE PREGNANCY

- It is a high-risk pregnancy
- Counselling about more frequent visits, nutrition, adequate rest, avoiding strenuous work
- Iron and folic acid supplementation throughout pregnancy to be given
- Anomaly scan and regular growth scans to be done

CASE 9 A CASE OF MULTIPLE PREGNANCY

- Timing of delivery—40% end in spontaneous or indicated pre-term birth
- If there are no complications, deliver by 38–40 weeks

Antenatal, Foetal and Intrapartum Complications in Multiple Pregnancy		
Antenatal Complications	**Foetal Complications**	**Intrapartum Complications**
Spontaneous abortion	IUGR	Uterine inertia
Anaemia	Prematurity	Cord prolapse
Hyperemesis	Discordant growth	Abruptio can happen after delivery of the first of the twin due to sudden decompression
Pre-eclampsia	Congenital anomaly of the foetus	
Gestational diabetes	IUD	
Polyhydramnios	Vanishing twin—multiple foetus identified in early USG, later one foetus dies and is re-absorbed	Increased operative interventions
Maternal pressure symptoms		Atonic PPH (due to over-distension)
APH (abruption, placenta previa)	Cord entanglement	Retained placenta
	Discordant growth	
PROM	Demise of one twin, TTTS, TRAP	
Pre-term labour	The PNMR is 6 times higher in twins than in singletons, mainly due to prematurity-related complications	
Malpresentation	It is higher in monochorionic than dichorionic twin pregnancies	

PPH, Post-partum haemorrhage.

UNIQUE COMPLICATIONS OF MONOCHORIONIC TWINS
- Twin-to-twin transfusion syndrome (TTTS)
- Twin reversed arterial perfusion (TRAP)
- Conjoint twin
- Acardiac foetus

INTRAPARTUM MANAGEMENT OF TWINS
- Both twins—vertex (Vx) presentation—vaginal delivery (if there are no other obstetric indications for caesarean)
- IV line to be started and blood to be cross-matched
- Epidural analgesia may be advocated
- Monitor FHR of both twins, CTG with twin tracing may be used
- Deliver the first twin after liberal episiotomy in usual manner
- Withhold oxytocin and methylergometrin
- Cord should be clamped at foetal and placental ends; keep the cord of the baby long

Preferable to have two obstetrician's clinicians for delivery and neonatologist and anaesthetist should be available at the time of delivery.

- *After delivery of the first twin*:
  - Palpate the abdomen and confirm the presentation with or without USG
  - Position and station of the second twin is confirmed by vaginal examination
- If the presentation of second twin is non-vertex, ECV is done (USG is helpful to assist ECV)
- *If second twin is in vertex presentation*:
  - Do ARM and start oxytocin drip, if there are inadequate contractions
  - Deliver the baby and clamp the cord
  - Active management of third stage of labour to be done
- *If second twin is in breech presentation*:
  - DO ARM and start oxytocin and conduct assisted breech delivery
- *If second twin is in transverse lie*
  - Do ECV and deliver as vertex
  - If ECV fails—take the patient to theatre
  - Under general anaesthesia—do internal podalic version and breech extraction.

Only place for internal podalic version and breech extraction in modern obstetrics is when second of twin is in transverse lie and ECV fails.

MANAGEMENT
MANAGEMENT OF TWIN GESTATION (Flow chart 9.1)

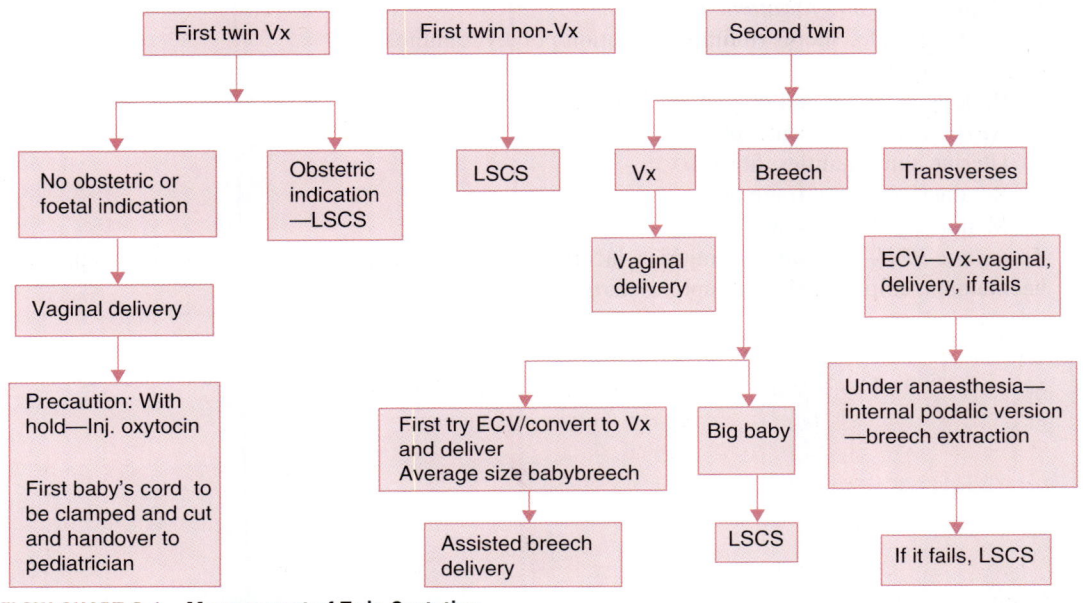

FLOW CHART 9.1 Management of Twin Gestation

INDICATIONS FOR LSCS IN TWINS
- First of twin is in non-vertex presentation
- Monoamniotic twins
- Discordant growth
- Conjoint twin
- Estimated weight of second twin is 500 g more than first twin
- Triplets
- Twins associated with other obstetric complications
- *Causes for post-partum haemorrhage (PPH) in multiple gestation*
  - Over-distension, large placenta, atonicity, retained placenta; it takes longer time for placenta to separate

CASE DISCUSSION IN POST-PARTUM HAEMORRHAGE
- **PPH** is defined as a blood loss of more than 500 mL from genital tract in the first 24 h after delivery of the foetus by vaginal delivery and 1000 mL following caesarean section
- Clinically PPH can be defined as any amount of blood loss that results in haemodynamic instability
- *Primary PPH*: bleeding which occurs within first 24 h
- *Secondary PPH*: bleeding which occurs after 24 h up to 6 weeks post-partum
- *Types and predisposing factors for PPH*:
  - Types: atonic and traumatic
- *Atonic PPH* is due to non-contraction and retraction of uterus, which prevents obliteration of blood vessels
- *Predisposing factors for atonic PPH*:
  - Over-distended uterus (multiple gestation/polyhydramnios)
  - Grand multi
  - Prolonged labour and precipitate labour
  - APH (abruptio placenta, placenta previa)
  - Uterine abnormalities, fibroid
  - Retained placental fragments
  - Mismanaged third stage
- *Traumatic PPH*—genital tract injuries, laceration of cervix, vagina, perineum, vulvovaginal haematoma, colporrhexis and rupture uterus

MANAGEMENT OF PPH (Flow chart 9.2)

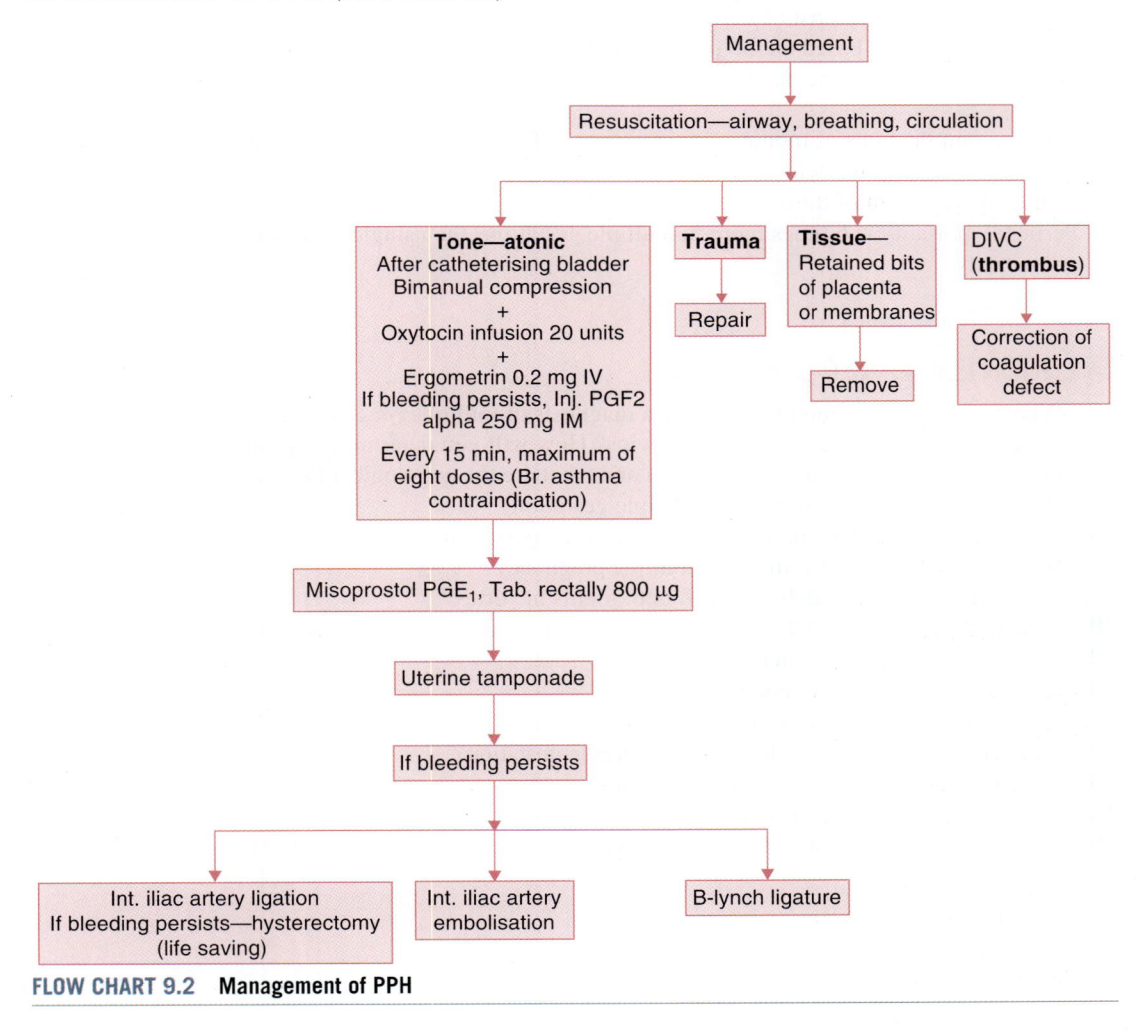

```
                        Management
                            │
                            ▼
          Resuscitation—airway, breathing, circulation
                            │
        ┌───────────┬───────┴───────┬──────────┐
        ▼           ▼               ▼          ▼
    Tone—atonic  Trauma         Tissue—       DIVC
  After catheterising            Retained bits (thrombus)
  bladder                        of placenta
  Bimanual compression    Repair or membranes
        +                                      │
  Oxytocin infusion                            ▼
  20 units                        Remove   Correction of
        +                                  coagulation
  Ergometrin 0.2 mg IV                     defect
  If bleeding persists, Inj. PGF2
  alpha 250 mg IM
  Every 15 min, maximum of
  eight doses (Br. asthma
  contraindication)
        │
        ▼
  Misoprostol PGE₁, Tab. rectally 800 µg
        │
        ▼
  Uterine tamponade
        │
        ▼
  If bleeding persists
        │
  ┌─────┼─────────┐
  ▼     ▼         ▼
Int. iliac    Int. iliac   B-lynch ligature
artery ligation  artery
If bleeding    embolisation
persists—
hysterectomy
(life saving)
```

FLOW CHART 9.2 Management of PPH

KEY POINTS

- Multiple pregnancy may be monozygotic (single ovum) or dizygotic (from two ova).
- The rate of monozygotic twins is relatively constant.
- The incidence multiple pregnancy is suspected when there is excessive vomiting or uterus is bigger for dates or if severe anaemia is present.
- All physiological changes during pregnancy are exaggerated.
- USG is very useful in determining chorionicity. Unique complications of monozygotic twins are detected early by USG.

CASE 9 A CASE OF MULTIPLE PREGNANCY

- Antenatal visits should be more frequent to detect complications early.
- Uncomplicated twins must be delivered by 38 weeks.
- Mode of delivery is based on the first twin presentation.
- Obstetrician, assistant, neonatologist should be available and blood bank facilities should be present.
- Unique complications of monoamniotic twins are TTTS, twin reversed arterial perfusion sequence (TRAPS) and conjoint twin.
- Active management of third stage is recommended.
- Perinatal mortality is 6 times more in multiple gestations than singleton and main cause is due to prematurity.

FREQUENTLY ASKED QUESTIONS

1. What are the early symptoms to make a diagnosis of multiple pregnancy?
2. What are monozygotic and dizygotic twins? How will you determine zygosity?
3. Frequency of which type of twin varies and what are the aetiological factors?
4. How will you diagnose clinically multiple gestation?
5. What are the antenatal complications in multiple gestation?
6. What is antenatal management of multiple pregnancy?
7. How will you conduct delivery with both foetus in vertex?
8. How will you conduct delivery if first twin is vertex and second twin is non-vertex presentation?
9. What are the foetal complications?
10. What are the intrapartum complications?
11. How will you assess chorionicity and what is its significance?
12. What are the various USG findings in multiple gestation?
13. Which type of twin has more complications?
14. What are the indications for caesarean section in multiple pregnancy?
15. What is the definition of PPH? How will you manage different types of PPH?

CASE

A CASE OF Rh NEGATIVE PREGNANCY

10

PATIENT'S DETAILS
Name.. Age.................. Address.......................... Occupation..............
Socioeconomic Class......................... Gravida, Para, Live, Abortion, (G......... P......... L......... A.........)
Booked/Unbooked........................ Immunization....................... LMP............ EDD

H/O............ months of amenorrhoea/period of gestation

PRESENT COMPLAINTS
Patient may present with period of amenorrhoea with following complaints:
   No specific complaints pertaining to Rh negative pregnancy if she is primi.
   If she is multi-H/O adverse foetal outcome in previous pregnancies may be present (foetal ascites neonatal jaundice, intrauterine death).

HISTORY
Present pregnancy
History of the following conditions that might increase the chance of foetomaternal haemorrhage resulting in Rh isoimmunisation should be elicited:

- Bleeding PV at any time either in early or late pregnancy
- Invasive procedure—Amniocentesis, Chorionic Villus Sampling (CVS)
- External cephalic version, trauma

   H/O indirect Coomb's test—elevated titres denote Rh isoimmunisation
   H/O antenatal Anti D prophylaxis—around 28–30 weeks given as prophylaxis
   H/O husband's Blood group and Rh type

MENSTRUAL HISTORY, MARITAL HISTORY, OBSTETRIC HISTORY, PAST MEDICAL AND SURGICAL HISTORY
- Refer Case 1.

To view the lecture notes log in to your account on www.MedEnact.com

CASE 10 A CASE OF Rh NEGATIVE PREGNANCY

Past obstetric history
Following history for severity of Rh isoimmunisation is to be elicited:
- H/O neonatal jaundice/anaemia in new born/exchange transfusion
- For baby/foetus with features suggestive of foetal hydrops/intrauterine death
- H/O bad obstetric history
- H/O taking anti D immunoglobulin injection—following spontaneous or medical abortion/MTP
- Antenatal or postnatal prophylaxis with anti D injection

PAST HISTORY
- H/O blood transfusion especially Rh positive blood

EXAMINATION
GENERAL EXAMINATION
- Refer Case 1

    Sometimes there may be associated pre-eclampsia in cases of Rh isoimmunisation (due to hyperplacentosis)

OBSTETRIC EXAMINATION
Polyhydramnios may be present and if present should be elicited by fluid thrill.

SUMMARY
- Mrs …age……. Rh Negative Gravida …..Para……EDD admitted with period of gestation…..If there is abortion and delivery, mention about administration of prophylactic inj-Anti D
- Mention about general, obstetric examination findings
- Mention about foetal lie, presentation and foetal heart rate

DIAGNOSIS
Rh Negative Gravida ….. Para…., period of amenorrhoea/gestation age with mention about single live foetus,…… presentation, ….foetal heart rate. If preeclampsia present mention that.

INVESTIGATIONS
Routine investigations
    Blood group and Rh type both for patient and husband

- *Indirect Coomb's test*
  - In non-immunized primi done at 28 weeks
  - In multi—done at first visit and repeat at 28 weeks, if negative give Anti D prophylaxis
  - In immunized mother, if ICT is positive repeat in dilutions every 4 weeks. Critical titre value—1:16
- *USG*
  - To find out condition of the foetus—all biophysical parameters are done/hydrops foetalis can be made out
  - Placental size—enlarged in isoimmunisation (hyperplacentosis)
  - Polyhydramnios
- *Obstetric Doppler done in the following foetal blood vessels*:
  - Umbilical artery
  - Middle cerebral artery Doppler velocity can detect foetal anaemia at earlier stage
  - MCA peak systolic velocity >1.5 MOM, for the gestation period is predictive of severe anaemia
  - Ductus venosus
- *Modified biophysical profile (AFI + NST) for foetal surveillance*
- *Amniocentesis*: Done to assess the bilirubin present in amniotic fluid. Optical density used for clinical management is 450 nm
  - Not done nowadays after the usage of Doppler of MCV
- *Cordocentesis*: Percutaneous umbilical blood sampling for foetal haematocrit and it is an invasive test
- *Investigations in new born*: Cord blood for—HB, PCV, blood group, Rh type, bilirubin level, direct Coomb's test

CASE DISCUSSION

Incidence: 1.5% of Indian population are Rh−ve.

IN Rh ISOIMMUNISATION OR ALLOIMMUNISATION

Rh negative woman develops antibodies to Rh antigen present in foetal RBCS in maternal circulation due to foetomaternal haemorrhage. IgM antibodies or saline agglutinin are produced which do not cross the placenta. In next pregnancy, if foetus is Rh positive, maternal IgG antibodies or albumin agglutinin A are produced which crosses placental barrier and may result in foetal anaemia, jaundice, leading to haemolytic disease of the foetus and new born.

Rh ISOIMMUNISATION DEPENDS ON

- Amount of foetomaternal haemorrhage
- Immune response of mother
- ABO incompatibility

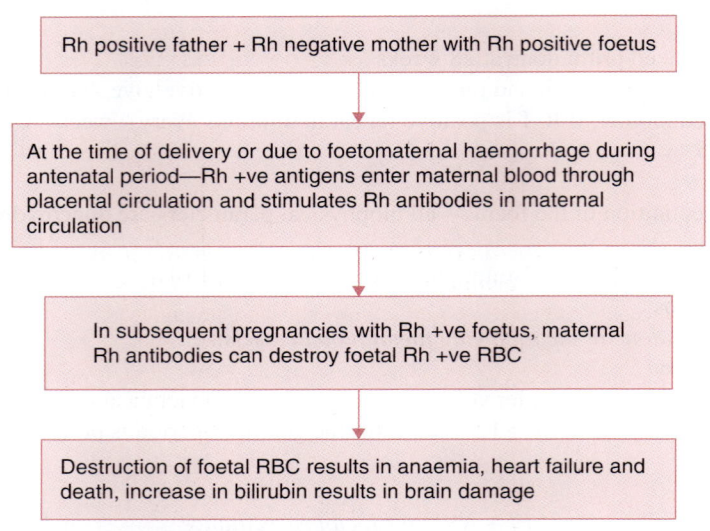

CASE 10 A CASE OF Rh NEGATIVE PREGNANCY

```
┌─────────────────────────────────────────────────────┐
│ Rh positive father + Rh negative mother with Rh positive foetus │
└─────────────────────────────────────────────────────┘
                          ↓
┌─────────────────────────────────────────────────────┐
│ At the time of delivery or due to foetomaternal haemorrhage during │
│ antenatal period—Rh +ve antigens enter maternal blood through     │
│ placental circulation and stimulates Rh antibodies in maternal    │
│ circulation                                                        │
└─────────────────────────────────────────────────────┘
                          ↓
┌─────────────────────────────────────────────────────┐
│ In subsequent pregnancies with Rh +ve foetus, maternal │
│ Rh antibodies can destroy foetal Rh +ve RBC            │
└─────────────────────────────────────────────────────┘
                          ↓
┌─────────────────────────────────────────────────────┐
│ Destruction of foetal RBC results in anaemia, heart failure and │
│ death, increase in bilirubin results in brain damage             │
└─────────────────────────────────────────────────────┘
```

FLOW CHART 10.1 Pathogenesis of Erythroblastosis Foetalis

ERYTHROBLASTOSIS FOETALIS

Occurs due to destruction of foetal RBCS, by Rh antibody present in maternal circulation. Hence there is presence of nucleated RBCS in circulation due to compensatory erythropoiesis (Flow Chart 10.1).

IN ABO INCOMPATIBILITY

If mother is O group, father is A or B group and the baby is A or B, major antigens react with mother's naturally present anti A or anti B antibodies before they are exposed to Rh antigen and thereby ABO incompatibility protects against Rh isoimmunisation.

Conditions which increase chances of foetomaternal haemorrhage which require Anti D Administration:

ANTI D ADMINISTRATION

- Threatened abortion, spontaneous abortion, missed abortion, MTP, ectopic gestation
- Chorionic villus sampling, amniocentesis, cordocentesis
- ECV/APH/IUD
- Delivery and caesarean/manual removal of placenta

USG FINDINGS IN HYDROPS FOETALIS

- Fluid collection in all cavities—foetal ascites, pleural effusion, pericardial effusion and scalp oedema (halo around the head-Buddha sign)

- Hepatosplenomegaly
- Large placenta (increased thickness of the placenta), polyhydramnios

Foetal anaemia nowadays is assessed by Doppler of middle cerebral artery—MCA

Middle cerebral artery—MCA-Peak systolic velocity value above 1.5 MOM (multiples of median) for the gestational age indicates anaemia
Liley's curve: Is based on the amount of bilirubin in amniotic fluid which gives clue to haemolysis (indirectly correlates with anaemia)
- Optical density of amniotic fluid containing bilirubin at wavelength 450 nm is measured. Based on the deviation at the 450 nm it is plotted in the Liley's chart

Degree of Manifestations in Erythroblastosis Foetalis *(haemolytic disease of foetus and new born)—HDFN*

Degree of Manifestation	Clinical Condition
1. Mildest form and anaemia develops slowly due to haemolysis-tolerated by foetus	1. Congenital anaemia of newborn
2. Newborn will be born alive. Jaundice will appear within 24 h	2. Icterus gravis Neonatorum
3. Severe form of Rh haemolytic disease. If no intervention is done, IUD may result.	3. Hydrops foetalis

Liley's zone 1—Foetus unlikely to be affected—pregnancy can be continued
  Zone 2—Repeat test every 2 weeks. If value goes up, do Cordocentesis—if haematocrit is less than 30%, intrauterine transfusion given
- If gestational age below 34 weeks—deliver after corticosteroids when indicated

Zone 3—Severely affected. Death is imminent. More than 34 weeks—deliver
- Below 34 weeks—intra uterine transfusion, give corticosteroids and deliver

Intra uterine transfusion:
- Indications—foetal haematocrit—below 30% by cordocentesis
- Transfusion with O negative blood
- Rate of transfusion—5–10 mL/min
- Amount—10 mL × gestational age in weeks min 20 = mL of blood transfused

  For example: 28 weeks − 20 = 8 × 10 mL = 80 mL to be transfused Route—Intra vascular (umbilical vein) or intraperitoneal

Precautions during antenatal period
- Invasive tests (CVS, amniocentesis), ECV—done only if absolutely indicated

CASE 10 A CASE OF Rh NEGATIVE PREGNANCY

Timing of delivery of a Rh negative mother
- Mother not immunised—pregnancy is allowed to continue upto 40 weeks
- Mother immunised—delivery time depends on the severity, antibody titre, MCA peak systolic velocity and the maturity of the foetus

The precautions taken during conduct of normal labour and LSCS to prevent Rh isoimmunisation:
- Intrauterine manipulation to be done only if absolutely indicated
- No prophylactic methylergometrin
- Early cord clamping
- LSCS: removal of blood from peritoneal cavity, mopping of blood to avoid spillage
- Avoid manual removal of placenta and uterine massage

Calculation of foetomaternal haemorrhage:
   Kleihauer Betke test—acid elution test: In 50 low power fields of maternal peripheral blood, if 80 foetal RBCs are present, it indicates 4 mL of foetomaternal haemorrhage.
- For 1 mL of foetal blood volume—10 μg of Rh immunoglobulin is given.

Coomb's test:
- **Direct Coomb's test (DCT):** The anti-human anti-globulin is added directly to the foetal RBCs and agglutination detects bound antibodies, denoting positive DCT. Direct Coomb's Test—Tests for the Rh antibodies bound to the foetal RBCs. Done in cord blood.
- **Indirect Coomb's test (ICT):** The free antibodies in the maternal serum are tested after incubating with RBCs of specific antigen type and then, the anti-human anti-globulin is added and agglutination detects Rh antibodies. Indirect Coomb's Test—Test for Rh antibodies circulating in maternal blood.

   Antenatal prophylaxis: To be given when ICT is negative 300 μg of Rh anti D immunoglobulin is given at 28 weeks and repeated after delivery
   Post-natal immunoprophylaxis following delivery: 300 μg of Rh anti D immunoglobulin is given, Within 72 h after delivery and if missed it can be given up to 28 days postpartum. 50 μg is to be given after abortion/MTP below 12 weeks.

Management of affected newborn:
- Phototherapy
- Phenobarbitone—enhances conjugation of bilirubin
- Exchange transfusion—cord length is kept long for cannulation

Exchange transfusion:
   Indications:
   Rh positive baby with DCT positive
   Cord blood—Hb <11 g/dL Cord bilirubin > 4 mg/dL. Serum bilirubin—20 mg/dL DCT positive
   Transfuse—Rh negative, same blood group of baby's group or O negative blood
   Total 160 mL/kg body weight, 15 mL to be withdrawn and 10 mL to be given

MANAGEMENT
MANAGEMENT Rh NEGATIVE PREGNANCY (Flow chart 10.2)

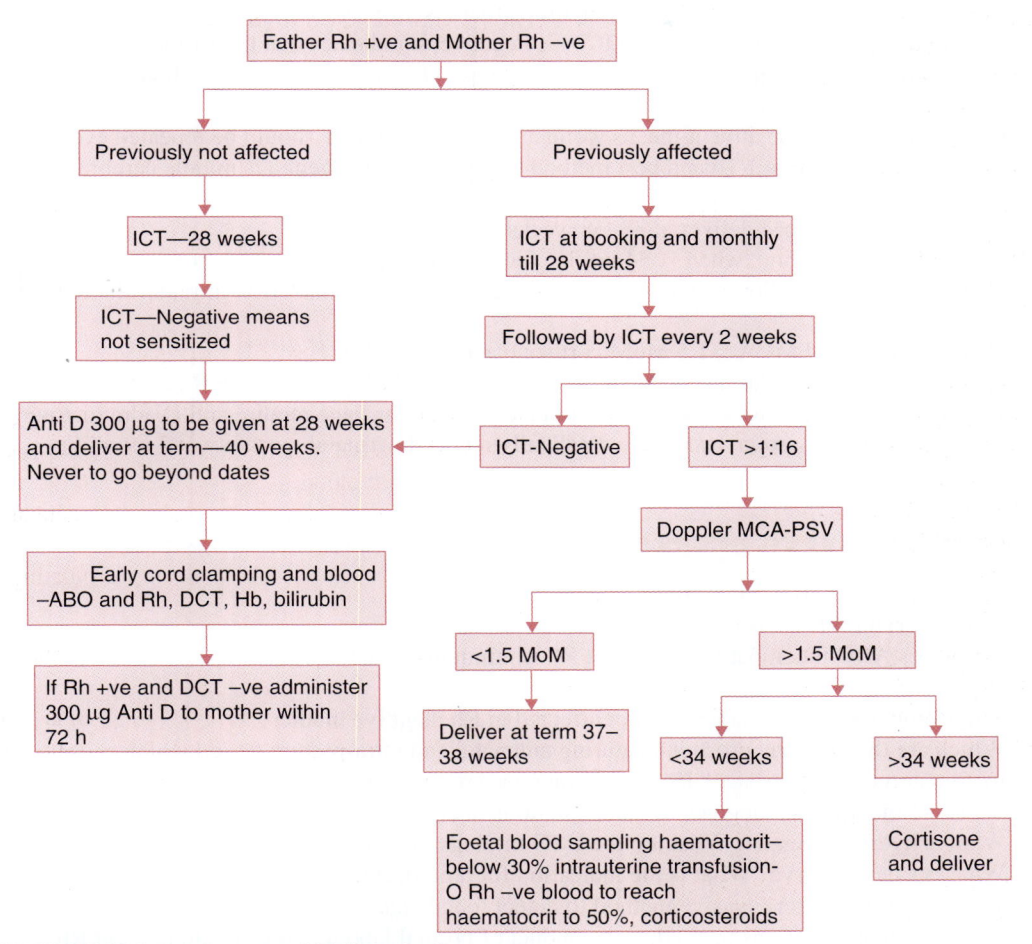

```
                    Father Rh +ve and Mother Rh –ve
                    ┌──────────────┴──────────────┐
              Previously not affected        Previously affected
                        │                            │
                   ICT—28 weeks            ICT at booking and monthly
                        │                       till 28 weeks
              ICT—Negative means                    │
                 not sensitized              Followed by ICT every 2 weeks
                        │                            │
   Anti D 300 µg to be given at 28 weeks   ┌─────────┴─────────┐
   and deliver at term—40 weeks.      ICT-Negative         ICT >1:16
   Never to go beyond dates                                    │
                        │                              Doppler MCA-PSV
          Early cord clamping and blood                        │
         –ABO and Rh, DCT, Hb, bilirubin              ┌────────┴────────┐
                        │                          <1.5 MoM         >1.5 MoM
      If Rh +ve and DCT –ve administer                │          ┌──────┴──────┐
      300 µg Anti D to mother within              Deliver at   <34 weeks  >34 weeks
                  72 h                            term 37–         │          │
                                                  38 weeks    Foetal blood  Cortisone
                                                              sampling...   and deliver
```

Foetal blood sampling haematocrit–below 30% intrauterine transfusion–O Rh –ve blood to reach haematocrit to 50%, corticosteroids

FLOW CHART 10.2 Management of Rh Negative Pregnancy

KEY POINTS

- In Rh isoimmunisation or alloimmunisation: Rh negative woman develops antibodies to Rh antigen present in foetal RBCS in maternal circulation due to foetomaternal haemorrhage. In next pregnancy, if foetus is Rh positive, maternal antibodies produced crosses placental barrier and may result in foetal anaemia, jaundice leading to haemolytic disease of the foetus and newborn.

- The degree of isoimmunisation varies depending on the volume of foetomaternal haemorrhage, 1/3 women are non-responders, ABO incompatibility of mother and foetus and strength of the antigenic stimulus.
- Degree of severity are mild degree—congenital anaemia of newborn, moderate degree—icterus gravis neonatorum and severe degree—hydrops foetalis.
- When maternal indirect Coombs test (ICT) is negative, it indicates that the woman is not immunised and test is repeated at 28 and antenatal prophylaxis anti D 300 µg should be given and deliver at term.
- When indirect test is positive it means woman is immunised, ICT should be repeated every 2 weeks. Critical titre is 1:16 and best method to assess foetal anaemia is middle cerebral artery Doppler (MCA).
- When MCA <1.5 MoM deliver at 37–38 weeks.
- When MCA >1.5 Mom , when < 34 weeks, foetal blood sampling is done from umbilical vein under USG guidance (Cordocentesis) and if haematocrit is less than 30%, intrauterine transfusion is done.
- When 34 weeks and MCA >1.5 MoM cortisone and deliver.
- Precautions to be taken during conduct of normal labour and LSCS to prevent Rh isoimmunisation.
- Conditions which increase chances of foetomaternal haemorrhage require anti D administration and antenatal anti D prophylaxis have drastically reduced perinatal mortality and morbidity.

FREQUENTLY ASKED QUESTIONS

1. What is isoimmunisation or alloimmunisation?
2. What is erythroblastosis foetalis?
3. How does ABO incompatibility protect Rh isoimmunisation?
4. When does foetomaternal haemorrhage occur?
5. Why some Rh positive babies are not affected in Rh negative mother?
6. Which are the obstetric procedures during antenatal and intra-partum period which cause foetomaternal haemorrhage? How will you measure for foeto maternal haemorrhage?
7. What are the different degrees of manifestations in erythroblastosis foetalis?
8. What is hydrops foetalis? What are the USG findings in hydrops foetalis?
9. What is Liley's curve? What is the indication for amniocentesis?
10. What is the other non-invasive method to detect foetal anaemia?
11. What are the precautions taken during conduct of normal labour and LSCS to prevent Rh isoimmunisation?
12. How will you calculate foetomaternal haemorrhage?
13. What is indirect Coomb's test and direct Coomb's test?
14. What are the investigations to be done with cord blood?
15. What is the dose of anti D immunoglobulin to be given following first trimester abortion?
16. What is antenatal immununo prophylaxis? What are the indications and dose?
17. What is post-natal immunoprophylaxis? What is the stipulated period and dose you can give?
18. What are the indications for intra-uterine transfusion?
19. What are the indications for exchange transfusion?

CASE 11

A CASE OF CEPHALOPELVIC DISPROPORTION

PATIENT'S DETAILS

Mrs................................ Age................. Coming from......................... Occupation..............
Socioeconomic Class......................... Gravida, Para, Live, Abortion, (G......... P......... L......... A.........)
Booked.......... Immunised........................ LMP............ EDD

H/O............ months of amenorrhoea/period of gestation

PRESENT COMPLAINTS

Patient may present with period of amenorrhoea with following complaints:
Woman may not have specific complaints pertaining to cephalopelvic disproportion. She may be admitted for safe confinement/pain/draining PV/bleeding PV.

MENSTRUAL HISTORY

- Refer Case 1.

MARITAL HISTORY

- Refer Case 1.

OBSTETRIC HISTORY

Past obstetric history

Nature of the delivery—if vaginal, following history is to be elicited:
- Prolonged labour with difficult forceps or vacuum delivery
- Perineal lacerations, complete perineal tear, PPH, rectovaginal fistula, vesicovaginal fistula
- Blood transfusion
- Size of the baby, whether baby cried immediately after birth/stillbirth/neonatal death or neurological sequelae

To view the lecture notes log in to your account on www.MedEnact.com

CASE 11 A CASE OF CEPHALOPELVIC DISPROPORTION

If LSCS—whether emergency or elective, indication, whether following prolonged labour due to CPD, H/O malpresentation, H/O blood transfusion

> Uncomplicated vaginal delivery of an average sized baby excludes contracted pelvis.

MEDICAL HISTORY
Pertaining to CPD, following history to be elicited:
- Rickets/osteomalacia/tuberculosis of hip, pelvic joints, spine/poliomyelitis of lower limbs

SURGICAL HISTORY (pertaining to CPD)
- Past history of fracture in spine, pelvis which might alter pelvic configuration
- Fracture in lower limbs—leading to shortening of lower limbs and contracted pelvis

FAMILY HISTORY
- Refer Case 1.

PERSONAL HISTORY
- Refer Case 1.

GENERAL EXAMINATION
- Refer Case 1.
- Short women are likely to have small pelvis which may lead to CPD and if foetus is also small, there may not be CPD

> Height: 145 cm or below is considered as short stature **in Indian women**.

Examination for other causes of CPD:
- Deformities in spine—kyphosis, scoliosis
- Deformities or tumour—in pelvic bone, hip joints
- Presence of rickety rosary
- Shortening of lower limbs

Dystocia dystrophy syndrome:
- Short stocky individual with male distribution of hair who may have android pelvis

Gait: look for limping/exaggerated waddling gait

OBSTETRIC EXAMINATION

It is done as in any other case.
    Specific points to be noted in CPD:
    Inspection: pendulous abdomen gives a clue that there may CPD due to inlet contraction
    Unengaged head/mobile head/malpresentation at term—suspect *CPD*

CLINICAL METHODS OF DIAGNOSING CPD

Abdominal method: It is a screening method but difficult to do in obese patient, deflexed head, floating head, thick abdominal wall (Fig. 11.1).
Procedure:
- Bladder should be empty
- Patient should be in dorsal position, thighs and knees semi-flexed and abducted
- With left hand, head is grasped
- Middle finger and index finger of right hand are placed above the pubic symphysis, keeping the inner surface of the middle finger in line with pubic symphysis
- Head is pushed downwards into pelvis
- The fingers of the right hand placed on the pubic symphysis will assess CPD

Interpretation:
- Head can be pushed down into the pelvis—*no CPD*
- Head is flush with symphysis pubis—*mild degree of CPD*
- Head cannot be pushed down at all and there is overriding of head over pubic symphysis—*major degree of CPD*

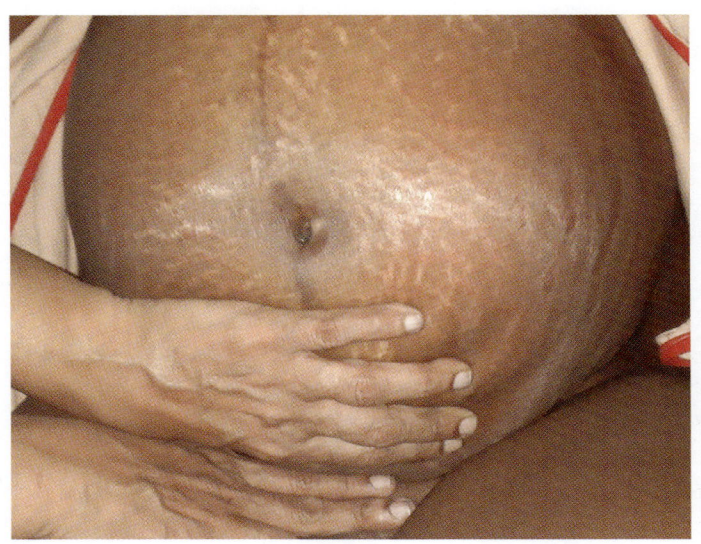

FIGURE 11.1 **Abdominal Method**

Ian Donald method (Fig. 11.3B):
- Patient lying in dorsal position; obstetrician stands on the right side of the patient
- Patient's knee not fully raised but fairly widely separated
- Using 3rd, 4th, and 5th fingers of both hands, head is grasped at sinciput and occiput
- Index finger reaches pubic symphysis
- Thumbs of both hands are kept on parietal eminence. Thumbs on parietal eminence press the head downwards and the index fingers on pubic symphysis can assess the degree of CPD

Abdomino-pelvic assessment by Munro Kerr–Muller method (Figs. 11.2 and 11.3A):

Munro Kerr described that thumb is to be placed over the pubic symphysis.

Muller described that the middle and index finger of right hand are to be placed at ischial spines, to find out whether head can be pushed up to the level of ischial spines.

Procedure: after emptying the bladder, woman is placed in dorsal position with thigh and knee semi-flexed

Obstetrician stands on the right side facing her and grasps the foetal head with the left hand and pushes it into pelvis brim, while middle and index fingers of right hand are kept at the level of ischial spine and thumb of the right hand is kept over the pubic symphysis.

Interpretation:
- When head can be pushed up to ischial spines and no overlapping of parietal bone occurs over the pubic symphysis—*no CPD*
- Head can be pushed little but not up to ischial spines and parietal bone is flush with pubic symphysis—mild degree CPD

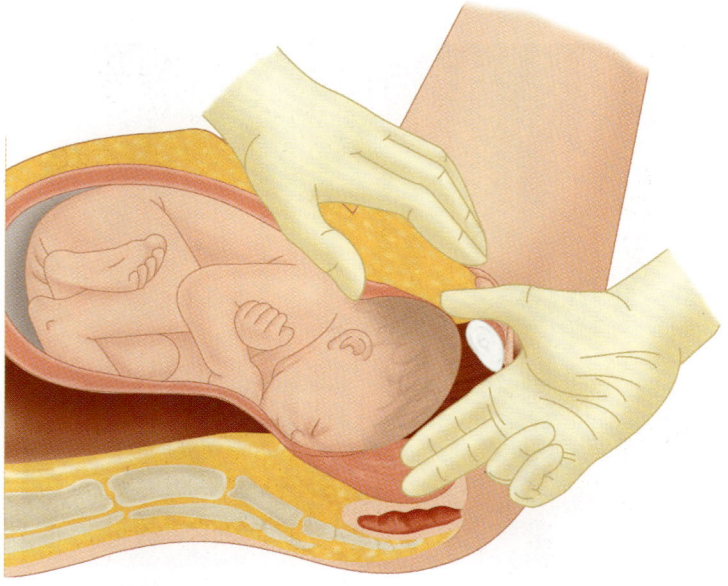

FIGURE 11.2 Munrokerr Muller Method

OBSTETRIC EXAMINATION 129

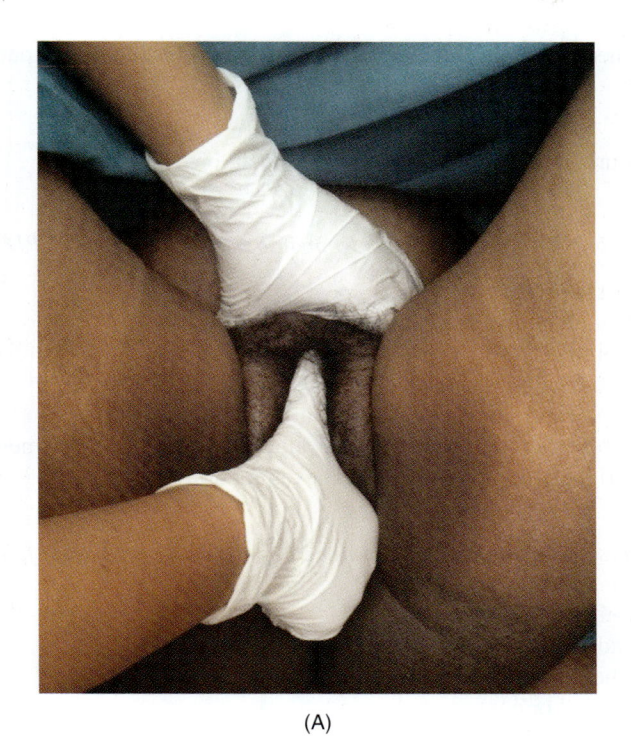

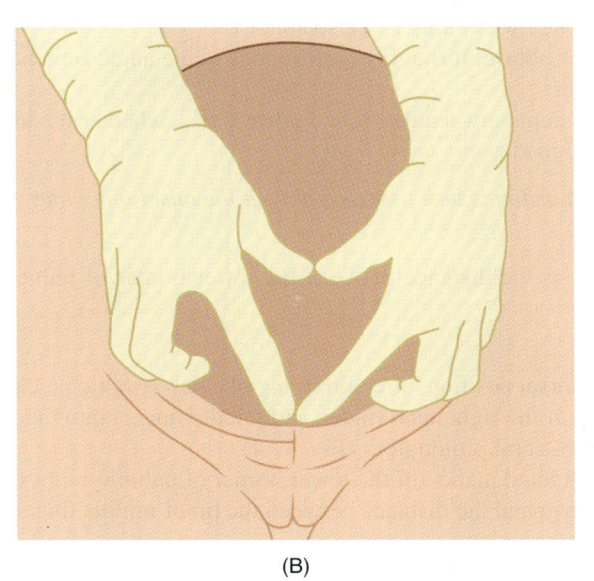

FIGURE 11.3

(A) Munro Kerr -Muller method. (B) Ian Donald method.

- Head cannot be pushed down and there is overriding of the parietal bone over pubic symphysis—*major degree CPD*

> Pitfall in the procedure: it can assess only contraction at the brim.

PV is done in cases of primi or nulliparous women to assess pelvis and CPD at 38 weeks.

Pre-requisites for assessing CPD:
- Explain to the patient about the procedure
- Bladder should be empty
- Patient should be in dorsal position
- Done under aseptic precautions; internal procedure should be gentle
- Pelvic capacity can be estimated clinically by evaluating various measurements with the middle and index finger of right hand during bimanual examination

To assess pelvis:
Index and middle fingers of right hand are introduced into vagina, to find out following details:
- Sacral promontory is reached easily or not
- Bay of sacrum is well-curved or not
- Sacrosciatic notch admits two fingers or not
- Beaking anteriorly behind pubic symphysis
- Pelvic side walls parallel or convergent
- Ischial spines are prominent or not
- Ischial spines are reached when fingers are spanned
- Pubic angle is acute or obtuse. It roughly corresponds to the angle subtended by fully abducted thumb and index finger
- When clenched fist is kept between the ischial tuberosities, whether it admits four knuckles or not
- Coccyx is mobile or tipped

Cephalopelvic disproportion is best assessed only at the onset of labour.

Clinical pelvimetry:
Diagonal conjugate—is the distance between the lower border of pubic symphysis to the sacral promontory: 12.5 cm

Procedure:
- Patient should be in dorsal position, after emptying bladder. Aseptic precautions are to be taken.
- Introduce two fingers of the right hand (index and middle finger) into the vagina until the middle finger impinges on the sacral promontory (Fig. 11.4).
- Index finger of the left hand marks off the lower border of pubic symphysis over the right hand. Right hand is withdrawn and the distance between the tip of middle finger and point marked is measured.
- This gives diagonal conjugate measurement, which is 12.5 cm.

Obstetric conjugate is estimated by detecting 1.5–2 cm (depending on the height, thickness and inclination of pubic symphysis) from diagonal conjugate; normal: 10.5 cm.

INVESTIGATIONS   **131**

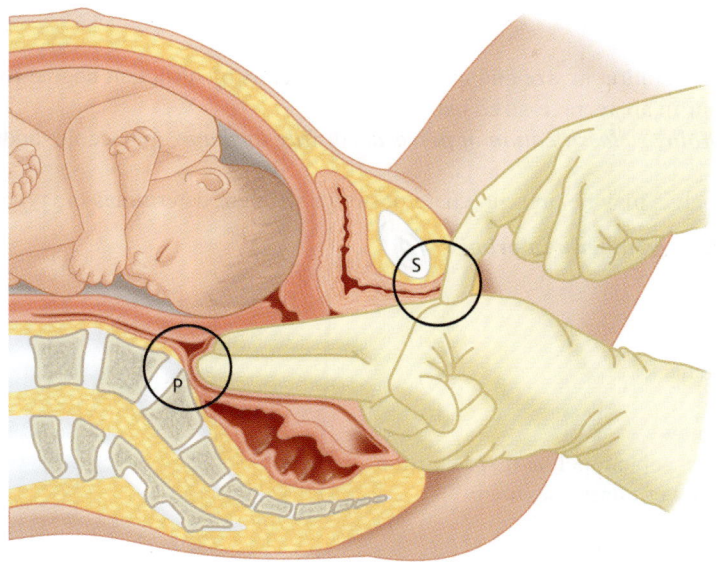

FIGURE 11.4   Clinical Pelvimetry

SUMMARY

Mrs … Age……..Gravida …..Para……EDD admitted with period of gestation——mention if there is LSCS.
  Mention about general/obstetric examination findings (undergraduates need not do PV examination)
  Mention about foetal lie, presentation and foetal heart rate

DIAGNOSIS

Gravida (if less than 145 cm, mention as short statured) ... Para...EDD with cephalopelvic disproportion—CPD

INVESTIGATIONS

Basic investigations:

  USG
  Cephalometry: bi-parietal diameter assessed by USG gives rough estimation of the probability of CPD. USG helps to find out relation of head to the plane of pelvis
  MRI: it can assess pelvis in all planes and gives information about foetal size and soft tissue; not done routinely

CASE 11 A CASE OF CEPHALOPELVIC DISPROPORTION

CASE DISCUSSION

Contracted pelvis: Alteration in size and or shape of the pelvis of sufficient degree to alter the normal mechanism of labour in an average-sized baby

Caldwell and Moloy's classification of pelvis according to shape: gynaecoid, android, anthropoid, platypelloid

Mixed type of pelvis may be present where posterior segment determines the type of pelvis.

Reasons for mobile head at term in primi:
- Wrong dates
- Prematurity
- Placenta previa
- Cord around the neck
- Polyhydramnios
- Multiple pregnancy
- Contracted pelvis, cephalopelvic disproportion
- Tumours in the lower uterine segment
- Foetal cause—hydrocephalus

Causes for contracted pelvis:
Developmental:
- Robert's pelvis—faulty development of both sacral alae
- Naegele's pelvis—faulty development of one sacral alae
- High and low assimilation pelvis
- Generally contracted pelvis (justo minor pelvis)

Deformity:
- Spines—kyphosis, scoliosis, spondylolisthesis
- Pelvic bone and joints—rickets, osteomalacia
- Tuberculosis, trauma and tumours
- Lower limbs—residual poliomyelitis
- Shortening of lower limbs due to fracture and surgery

Various methods to assess CPD:
  Clinical assessment of pelvis
  Imaging pelvimetry
  Assessment of foetal weight

Trial labour is conducted in a woman with minor degree of CPD with vertex presentation, with no other obstetric or medical complications in an attempt to deliver vaginally
- Should be conducted in an institution with facilities for LSCS
- Counselling of the woman (regarding advantages and disadvantages of trial labour and that it may end up in LSCS)
- Monitor with partogram
- No time limit for trial labour, and it is decided by effectiveness of uterine contractions and progress of labour (Table 11.1)

Trial labour is dependent on three factors that cannot be assessed before labour:
- Uterine contractions

Table 11.1 Indication and Contraindication for Trial of Labour

Indication for Trial of Labour	Contraindication for Trial of Labour
Minor or first degree CPD	Elderly woman
Average size foetus	Outlet contraction
No obstetric complication	Obstetric conjugate less than 9 cm
	Medical and obstetric complications of pregnancy

- Moulding of the foetal head leading to decrease in diameters of the foetal head
- Yield of the pelvis at the sacroiliac joints and pubic symphysis with resultant increase in pelvic dimensions and giving up of perineum

Successful trial labour: vaginal delivery, normal or assisted with forceps or vacuum with good maternal and foetal outcome

Failed trial labour: LSCS or vaginal delivery with poor maternal or foetal outcome

Conduct of trial labour: *during trial labour, adequate hydration, nutrition and analgesia should be maintained*

- Informed consent
- Nil oral, only IV fluids
- Analgesia—epidural can be advocated
- Progress of labour monitored by partogram
- If inadequate uterine contractions—oxytocin drip can be started
- Apply forceps when necessary
- Active management of third stage of labour

Termination of trial labour by LSCS: if there is foetal or maternal distress, inadequate progress of labour (Table 11.2)

Complications of CPD:
Maternal:
- PROM, cord prolapse
- Prolonged labour
- Increased chances for operative delivery
- PPH (both atonic and traumatic)
- Obstructed labour can cause dehydration, ketoacidosis and sepsis. If unattended, leads to rupture uterus, VVF

Table 11.2 Favourable and Unfavourable Sign of Progression of Trial Labour

Favourable Sign	Unfavourable Sign
Good uterine contractions—3 contractions in 10 min, each contraction 30–45 s	Ineffective uterine contractions
	Head remaining high at full cervical dilatation
Early engagement of head occipito-anterior position	Loosely hanging cervix not applied to head
Closely applied cervix	Rupture of membrane before full dilatation of cervix
Rupture of membrane after full dilatation of cervix	

Foetal: asphyxia, hypoxia, intrapartum death, tentorial tear, multiple fractures, cephalhaematoma, hypoxic encephalopathy

Trial forceps: tentative attempt at forceps delivery in the presence of mild CPD
- It should be attempted in operation theatre after informed consent, to expedite the delivery.
- If there is difficulty in application, locking or traction, procedure is abandoned.
- In these situations, we have to inform the patient and caesarean section has to be done.

Failed forceps:
- Error in judgment of CPD
- After applying forceps, the obstetrician fails to deliver the foetus vaginally

Role of elective LSCS in CPD:
- Major degree of CPD
- CPD associated with BOH, APH, pre-eclampsia, GDM, FGR, prolonged pregnancy

MANAGEMENT
MANAGEMENT OF CEPHALOPELVIC DISPROPORTION (Flow chart 11.1)

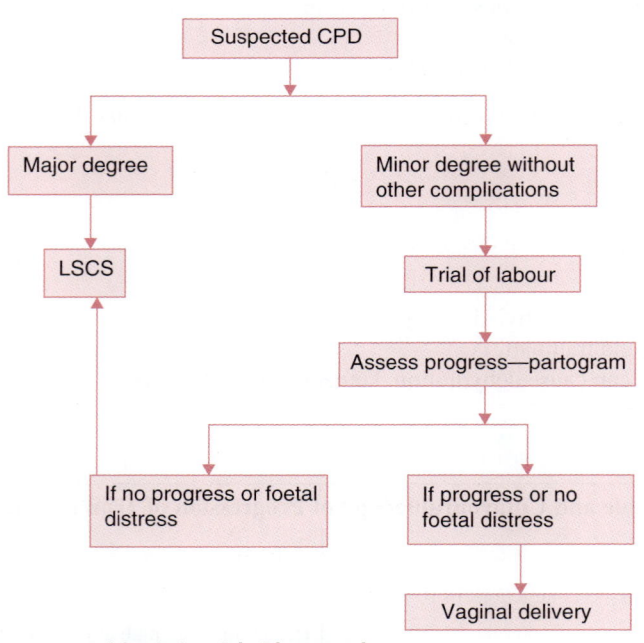

FLOW CHART 11.1 Management of Cephalopelvic Disproportion

KEY POINTS

- Contracted pelvis is alteration in size and/or shape of the pelvis of sufficient degree to alter the normal mechanism of labour in an average-sized baby.
- Various clinical methods for assessing CPD are abdominal method, Ian Donald method and Munro Kerr–Muller method.
- Cephalopelvic disproportion is best assessed only at the onset of labour.
- Trial of labour is the preferred mode of management in minor degree CPD without other complication.
- Trial of labour should be terminated, when there is no progress in cervical dilatation, failure of descent or foetal or maternal distress.
- Following trial of labour, vaginal delivery, normal or assisted with forceps or vacuum with good maternal and foetal outcome is successful trial labour.

FREQUENTLY ASKED QUESTIONS

1. What is the definition of contracted pelvis?
2. What are the different varieties of pelvis?
3. What are the common causes of CPD?
4. How will you asses CPD clinically?
5. What are the methods to assess pelvis?
6. What are the different methods of management in CPD?
7. Define trial labour.
8. What are the contraindications for trial labour?
9. How will you conduct trial labour?
10. What are the unfavourable factors in trial labour?
11. What are the factors in trial labour for successful outcome?
12. What is successful trial labour?
13. What are the causes for mobile head at term in a primi?
14. What are trial forceps and failed forceps?

A CASE OF DIABETES COMPLICATING PREGNANCY

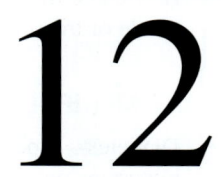

CASE 12

PATIENT'S DETAILS

Mrs................................. Age.................. Coming from.......................... Occupation..............
Socioeconomic Class......................... Gravida, Para, Live, Abortion, (G......... P......... L......... A.........)
Booked........................ Immunised...................... LMP............ EDD

H/O............ months of amenorrhoea/period of gestation

Age—older age group—prone for GDM

Higher socioeconomic class—prone for GDM

PRESENT COMPLAINTS

Patient may present with period of amenorrhoea with following complaints:
- Woman may give history of increased blood sugar level detected by random blood sugar or GCT or GTT
- Period of pregnancy at which GDM was diagnosed and how
- H/O repeated urinary tract infection, symptoms like frequency burning and pain during micturition
- Recurrent curdy white vaginal discharge and itching (moniliasis)
- Excessive weight gain (due to big baby, polyhydramnios, development of pre-eclampsia)
- Excessive enlargement of uterus (due to big baby, polyhydramnios)
- H/O treatment taken (meal plan/insulin)
- USG findings that has been done in this pregnancy

HISTORY

MENSTRUAL HISTORY AND MARITAL HISTORY
- Refer Case 1.

PAST OBSTETRIC HISTORY
- Previous H/O abortion/polyhydramnios/unexplained intra-uterine death/big baby/anomalous baby, neonatal death/wound infection/puerperal infection

To view the lecture notes log in to your account on www.MedEnact.com

- *H/O GDM in past pregnancy*: period of gestation at which it was diagnosed
- Mode of treatment/type of delivery/weight of baby at birth and present condition of baby

PAST MEDICAL HISTORY
- Diabetes—type of drug she was on, oral/insulin dose/previous blood sugar range/HbA1C/H/O hypertension

FAMILY HISTORY
- Diabetes in the family—mother, father, siblings, uncle, aunt, grandparents

PERSONAL HISTORY
- Refer Case 1.

GENERAL EXAMINATION
Refer Case 1.
- Pregnant woman may be obese.

OBSTETRIC EXAMINATION
As in Case 1.
- Height of the uterus may be bigger than period of amenorrhoea (due to polyhydramnios or big baby)
- If polyhydramnios is present, confirm with fluid thrill and rule out malpresentation
- Rarely FGR may occur in pregnancy with overt diabetes with vasculopathy

SUMMARY
- Mrs ……Age…..Gravida, Para …Booked, Immunised, Socioeconomic class….admitted for…. months of amenorrhoea/period of gestation and her LMP and EDD…….with her complaints
- Period at which she was diagnosed as diabetic and treatment given—meal plan/insulin she is on; examination details of both general and obstetric examination and available report of investigations

DIAGNOSIS
- Gravida, Para with GDM/pre-existing diabetes complicating pregnancy with …. weeks of pregnancy with single foetus, live in cephalic or podalic presentation.

  Mention about polyhydramnios, if present.

INVESTIGATIONS
- *Routine basic investigations*
- *Specific investigations*:
  - *Urine*—alb, sugar, deposits, culture and sensitivity
  - *Blood sugar*—fasting and post-prandial, HbA1C/glycaemic profile
  - *Diagnosis not established*—OGCT/OGTT or glycaemic profile
  - *Blood urea, serum creatinine, and uric acid* (when pre-eclampsia is associated)
  - Optic fundus examination—done in overt diabetes/when GDM is associated with pre-eclampsia
  - Thyroid function test (thyroid dysfunction can co-exist)
- *USG*:
  - Early scan, target scan, growth scan
  - Rule out polyhydramnios and macrosomia
  - Best parameter to detect macrosomia is abdominal circumference (AC) more than 95th percentile for that gestational age. Truncal skin fat and skin thickness above the scapula are also to be measured
  - Large placenta
- *Obstetric Doppler*

CASE DISCUSSION
GDM
- *Definition of gestational diabetes*: it is defined as carbohydrate intolerance of variable severity with onset or first recognition during present pregnancy.
- *High risk factors for GDM*:
  - Family H/O diabetes
  - Obesity
  - Older age group
  - Previous big baby
  - Anomalous foetus
  - Ethnicity—Indian, South East Asian
  - Previous IUD, stillbirth
  - Polyhydramnios
  - Previous H/O GDM
  - PCOD/metabolic syndrome
  - Present pregnancy—repeated UTI, monilial infection, polyhydramnios, macrosomia

Pregnancy is diabetogenic due to the following:
- Insulin resistance caused by:
  - Production of placental somatomammotropin (human placental lactogen)
  - Increased production of cortisol, oestriol and progesterone
  - Increased insulin destruction by kidney
  - Production of enzymes like placental insulinase

- Increased lipolysis
  - The mother uses fat for her caloric needs and saves glucose for foetal needs
- Change in gluconeogenesis
  - The foetus uses preferentially alanine and other amino acids and deprives the mother of a major gluconeogenic source

> In pregnancy, there is facilitated anabolism and accelerated starvation.

- *Screening test*: OGCT is done around 24–28 weeks
  - In high risk patients, OGCT is done at first visit and if negative, repeated at 28 weeks and 32–34 weeks
  - Irrespective of previous meal, after giving 50 g of glucose, blood sugar is checked after 1 h. Value of 140 mg/dL or more will identify 80% of women with GDM. Nowadays many use 130 mg/dL as cut off and this test has to be followed by oral GTT to confirm GDM—two-step procedure
- *Diagnostic test*: oral GTT—normal diet to be taken on the previous day; fasting blood sugar to be taken after 8–10 h of fasting
- *As per WHO criteria*: 75 g of glucose in 200 mL of water to be given and venous blood to be taken after 2 h
- *GDM*—if fasting blood sugar is >110 mg/dL and after 2 h, it is > 140 mg/dL
- *Overt or pre-gestational diabetes*:
  - Fasting blood sugar: > 126 mg.%
  - After 2 h: >200 mg.%
- *As per NDDG*—National Diabetes Data Group and Carpenter and Coustan—100 g of glucose in 200 mL of water is given. Venous samples are taken for fasting and 1, 2 and 3 h after glucose intake (Table 12.1)

The diagnosis of GDM is made when any two values are abnormal.
- *Diabetes in pregnancy study group of India (DIPSI) criteria*: one-step test
  - This test is done around 24–28 weeks or at the first visit in high-risk group. Irrespective of previous meal, 75 g glucose is given mixed with 200 mL of water
  - Blood sugar is checked after 2 h. If value is 140 mg/dL or more, treat as GDM; values 120–140 mg/dL, decreased or impaired glucose tolerance

Table 12.1 To Diagnose GDM

Time	Carpenter and Coustan (mg/dL)	NDDG (mg/dL)
Fasting	95	105
1 h	180	190
2 h	155	165
3 h	140	145

- *HbA1C—glycosylated haemoglobin—gives an idea about glycaemic control over 3 months prior to date of testing. Normal: < 6*

Maternal, Foetal and Neonatal Complications in GDM		
Maternal Complications	**Foetal Complications**	**Neonatal Complications**
Abortion—uncontrolled diabetes	Macrosomia	RDS, hyperbilirubinaemia, hypoglycaemia, hypocalcaemia, hypothermia, polycythaemia, hyper-viscosity due to increased erythropoiesis which in turn results in renal vein thrombosis and necrotising enterocolitis. Hypertrophic cardiomyopathy which may progress to heart failure
Ketoacidosis occur due to hyperemesis gravidarum, infections	Shoulder dystocia	
Polyhydramnios in 10% of GDM (amniotic fluid >2000 mL—due to foetal polyuria and hyper-osmosis due to hyperglycaemia)	Unexplained foetal death	
Increased risk of abruptio placenta	Four- to eightfold increased risk of congenital anomalies like caudal regression syndrome, sacral agenesis, congenital heart disease (ASD, VSD, transposition of great vessels) NTD, also renal and GI defects	
Pre-term labour Polyhydramnios Post-partum uterine atony—PPH		
Increased risk of pre-eclampsia—24%		
Increased risk of infection, for example vaginal candidiasis, UTI, endometritis or wound infection, puerperal sepsis		
Increase in instrumental delivery and LSCS rate		
NTD, Neural tube defects.		

- *Foetal macrosomia*: explained by Pederson's hypothesis below

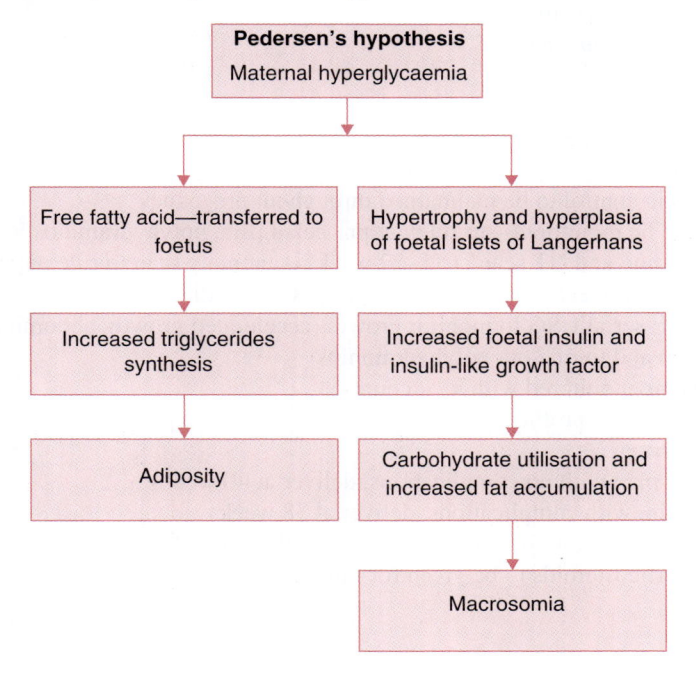

```
              Pedersen's hypothesis
              Maternal hyperglycaemia
              /                    \
Free fatty acid—transferred    Hypertrophy and hyperplasia
        to foetus              of foetal islets of Langerhans
            │                           │
Increased triglycerides         Increased foetal insulin and
       synthesis                insulin-like growth factor
            │                           │
        Adiposity              Carbohydrate utilisation and
                                increased fat accumulation
                        \      /
                      Macrosomia
```

- Gabbe rule of 15 in GDM:
  - 15% of positive GCT will have GDM
  - 15% GDM will require insulin
  - 15% GDM will have macrosomia
  - 15% GDM will have Type 2 DM after delivery
- Glycaemic profile targets during pregnancy:
  - Blood samples are taken fasting, post-breakfast, pre-lunch, post-lunch, pre-dinner, post-dinner and preferably at 3 a.m.
  - It is desirable to maintain pre-prandial blood sugar <90 mg/dL, post-prandial <120 mg/dL
  - HbA1C < 6 during pregnancy
- *Control of blood sugar*:
  - Diet and judicious use of exercise
  - Diet or medical nutrition therapy is the initial treatment of choice
  - Meal plan by nutritionist—**medical nutritional therapy**—24–30 kcal/kg: avoid sweets, take high fibre, low-fat food, with calories distributed by three meals and two snacks
  - If diet therapy fails to maintain fasting blood sugar <90 mg and post-prandial blood sugar <120 mg and these targets are not attained, within 2 weeks insulin therapy started
  - Exercise—brisk walk for 45–60 min/day
  - Insulin therapy is recommended for all overt diabetics
  - Regimes vary with woman's requirement
  - A mixture of short and intermediate acting insulin given in divided doses
  - Nowadays oral anti-glycaemic agent, metformin is also used
- *Principles of management*:
  - Tight glycaemic control with diet/exercise/insulin
  - Antepartum foetal surveillance
  - Daily foetal movement chart
  - Ideal timing of delivery
  - Good neonatal care
  - Counselling for the future
- *Antenatal monitoring*:
  - Strict glycaemic control to be maintained throughout pregnancy
  - Weight gain to be monitored—to rule out pre-eclampsia, polyhydramnios, macrosomia
  - Ultrasound: dating and NT scan/at 18–22 weeks—anomaly scan to rule out major malformations/foetal echocardiogram—24 weeks for cardiac evaluation
  - Third trimester: serial USG to monitor growth (accelerated growth, abdominal: head circumference) and to rule out polyhydramnios
  - Foetal wellbeing monitored with kick counts
  - Modified biophysical profile
- *Induction and delivery*:
  - GDM on meal plan with no complications, deliver at 40 weeks
  - GDM on insulin, with complications, deliver at 38 weeks
  - Pre-diabetes complicating pregnancy, deliver at 38 weeks
  - A course of corticosteroids to be given for lung maturity

- Day of induction or caesarean—withhold insulin
- IV fluids to be started and insulin given as per glucose level checked every 2 h
- Small risk of late IUD is present even with good glycaemic control
- Deliver at 38 weeks because beyond 38 weeks, there is increased risk of IUD
- *Vaginal delivery:*
  - Preferred, if there is no maternal or foetal complications
  - Average-sized baby
  - No CPD
  - Cervix is favourable
  - Labour monitored by partogram
  - Resort to emergency CS in cases of foetal distress or prolonged labour
  - In labour, omit long acting insulin; regular insulin is given as infusion 1 μm/h, maintaining blood sugar value at 90–100 mg.
- *Elective caesarean section is done* in cases of macrosomia, CPD, BOH and other obstetric indications
- *Post-partum follow up*:
  - Soon after delivery, the need for insulin is decreased or absent in GDM and dose is decreased in overt diabetics
  - Post-partum, 95% of GDM mothers return to normal glucose tolerance and require no further insulin in the post-partum period
  - Check blood sugars before discharge
  - OGTT done at 6–12 weeks post-partum
- *Common foetal anomalies*:
  - Cardiac—ASD, VSD, transposition of great vessels
  - Neural tube defects (NTD) like anencephaly, spina bifida, orofacial defects, omphalocoele
  - Caudal regression syndrome

MANAGEMENT OF GDM

Management of GDM is given in Flow chart 12.1.

POLYHYDRAMNIOS

Twenty per cent of GDM will develop polyhydramnios.

- Definition: defined as an excess of amniotic fluid >2000 mL or AFI > 25 cm or single pocket > 8 cm
- Causes:
  - Maternal—diabetes mellitus
  - Foetal—multiple pregnancy, foetal malformations like open NTD namely anencephaly, meningocoele, meningomyelocoele (due to increased transudation of fluid from exposed meninges)
  - Oesophageal atresia causes impaired foetal swallowing
  - Placental—chorioangioma of the placenta

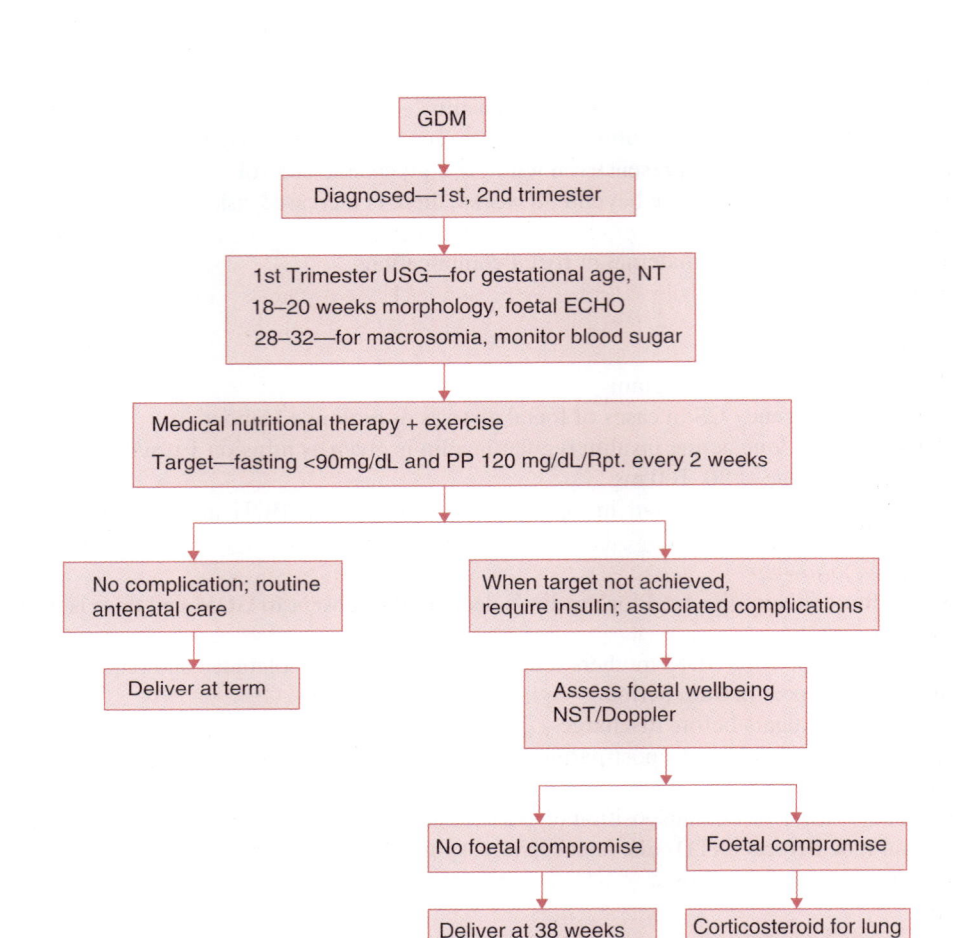

CASE 12 A CASE OF DIABETES COMPLICATING PREGNANCY

```
                          ┌─────────┐
                          │   GDM   │
                          └────┬────┘
                               ▼
                  ┌────────────────────────────┐
                  │ Diagnosed—1st, 2nd trimester│
                  └────────────┬───────────────┘
                               ▼
        ┌──────────────────────────────────────────────┐
        │ 1st Trimester USG—for gestational age, NT    │
        │ 18–20 weeks morphology, foetal ECHO          │
        │ 28–32—for macrosomia, monitor blood sugar    │
        └──────────────────────┬───────────────────────┘
                               ▼
        ┌──────────────────────────────────────────────┐
        │ Medical nutritional therapy + exercise       │
        │ Target—fasting <90mg/dL and PP 120 mg/dL/    │
        │ Rpt. every 2 weeks                           │
        └──────────┬──────────────────────┬────────────┘
                   ▼                      ▼
      ┌────────────────────┐   ┌──────────────────────────────┐
      │ No complication;   │   │ When target not achieved,    │
      │ routine antenatal  │   │ require insulin; associated  │
      │ care               │   │ complications                │
      └─────────┬──────────┘   └──────────────┬───────────────┘
                ▼                             ▼
        ┌──────────────┐              ┌──────────────────┐
        │ Deliver at   │              │ Assess foetal    │
        │ term         │              │ wellbeing        │
        └──────────────┘              │ NST/Doppler      │
                                      └────┬────────┬────┘
                                           ▼        ▼
                              ┌─────────────────┐  ┌──────────────────┐
                              │ No foetal       │  │ Foetal compromise│
                              │ compromise      │  └────────┬─────────┘
                              └────────┬────────┘           ▼
                                       ▼          ┌────────────────────┐
                              ┌─────────────────┐ │ Corticosteroid for │
                              │ Deliver at 38   │ │ lung maturity and  │
                              │ weeks           │ │ deliver            │
                              └─────────────────┘ └────────────────────┘
```

FLOW CHART 12.1 Management of GDM

- Types:
  - Acute—more common in monochorionic twin; it occurs by 20 weeks and usually results in pre-term labour
  - Chronic—occurs after 32 weeks; pressure symptoms occur
- Clinical features:
  - Uterine height bigger than period of amenorrhoea
  - Abdominal skin may be stretched and shiny, uterus tense but not tender
  - Fluid thrill may be elicited
  - Foetal parts difficult to palpate
- Differential diagnosis: multiple pregnancy, concealed abruption, maternal ascites, pregnancy with ovarian cyst
- Diagnosis: USG

MANAGEMENT OF POLYHYDRAMNIOS
- Rule out—anomaly/maternal diabetes
- Mild form—no treatment
- Indomethacin—1.5–3 mg/kg/day; must be used with caution as it causes premature closure of the foetal ductus arteriosus
- When patient is in distress—slow amniocentesis under USG guidance is done
- At a time, not more than 1000–1500 mL of amniotic fluid is withdrawn
- During labour—controlled ARM, careful monitoring of labour and active management of third stage of labour

KEY POINTS
- Gestational diabetes is defined as carbohydrate intolerance of varying severity recognised first time during pregnancy.
- Pregnancy is a diabetogenic state due to physiological insulin resistance state.
- Antenatal screening of all pregnant women should be done at first visit and if negative repeated at 24–28 weeks.
- Tight glycaemic control—fasting <90 mg/dL and post-prandial <120 mg/dL is the cornerstone of management.
- Foetal surveillance should be done to assess foetal wellbeing, to predict macrosomia and detect polyhydramnios.
- With medical nutritional therapy and exercise, if optimal glycaemic control is obtained they can deliver at term.
- Those who require insulin and are with complications, deliver by 38 weeks.
- Insulin requirement falls sharply after delivery.

FREQUENTLY ASKED QUESTIONS
1. What is gestational diabetes? What is pre-gestational diabetes mellitus?
2. How will you classify diabetes in pregnancy?
3. Why pregnancy is considered as diabetogenic state?
4. What are the risk factors for gestational diabetes?
5. What is the importance of HbA1C and what is the optimal value in pregnancy?
6. What is the time of universal screening? Why?
7. What is glucose challenge test?
8. What is glucose tolerance test?
9. What is DIPSI guideline?
10. What is the ideal blood sugar level to be maintained in pregnancy?
11. What is the effect of diabetes on mother and foetus?
12. How does diabetes cause macrosomia? What are the causes of macrosomia?
13. How will you manage a pregnancy with GDM?

14. How will you control blood sugar level?
15. How will you do antenatal foetal monitoring?
16. Why is there increased requirement of insulin during pregnancy?
17. How will you adjust insulin during labour, LSCS and after delivery?
18. How will you manage labour in a woman with GDM?
19. What are the common foetal anomalies in GDM?
20. What are the neonatal complications in GDM?

A CASE OF RECURRENT PREGNANCY LOSS

CASE 13

PATIENT DETAILS

Mrs... Age.................. Coming from.........................Occupation..............
Socioeconomic Class......................... Gravida, Para, Live, Abortion, (G......... P......... L......... A.........)
Booked........................ Immunised....................... LMP............ EDD

H/O............ months of amenorrhoea/period of gestation

PRESENT COMPLAINTS

Patient may present with period of amenorrhoea with following complaints:
- Usually woman may not have complaints.
- She will be admitted in view of her previous pregnancy loss—loss like abortion or foetal death or immediate neonatal death.
- She will be admitted for evaluation and management or safe confinement.

HISTORY
MENSTRUAL HISTORY AND MARITAL HISTORY
- Refer Case 1

PRESENT OBSTETRIC HISTORY
- Whether spontaneous conception or assisted/medication for medical illness like thyroid, diabetes, renal disease
- Surgical procedure—previous/like cerclage for incompetent os during previous/present pregnancy
- If Rh negative woman—H/O Rh antenatal prophylaxis and previous postpartum prophylaxis
- History of investigations done and treatment given so far

Past history
Following details are elicited if there is history of abortion:
- Gestational age at the time of abortion
- Spontaneous abortion/induced/certified by doctor

CASE 13 A CASE OF RECURRENT PREGNANCY LOSS

- Whether USG was done and if so whether foetal loss occurred before or after cardiac activity. If there was no foetal pole made out it means blighted ovum
- Whether curettage was done or medical abortion done
- Post-abortal period—H/O fever, blood transfusion
- Histopathology evidence for abortion
- Preceding event like fever, infection, trauma, drug intake or long travel
- Period of gestation at which it occurred and method of termination, histopathology report if available should be asked for
- H/O repeated first trimester abortion—may be due to submucous fibroid
- Exposure to teratogens in early pregnancy

History suggestive of Incompetent os:
- Painless expulsion of foetus around 16–18 weeks/repeated second trimester loss
- Watery discharge PV and rupture of membranes followed by abortion, pre-term deliveries (whether foetus was born alive)
- If history is suggestive of incompetent os, take detailed history regarding previous D&C or MTP, surgeries in the cervix like amputation, conisation/previous instrumental delivery

Previous intrauterine death:
- H/O intrauterine death—period of gestation at the time of foetal death
- History suggestive of APH, preeclampsia, GDM, trauma, fever drug intake
- Whether foetal movements were absent in the antenatal period or intrapartum period
- Mode of delivery
- Size of the baby/term or pre-term/macerated/any obvious congenital anomaly/foetal autopsy done/X-ray taken for foetus
- Details about placenta—infarcts, circumvallate, marginate and true knots in the cord can be obtained by old records
- Puerperium—fever, foul smelling discharge
- History of blood transfusion.
- History suggestive of hydrops foetalis, neonatal jaundice, exchange transfusion

Recurrent malpresentation—indicates uterine malformation which may lead to PROM, pre term labour prolonged labour which increases foetal loss

Previous intrapartum/early neonatal death:
- Period of gestation
- Booked or unbooked
- Place of delivery—home/institution
- Referred to higher institutions
- PROM or spontaneous rupture of membranes/meconium stained liquor
- Induction or augmentation of labour
- Duration of labour—prolonged or precipitate labour
- Mode of delivery—natural/instrumental delivery/caesarean

- Baby—alive or dead born/anomaly/weight of the baby/Apgar score/H/O NICU admission/if dead born—fresh death or macerated/anomalies

History suggestive of APLA syndrome:
- Early onset of preeclampsia, APH, FGR, IUD, H/O arterial or venous thrombosis

H/O CONSANGUINITY
- First degree, second or third degree

PAST MEDICAL HISTORY
- H/O GDM, preeclampsia, hypertension, diabetes mellitus, hypo- or hyperthyroidism, chronic renal disease, systemic lupus erythematosus, history suggestive of APLA syndrome any other medical disease and medications

PAST SURGICAL HISTORY
- Dilatation and curettage (D&C), cerclage, myomectomy

FAMILY HISTORY
- Routine—H/O diabetes, hypertension, tuberculosis, congenital anomalies in the family

PERSONAL HISTORY
- Alcoholism/drug abuse/smoking

GENERAL EXAMINATION AND OBSTETRIC EXAMINATION
- Refer Case 1
- Look for signs of thyroid disorder and other endocrine disorder.

SUMMARY
- Name......................... age........... gravida, para,.......................... booked, immunized, socioeconomic class......................... mention about H/O amenorrhoea period of gestation/previous obstetric history, abortion/foetal loss in..........................weeks with fresh death or macerated foetus any investigations done.
- Mention—if woman underwent any medication during antenatal period or cerclage at what period of gestation/positive family history/positive general examination and obstetric examination findings are to be included.

CASE 13 A CASE OF RECURRENT PREGNANCY LOSS

DIAGNOSIS

- Age............ Gravida............ Para............ with............ weeks of gestation with single live foetus/foetal heart rate—in cephalic/podalic presentation/with recurrent pregnancy loss (RPL) for evaluation

INVESTIGATIONS

Routine investigations

- HB, VDRL, HIV, blood group, Rh type—if negative and if husband's Rh type is positive indirect coomb's test should be done.

Specific investigations based on the history
- Immunological—anti-phospholipid antibody (lupus anticoagulant, anti-cardiolipin antibody)
- Thyroid function test
- Thrombophilia screening—factor V Leiden mutation
- Hyperhomocysteinaemia, protein C and protein S deficiency
- USG for uterine anomalies, location of placenta, diameter of internal os and length of cervix, presence of leiomyoma
- In case of previous incompetent os—USG is done during pregnancy. Look for cervical length <3 cm, internal os diameter >1.5 cm, bulging of membrane through os (Fig. 13.1)

Test in non-pregnant state: cervix internal—os admits No-8 Hegar's dilator without pain and resistance/Foley's catheter without difficulty and HSG—will show funnelling when there is incompetent os.
- Glucose challenge test and GTT
- Blood VDRL
- Karyotyping for parents—especially, in recurrent first trimester abortions
- High vaginal swab for culture and sensitivity
- Uterine anomalies can be made out
    - In non-pregnant state—HSG, USG, hysteroscopy
    - During pregnancy—USG

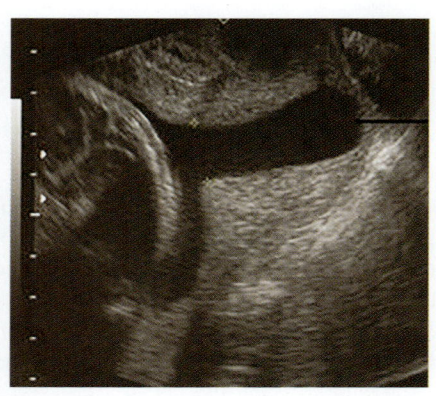

FIGURE 13.1 USG—Cervical os Incompetence

CASE DISCUSSION
- *RPL defined* as three or more consecutive pregnancy loss. Recently, redefined as two or more consecutive pregnancy loss at any gestational age
- *Incidence*—1% of pregnancy
- *BOH*—bad obstetric history—is where present obstetric outcome is likely to be affected adversely by the previous obstetric mishap (disaster)

CAUSES FOR RPL
- *Genetic factors*—70% first trimester losses are due to chromosomal abnormalities, like autosomal trisomy, monosomy, triploidy, tetraploidy, translocation
- *Environmental*
- *Endocrine factors*—Thyroid disorders, diabetes, luteal phase defect
- *Anatomic causes*—Cervical incompetence
- *Mullerian anomalies*—Septate uterus, bicornuate, unicornuate uterus, etc.
- *Others*—Large fibroids, polyps, Asherman's syndrome
  - DES exposure
  - Infectious causes
- *Thrombophilias*—Protein S and protein C deficiency, factor V Leiden mutation
- *Immunologic problems*—APLA syndrome
- Unexplained

MANAGEMENT
MANAGEMENT OF ANTI-PHOSPHOLIPID ANTIBODY SYNDROME
- Offer low dose aspirin and low molecular weight heparin as soon as cardiac activity is seen and continue up to 34 weeks.

INCOMPETENT OS CAUSES & MANAGEMENT
- *Causes*: It can be acquired or congenital.
  - *Acquired causes:* Forceful dilatation of cervix during abortion/D&C/MTP and surgeries on cervix—Fothergill's, conisation or amputation of cervix
  - *During previous delivery*—Cervical tear not repaired, instrumental delivery
  - *Typical history of Incompetent os:* Sudden rupture of membranes in second trimester with painless expulsion of foetus
  - Recurrent mid trimester loss
- *Diagnosis during pregnancy*:
  - USG—Cervical length less than 3 cm, funnelling of upper cervix with bulging of the foetal membrane
  - In TVS—Late first trimester scan, opening of the cervical os at rest or in response to fundal pressure is an early feature of incompetent os

CASE 13 A CASE OF RECURRENT PREGNANCY LOSS

- *Management of incompetent os*:
  - USG done before procedure
    - To confirm viability
    - To rule out anomaly and for placental location
  - Cerclage done around 14 weeks
    - *McDonald's cerclage*: Non-absorbable material is used to place purse string suture around cervix at the level of internal os and suture is tied anteriorly
    - Removal of suture at 37-completed weeks or
    - Whenever there is pain/draining or bleeding PV/foetal demise
    - *Advantage of McDonald's cerclage*: Simple easy procedure. No need for bladder reflection
  Infection and bleeding is less. Vaginal delivery is possible.
  Complications: Rupture of membranes, chorioamnionitis, bleeding PV, failure of the procedure resulting in abortion
  Other cerclage procedures: Shirodkar and Wurm's methods

ANTENATAL FOETAL SURVEILLANCE OF RPL

Daily foetal movement counts or kick chart:
- Normal—3 kick/1 h.
- Foetal alarm signal—less than 10 FM/12 h indicates foetal compromise and needs further evaluation.
- Less than 4 FM/12 h, may go for IUD—immediate delivery is advised.

Cardiff count to 10:
- After a meal, patient is given a piece of string and asked to put knot whenever she perceives a foetal movement till 10 movements are perceived. Starting time and ending time are noted.
- If < 10 FM are perceived in 12 h—foetal compromise. Practical difficulty in this method, woman has to notice FM from 9 a.m. to 9 p.m.

Hence she is advised to put FKC for 1 h in the morning, afternoon and evening.

Manning's biophysical profile:
- Foetal hear rate acceleration, foetal breathing movements, foetal gross body movements, foetal tone and AFI
- Each component is given a score of 2
- Since it takes minimum of 30 min to finish the test, it is not done nowadays

Modified biophysical profile is used nowadays (NST+ AFI) biweekly:
- NST—basis—autonomic influences mediated by sympathetic and parasympathetic impulses have impact and affect the foetal heart rate which results in beat to beat variability.
- There is acceleration of foetal heart rate with foetal movements when the foetus is not hypoxic.

Interpretations:
- NST reactive: Baseline rate 110–160 bpm
  - Normal beat to beat variability 5–15 beats/min
  - Two or more accelerations of 15 beats/min lasting for 15 s in response to foetal movement over a period of 20 min
  - Absence of late or variable decelerations

- NST non-reactive: Anything which does not meet the aforementioned criteria.
  - In foetal sleep cycle, absence of foetal heart rate accelerations may be there, so extend the duration of NST for further period of 20 min or stimulate the foetus by vibro acoustic stimulation test (VAST)
  - Reactive NST denotes foetal well being
  - Non-reactive NST needs further evaluation with Doppler study of foetal umbilical artery and MCA, and Ductus venosus

Amniotic fluid index: It is a measurement done with USG.
- It is the sum of the largest vertical pockets of amniotic fluid measured in four quadrants of the uterus
- Oligohydramnios denotes placental insufficiency
- Oligohydramnios—AFI < 5 cm
- Polyhydramnios—AFI > 25 cm

Doppler velocimetry: Whenever foetus is at risk of hypoxia, Doppler will show sequential changes in foetal blood vessels.
- Doppler study is done in the umbilical artery, middle cerebral artery and ductus venosus.
- When all three vessels show normal S/D ratio—no foetal hypoxia.
- When umbilical artery show—reduced diastolic flow/absent/reversed flow—foetus is hypoxic. Reversed flow—ominous sign.
- Middle cerebral artery—shows changes due to preferential cerebral flow (brain sparing effect) to compensate hypoxia.
- Ductus venosus—changes occur when foetus goes for cardiac failure and death is imminent.

BASIC PRINCIPALS IN THE MANAGEMENT OF RPL
- Treat the underlying cause
- Frequent USG for growth assessment
- Antenatal foetal surveillance
- Timely delivery and LSCS for obstetric indications

KEY POINTS
- When miscarriage occurs consecutively more than two or three times it is termed RPL.
- Various causes for RPL are systemic causes like diabetes, chronic nephritis, essential hypertension, syphilis, endocrine causes like luteal phase defect, thyroid dysfunction, anatomical factors, such as cervical insufficiency, uterine anomalies, immunological cause like anti-phospholipid syndrome.
- In first trimester RPL commonest cause is due to chromosomal abnormalities.
- In second trimester recurrent miscarriage commonest cause is due to cervical insufficiency.
- Treatment of RPL depends on the underlying cause and reassurance.
- For RPL due anti-phospholipid syndrome, low dose aspirin 50–100 mg/day to be started at the earliest confirmation of pregnancy. Unfractionated heparin or low molecular weight heparin is started as soon as foetal cardiac activity is seen in USG.

CASE 13 A CASE OF RECURRENT PREGNANCY LOSS

FREQUENTLY ASKED QUESTIONS
1. What is the definition of RPL?
2. What are the common causes of RPL in first trimester and second trimester?
3. What are the causes for cervical incompetence?
4. How will you manage cervical incompetence? What are the complications of cerclage operation?
5. When will you remove the cerclage sutures?
6. What are the causes of stillbirth?
7. How will you do antenatal foetal surveillance?
8. How will you manage a case of RPL antenatally? What are the causes for cervical incompetence?
9. How will you manage cervical incompetence? What are the complications of cerclage operation?
10. When will you remove the cerclage sutures?
11. What are the causes of stillbirth?
12. How will you do antenatal foetal surveillance?
13. How will you manage a case of RPL antenatally

A CASE OF FOETAL GROWTH RESTRICTION

CASE 14

PATIENT'S DETAILS

Mrs.................................. Age................ Coming from......................... Occupation.............
Socioeconomic Class........................ Gravida, Para, Live, Abortion, (G......... P......... L......... A ....)
Booked, Immunised........................ LMP............ EDD

H/O months of amenorrhoea/period of gestation......

PRESENT COMPLAINTS

- Usually, she will not have complaints
- She may notice size of uterus is small or her relatives may tell her that her uterus appears small
- H/O reduced weight gain/diminished foetal movements
- Admitted in view of FGR, for evaluation and management

HISTORY

MENSTRUAL HISTORY AND MARITAL HISTORY

- Refer Case 1

PRESENT OBSTETRIC HISTORY

- LMP to be ascertained—for reliability of EDD—refer case prolonged pregnancy
- H/O persistent hyperemesis/reduced weight gain/diminished foetal movements/loss of foetal movements
- History suggestive of anaemia/malnutrition/preeclampsia if present to be elicited which may be the cause for FGR
- Enquire about dating scan/serial growth scan/growth lag between scans

PAST OBSTETRIC HISTORY

- History suggestive of anaemia, heart disease complicating pregnancy, preeclampsia, malnutrition
- Period of gestation at the time of delivery, mode of delivery, weight of previous babies at birth and their present condition
- History of previous growth restricted baby

PAST MEDICAL HISTORY
- Hypertension, chronic infections, heart disease, renal disease, collagen disorder, diabetes with vascular involvement, intake of anticonvulsants

FAMILY HISTORY
- Refer Case 1

PERSONAL HISTORY
- Alcoholism, drug abuse, smoking

GENERAL EXAMINATION

Special attention to be paid for the following details:
- Anaemia, malnutrition, features of preeclampsia, cyanotic heart disease.
- BMI—may be low.
- Decrease weight gain during pregnancy.
- CVS/RS *examination*.

OBSTETRIC EXAMINATION

As in Case 1

Specific points to be noted:
- If fundal height is lesser than the period of gestation.
- If SFH is <4 cm for GA.
- If abdominal girth is lesser than expected.
- If serial growth curve by palpation, SFH and USG—shows lag.
- If liquor is diminished both by palpation & in USG.

} suspect IUGR

SUMMARY
- Name…..age….. gravida, para,…..booked, immunized, socioeconomic class…..
- Mention about previous relevant obstetric history if present
- Mention about positive general examination findings
- Mention about…..obstetric examination findings…..height of uterus in…..weeks lesser than period of gestation by palpation/by dates/by USG…..single foetus/cephalic/podalic presentation/ with…..foetal heart rate
- Mention—positive medical history which may be a probable cause for FGR

DIAGNOSIS
- Age…..Gravida…..Para.....of gestation by dates, but by palpation.....weeks.....
- If some investigation findings are available, mention it.....hence FGR for evaluation

INVESTIGATIONS

Routine investigations

Specific for FGR:
- Serial USG—record serial BPD, FL, abdominal circumference (AC), head circumference (HC)
  - The aforementioned parameters can be used to calculate foetal weight
  - HC: AC ratio, amniotic fluid index (AFI), congenital anomalies
- Doppler: umbilical artery, middle cerebral artery, ductus venosus
- Daily foetal movement count—for assessment of foetal wellbeing (3 per 1 h or >10 in 12 h—normal)
- Modified biophysical profile (AFI + NST)—AFI (oligohydramnios indicates chronic foetal distress) + NST (non-stress test—non-reactive indicates acute foetal distress)
- Maternal biochemical test—to rule out diabetes/preeclampsia/APLA syndrome/renal diseases

CASE DISCUSSION
FGR

- Failure of foetus to grow to its genetic growth potential for that gestational age
  - Estimated weight < 10th percentile for given gestational age
- *Definition* of SGA: Small for gestational age—infants with weight < 10th percentile for their gestational age. Infants with weight < 2 SD of the mean weight, for their gestational age

TYPES OF FGR
- Early and late onset FGR or symmetrical and asymmetrical FGR

CAUSES
- *Early onset FGR*—symmetrical FGR. Early insult affects cell division
  - It can be due to chromosomal aberration, congenital anomaly, viral infection, idiopathic, exposure to teratogen
- *Late onset FGR*—asymmetrical—due to placental insufficiency
  - Maternal factors—extremes of age, low socioeconomic class, malnutrition, anaemia, PE, diabetes, heart disease, renal disease, smoking, tobacco chewing, alcohol and drug abuse (Table 14.1)

DIAGNOSIS OF FGR
- Decreased weight. gain, fundal height—lag by 4 weeks, SFH—lag of 4 cm, diminished liquor, decrease abdominal girth
- *USG*: By serial scans—BPD, HC, AC—altered HC/AC ratio, AFI

Table 14.1 Difference Between Symmetrical FGR and Asymmetrical FGR	
Symmetrical FGR—Type 1 *(Intrinsic) (20%–30%)*	**Asymmetrical FGR—Type 11** *(Extrinsic) (60%–70%)*
Early onset affects cell hyperplasia	Late onset affects cell hypertrophy
Organs are symmetrically small	Brain and long bones spared
Aetiology—chromosomal	Aetiology—placental
Infection	Insufficiency
HC/AC and FL/AC ratio—normal	HC/AC and FL/AC ratio increased
Ponderal index—normal	Ponderal index—low
Long-term growth delay and neurological problems	Early neonatal problem, no long-term problems if treated properly

AC, abdominal circumference; HC, head circumference.

- *Normal HC/AC*:
    - HC/AC ratio—more than 1 before 32 weeks, HC/AC ratio—1 between 32 and 34 weeks
    - HC/AC ratio—less than 1 after 34 weeks
- In asymmetrical FGR: HC/AC ratio is elevated and in symmetrical FGR—HC/AC ratio is normal

Abdominal circumference (AC) is the single most sensitive predictor for FGR. Increase in AC of less than 10 mm over 2 weeks—is suggestive of FGR

ANTENATAL FOETAL ASSESSMENT OF FGR
Serial USG, NST, AFI, Doppler study of uterine artery, umbilical artery, MCA, ductus venosus (Flow chart 14.1)
- Refer Case 5.

INDUCTION OF LABOUR AND CONDUCT OF LABOUR IN FGR
- Assess Bishop's score—if it is less than 6, cervical ripening is done by PGE2 gel
- Early ARM in active phase (look for meconium staining of liquor)
- Monitor progress of labour by partogram
- Monitor FHR by continuous CTG
- If there is good progress—allow for vaginal delivery
- When there is evidence of foetal distress by CTG having ominous trace, persistent late deceleration, loss of beat to beat variability and meconium stained liquor it warrants emergency LSCS

KEY POINTS

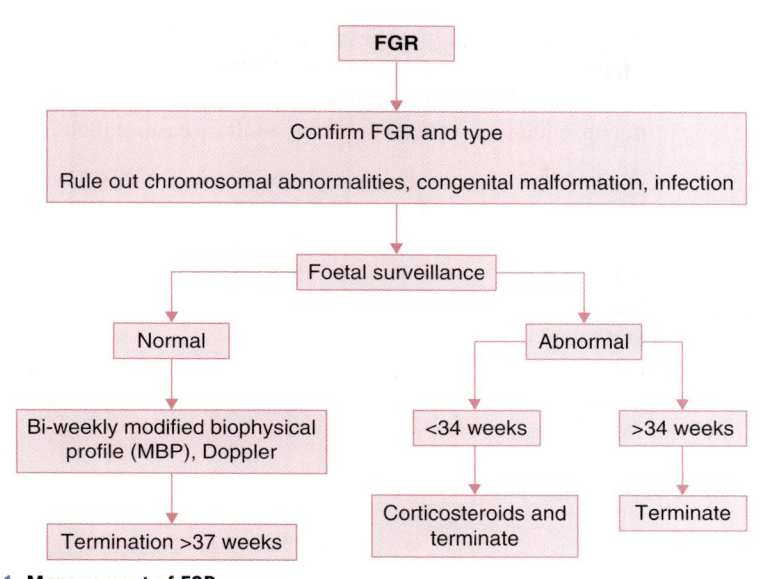

```
                    FGR
                     │
                     ▼
        Confirm FGR and type
  Rule out chromosomal abnormalities,
  congenital malformation, infection
                     │
                     ▼
          Foetal surveillance
           │              │
        Normal         Abnormal
           │           │       │
           ▼       <34 weeks  >34 weeks
  Bi-weekly modified    │       │
  biophysical profile   ▼       ▼
  (MBP), Doppler    Corticosteroids  Terminate
           │        and terminate
           ▼
  Termination >37 weeks
```

FLOW CHART 14.1 Management of FGR

INDICATIONS FOR ELECTIVE LSCS
- FGR with abnormal biophysical profile/abnormal Doppler study/FGR with associated maternal complications.

COMPLICATIONS OF FGR
- *Antenatal*—chronic foetal distress and death
- *Neonatal*—immediate-asphyxia, RDS, hypoglycaemia, hypothermia, meconium aspiration syndrome (MAS), polycythaemia, hyperviscosity, necrotizing enterocolitis
- *Late*—retarded neurological and intellectual development
- *Barker's hypothesis*—(intrauterine origins of adult disease). In utero malnutrition results in type 2 diabetes, cardiovascular disease, hyperlipidaemia in adulthood

KEY POINTS
- FGR is characterised by reduced foetal growth and aetiology is not clear.
- There are two types of FGR—symmetrical and asymmetrical.
- FGR may occur due to maternal, placental, foetal causes; in 50% of cases no obvious cause may be found.
- FGR can be suspected clinically and it is confirmed by serial USG.
- When FGR is suspected, monitor serially and decide on appropriate time to deliver.

- Best time to plan delivery of the foetus is when intrauterine existence becomes hazardous.
- Every effort is made to deliver vaginally but rate of LSCS is increased in FGR.
- FGR is prone to number of complications after delivery.
- FGR can have long term consequences—foetal origin of adult diseases called Barker's hypothesis.

FREQUENTLY ASKED QUESTIONS

1. What is the definition of FGR?
2. What are the types of FGR and how do you differentiate between them?
3. What are the maternal and foetal causes for FGR?
4. How will you diagnose FGR?
5. Management of FGR before 37 weeks?
6. Management of FGR after 37 weeks?
7. Indications for LSCS in FGR?
8. Complications of newborn with FGR?

CASE 15

NORMAL PUERPERIUM AND POSTNATAL CARE

PATIENT'S DETAILS
Name……………………………... Age…………… Para………… Socioeconomic Class……………
Postnatal Day………… Mode of Delivery…………… Baby Condition

HISTORY
- Mode and date of delivery and which postnatal day?
- If LSCS indication for the same
- H/O fever, pain in the abdomen or perineum
- H/O excessive bleeding PV or unhealthy discharge PV, foul smelling lochia/colour of lochia
- Micturition problems
- Constipation
- H/O pain in the breast, engorgement, cracked nipple, retracted nipple and difficulty in feeding the baby
- Diet and oral fluids taken
- In case of LSCS-1st post-op day-H/O distension of abdomen, vomiting, headache/2nd post-op day whether she has passed flatus, voided urine/3rd post-op day whether she has passed stools
- Is she on medication which is contraindicated during lactation

EXAMINATION
EXAMINATION OF THE MOTHER
GENERAL EXAMINATION
- Refer Case 1

Special attention for the following details to be made
- Pallor, oedema, blood pressure
- Calf muscle tenderness, tenderness over veins in the leg
- Examination of breast for engorgement, retracted/cracked nipple, mastitis

ABDOMINAL EXAMINATION
Inspection—In case of LSCS distension of abdomen, soakage of dressing with blood/wound infection/wound gaping
    Palpation—Height of fundus whether uterus is well contracted/involuted, distended bladder

161

EXAMINATION OF PERINEUM

Following points to be noted:
   Undue bleeding, PV/vulval haematoma, colour and nature of lochia/episiotomy wound infection/gaping

SUMMARY

- Mrs.......................... age........... para........... delivered on ...by labour natural with or without episiotomy/LSCS on........... male/female baby/post natal day /general examination findings/uterus involuting, lochia healthy/episiotomy wound/LSCS wound healthy.

CASE DISCUSSION
DEFINITION OF NORMAL PUERPERIUM

- It is the period following childbirth during which the pelvic organs and other systems revert back to almost pre-pregnant state both anatomically and physiologically. It takes up to 6 weeks (42 days), immediate 24–48 h, early upto 7 days and remote upto 6 weeks.

FOLLOWING PHYSIOLOGICAL CHANGES OCCUR IN NORMAL PUERPERIUM

- Changes in genital tract
- Changes in other systems
- Changes in breast and lactation
- Changes in genital tract are involution of the uterus, appearance of lochia, involution of other pelvic organs and menstruation (Table 15.1 and Fig. 15.1)

Table 15.1 Process and Rate of Uterine Involution

Process of Uterine Involution	Rate of Involution	Causes for Sub-Involution
Immediately after delivery uterus measures and weighs 1000 g. Involution occur in post-partum period and uterus returns to pre-pregnant state by autolysis due to withdrawal of oestrogen and progesterone and at the end of 6 weeks weighs 60 g. During this period, number of muscle fibres are not decreased but myometrial size decreases. Uterine involution is aided by release of oxytocin in breast-feeding women. Uterine contractions occlude blood vessels formerly supplying placenta.	Immediately after delivery of the placenta, the fundus is midline and just below the level of umbilicus. Uterine size reduces 1.25 cm per day and, no longer palpable per abdomen by 14 days. By end of 2nd week, the internal os closes but external os remains open permanently called patulous (parous cervix).	Uterine infection Retained products of conception Presence of fibroids Due to broad ligament haematoma

EXAMINATION 163

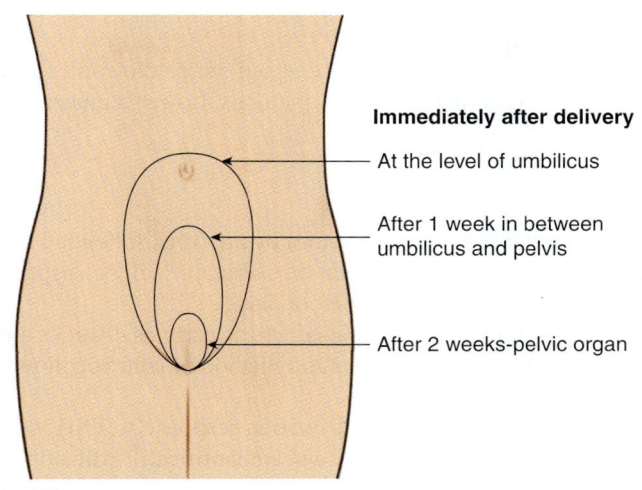

FIGURE 15.1 Involution of Uterus

- Immediately after delivery
- At the level of umbilicus
- After 1 week in between umbilicus and pelvis
- After 2 weeks-pelvic organ

AFTER PAINS

Puerperal uterus tends to remain contracted. Uterus often contracts vigorously at intervals and gives rise to pain but less severe than labour pains. This pain is called after pains .This will be more appreciated as the parity increases and it worsens during suckling of the infant due to release of oxytocin. Usually this pain decreases after third day.

ENDOMETRIAL AND PLACENTAL CHANGES

By 10th day endometrial regeneration is complete. Two superficial layers namely zona compacta and spongiosa will shed in lochia once it becomes necrotic. New endometrium will form from zona basalis and is completed with endometrial glands in about 14 days.

Placental site takes longer time to recover. It takes 6 weeks to involute and regenerate. Arteries get obliterated by endarteritis and veins undergo thrombosis.

LOCHIA

It is bloodstained uterine discharge (blood + necrotic decidua + leukocytes + exudates). Duration of lochial discharge is 6–8 weeks (Table 15.2).

Table 15.2 Changes in Lochia

Lochia Rubra	Lochia Serosa	Lochia Alba
First few days after delivery lochia will be red called lochia rubra.	After 5 days gradually lochia changes to pink becomes thinner called lochia serosa.	Lochia will be pale yellowish white called Lochia alba consists of exudate and leukocytes.
Has fishy odour.	Has fishy odour.	Duration: upto 6–8 weeks
Duration: 4–5 days.	Duration: 2–3 weeks	

CERVIX

Though cervix contracts immediately after delivery, it will be patulous till first few days. Changes in cervical canal only by 6 weeks. External os remains patulous. Lower segment contracts by 6 weeks and will form isthmus.

MENSTRUATION AND OVULATION

If patient does not breast-feed her baby, periods return by 6th week following delivery in 40%, by 12th week in 80%. If patient breast-feeds her baby then menstruation will be suspended in 70% till breast-feeding is stopped. In 30% variable starts even before that.

Ovulation: In non-lactating mothers ovulation occurs as early as 4 weeks and in lactating mothers about 10 weeks after delivery. Lactation is the natural method of contraception. But not fool proof. So advice regarding contraception should be given

Breast-feeding ↑ prolactin which will inhibit ovarian response to FSH which in turn causes less follicular growth resulting in hypoestrogenic state and amenorrhea. ↑ Prolactin will suppress release of LH and there is no LH surge, hence results in anovulation.

OTHER PELVIC ORGANS

Vagina markedly relaxed. Hymen is torn completely and represented as carunculae myrtiformes. Pelvic floor and perineum will be relaxed and regain the tone gradually (Table 15.3).

PERITONEUM AND ABDOMINAL WALL CHANGES

It takes longer time for broad and round ligaments to recover. Abdominal wall will be flabby and this laxity remains permanently. Divarication of recti can happen.

Table 15.3 Changes in Other systems

Urinary System	GIT and Weight Loss	Circulation, Haematological, Coagulation System and Hormonal Changes
Urinary tract—edematous and hyperemic. Bladder—over distended. Kidney/ureter normalize in 8 weeks. Diuresis—2nd–5th day. Bladder is insensitive due to trauma sustained by the nerve plexus and causes incomplete emptying of bladder but it is transient.	↑ Thirst/constipation due to intestinal paresis. Weight loss—2nd–5th day loss of 2 kg (Diuresis). Fluid loss—2 L in 1st week and 1.5 L during next 5 weeks. After 6 months women attain pre-pregnancy weight.	Hb. rises and reaches non-pregnant values by 6 weeks. Total leukocyte increases. Platelets increases and increased adhesiveness. Fibrinogen remain elevated till first week, this increases chances of deep vein thrombosis. Diuresis—2nd–5th day post-delivery. Cardiac size returns, stroke volume, cardiac output decreases slowly—1 week. Pulse slows down, peripheral resistance raises rapidly. Temperature should not be above 37.2°C (99°F) within first 24 h. On 3rd day breast engorgement—slight rise in temperature. Within 48 h human placental lactogen, human chorionic gonadotropin and oestradiol decreases and in 2–8 weeks to non-pregnant level.

CHANGES IN BREAST AND LACTATION

Mammogenesis (Mammary duct-gland growth and development occur during pregnancy). Lactogenesis (initiation of milk secretion in alveoli). Galactokinesis—Ejection of milk Galactopoiesis (maintenance of lactation).

Milk secretion establishes by 2–3 days of the puerperium. Colostrum is secreted within 24 h. It is rich in immunoglobulin, minerals and proteins and it declines in about 4 days.

PHYSIOLOGY OF LACTATION (Fig. 15.2)

It involves complex mechanisms of humoral and neural. Suckling sends afferent impulses to hypothalamic-pituitary axis which releases prolactin from anterior pituitary which acts on secretory cells of alveoli and stimulate synthesis of milk proteins. Prolactin release is controlled by prolactin inhibitory factor (Dopamine). Repetitive stimulus (sucking) controls intensity and duration of lactation. Progesterone, oestrogen, placental lactogen decreases abruptly after delivery and along with prolactin serves to stimulate lactation. Expression of milk from breast is caused by pulsatile release of oxytocin from neuro-hypophyis which stimulates the expression of milk. Suckling initiates reflex and stimulates the release of oxytocin which causes ejection of milk or letting down of the milk.

Breast-feeding should be started immediately after vaginal delivery and after caesarean section as soon she recovers from anaesthesia.

Advantages of breast-feeding:
- Ideal food
- Has immunologic and antibacterial property
- Helps in better IQ, mental and psychological development

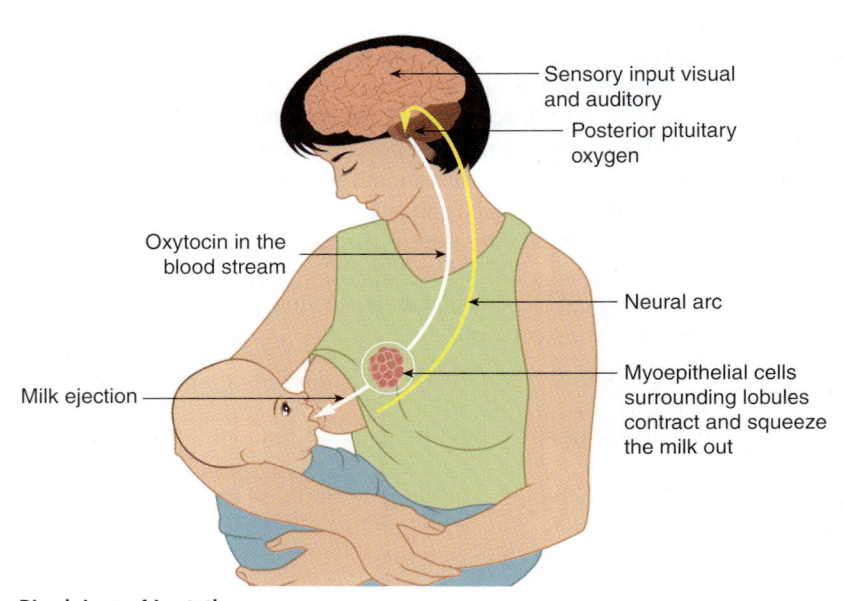

FIGURE 15.2 Physiology of Lactation

- Increases emotional bonding
- Cost effective

Indications for suppression of lactation:
- Following intra-uterine death:
- Active maternal tuberculosis
- Mother on cytotoxic drugs
- Mother undergoing breast cancer treatment
- Mother who is on illicit drugs
- Simple remedy to suppress milk is by breast binding and lactation slowly decreases and stops. Finally, if stimulation is not initiated for lactation and not manually emptied periodically then lactation will be suppressed.

Drugs used for suppression of lactation:
- Tablet Bromocriptine—2.5 mg once or twice daily for week
- Tablet Cabergoline—to inhibit Lactation—1 mg as single dose on the first day to suppress lactation 0.25 twice daily for 2 days
- Tablet Pyridoxine 40 mg twice daily for a week

Contra indication for breast-feeding:
- Maternal HIV
- Mother having illicit drugs habit or drugs secreted in breast milk
- Mother with active tuberculosis, undergoing treatment for breast cancer, maternal CCF, puerperal psychosis

Problems faced in breast-feeding:
- Retracted nipple: Should be recognized during antenatal period. Nipple should be pulled out by fingers or by inverted syringe technique
- Cracked nipple: Proper technique of breast-feeding advised. Nipple should be cleaned before and after feed. To soothen the painful nipples, emollients can be applied
- Engorgement: It is due to excess milk secretion. It can be treated with frequent breast-feeding, pumping of milk, analgesics and firm support of breast with proper underclothes
- Mastitis: It is caused from infection of infant's mouth. Woman will have fever, breast tenderness and redness. Breast-feeding to be continued and analgesics to be prescribed
- Breast abscess: Mastitis will lead to breast abscess. Breast will be red, tender and indurated.
- USG guided aspiration or surgical incision and drainage along with antibiotics. Commonest infection is staphylococcal or streptococcal

CARE OF NORMAL PUERPERIUM

- *Immediate care*
- *Early puerperium care*
- *At discharge advice*
- *Subsequent post-natal visit-care*

Immediate:

After delivery, patient will be observed for 2 h in the labour ward. Patient can be shifted to postnatal ward, if vitals are stable, if uterus is well contracted with no undue bleeding, if she passed urine and after examining perineum and the episiotomy wound. Antiseptic dressing to be applied to episiotomy wound before shifting. Patient is allowed to meet relatives and encouraged to feed the baby (Table 15.4).

Table 15.4 Care of Early Puerperium

Care Given	Why and What Care to be Given
Early ambulation within few hours Sleep and rest.	To facilitate bowel movement, to prevent venous thrombosis. Adequate sleep and rest woman should have. Rooming-in should be encouraged to promote bonding with baby.
Uterine involution	Uterus involution to be assessed daily. It involutes by 1 cm per day. After 2 weeks, it is not palpable per abdomen. Sub-involution indicates sepsis and other cause of sub-involution also to be ruled out.
Care of bowel and bladder	Urinary retention is common due to reduction in bladder sensation and perineal pain or epidural analgesia. Timely, aseptic indwelling catheter should be left in place for 24 h. There may be reduced urine output due to dehydration and overdose of oxytocin's anti-diuretic effect. Hence women should be encouraged to take adequate liquids and to void. Constipation is common. High fibre diet, plenty of fluids, sometimes mild laxatives may be required.
Care of perineum	Perineum should be kept dry and covered with antiseptic dressing. Woman should be advised to clean vulva from anterior to posterior to reduce chances for infection. Analgesics can be given for pain. Severe pain may be due to infection or haematoma.
Care of breast	Woman should be taught for proper positioning of the baby and to clean the nipples before and after each feed. If demand feeding is practiced, it will prevent sore nipples or breast congestion.
Diet, supplements and mood changes	After 2 h of vaginal delivery, normal diet can be started. Plenty of fluids, fresh green leafy vegetable, milk and extra calorie 500 kcal and protein 25 g of protein is recommended. Oral iron and calcium are continued. In early puerperium, mood changes are common termed *post-partum blues* which may lead to post-partum depression. Hence reassurance and family members support are vital.
Immunisation	Within 72 h anti D 300 μg can be given to non-sensitized Rh negative women. Rubella vaccine or MMR vaccine can be given, who are not immunized against rubella.
Care of newborn	Neonate should be kept warm, umbilical cord should be clean and demand feeding encouraged. Before discharge BCG vaccine to be given.

At discharge advice:
After physical examination of mother and baby following advice to be given:
- Advise regarding post-natal and pelvic exercise is given which can be started after 1 week to tone up the abdominal and back muscle and can prevent urinary incontinence. Exercise should be done 3–4 times/day.
- Discussion regarding temporary contraception methods, emergency contraception and permanent sterilization is done based on the parity. Proper counselling to be given.
- Oral iron and calcium are continued throughout lactating period.
- Woman should be told to avoid medications, since all medications may be secreted in breast milk.
- Rooming in and demand feeding to be encouraged

Subsequent post-natal visit-care:
- Woman is asked to come for follow-up after 6 weeks with her baby.
- Enquiry regarding breast problems, lochia, wound infection and mental health are made.
- Clinical examination, blood pressure, breast examination, abdominal and pelvic examination is done.
- Urine, haemoglobin examination and special investigations, like 75 g GTT incase of gestational diabetics should be done.
- When pre-existing or persistent medical problems are present woman should be referred to physician.
- Woman is advised regarding weight reduction by proper diet and exercise.
- Advise regarding sexual activity should be given. Woman can resume sexual activity whenever she is comfortable.

KEY POINTS

- Puerperium is the period between delivery of placenta to 6 weeks post-partum, during which all the organs revert back to pre-pregnant state.
- Mother should be monitored closely in the immediate post-partum period.
- During this period physiological changes occurs both in urogenital system and other pelvic organs.
- Uterus involute and lactation is established.
- Lochia is the uterine discharge consisting of blood, decidua, leukocytes and exudates.
- If patient breast-feeds her baby then menstruation will be suspended in 70% till breast feeding is stopped.
- In non-lactating mothers ovulation occurs as early as 4 weeks and in lactating mothers about 10 weeks after delivery.
- Early ambulation, normal diet with extra 500 kcal and breast and perineal care should be given.
- Rooming in and demand feeding should be encouraged.
- Any problems arising due to delivery and restoration of maternal health are the objective of management of puerperium.
- Advice on baby care, contraception and immunisation should be given at discharge.
- Women should come for follow-up with baby after 6 weeks. During this visit clinical examination namely breast, abdominal and pelvic examination with specific investigations are done.
- Advice regarding breast care, contraception, sexual activity should be given.

FREQUENTLY ASKED QUESTIONS

1. Define puerperium?
2. Discuss physiological changes in genital system?
3. Discuss physiological changes in other systems?
4. What is Lochia and it's different type?
5. What are the causes for sub-involution?
6. What is the physiology of lactation?
7. Contraindications for lactation?
8. When and how will you suppress lactation?
9. What are the advantages of breast-feeding?
10. Write about care of mother during puerperium?

CASE 16

VIVA VOCE (ORAL EXAM)

The following instruments, drugs, specimens, USG pictures are few examples which can help the student to answer during viva voce (oral exam).

- After identification of the previously mentioned, relevant questions regarding their use, steps of surgery and about the obstetric conditions can be asked.
- Brief details regarding drugs commonly used in obstetric and gynaec practice is written in this chapter. More importance is given to indications, contraindications, dose, side-effects and complications of the drugs.
- During discussion of a pathological specimen, student should describe briefly the gross appearance of the specimen followed by diagnosis.
- Based on this, questions may be asked regarding aetiology, clinical features, investigations, management and steps of surgery.
- During the USG pictures discussion, describe the ultrasonic appearance and then come to diagnosis.
- This section deals with commonly used instruments, USG pictures and specimens seen in clinical practice.
- This chapter will help the student to describe instrument, USG findings, specimen and able to interpret and answer confidently.
- In addition, mechanism of labour in vertex (occipito-anterior and posterior position) and breech, should be learnt from textbooks. Student should be able to demonstrate the mechanism of labour with dummy and pelvis.

BONY PELVIS AND FOETAL SKULL

In women the pelvis has special form that adapts to child bearing. It is composed of four bones.

Bony pelvis consists of the following bones:
- The sacrum, coccyx and two innominate bones.
- The innominate bone is formed by the fusion of the ilium, ischium and pubis.
- These bones are united together by four joints namely two sacroiliac joints, sacrococcygeal joint and the pubic symphysis.

Difference Between Major and Minor Pelvis

False (Greater/Major) Pelvis	True (Lesser/Minor) Pelvis
It lies above the linea terminalis (pelvic brim) bounded by lumbar vertebrae posteriorly, iliac fossa bilaterally and abdominal wall anteriorly	It lies below linea terminalis (pelvic brim)
	It has inlet, cavity and outlet
It forms a support for the pregnant uterus	Inlet is an oval space and it is bounded posteriorly by sacrum, alae of the sacrum and pectineal line at the sides, anteriorly by the upper margin of the pubic bone (tubercle and the crest); below by the pelvic outlet
It has no obstetrical significance	
	In true pelvis, ischial spine has important role in childbirth
	In true pelvis inter-ischial spine distance is of great obstetrical importance because it is the shortest pelvic diameter and has a valuable landmark in assessing the level of the presenting part of the foetus
	When presenting part is at the level of ischial spines it means -0- station and engagement of presenting part
	At the level of ischial spine, internal rotation occurs

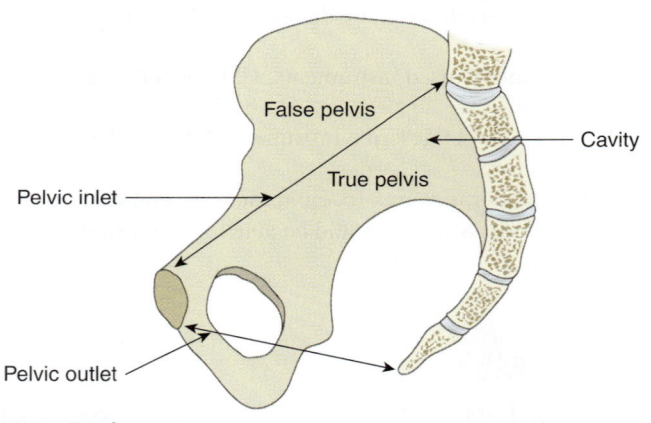

FIGURE 16.1 True and False Pelvis

Pelvis is arbitrarily divided into pelvic brim, cavity and outlet (Fig. 16.1).

THE PELVIC BRIM

The pelvic brim is the inlet of the pelvis, which divides the pelvis into true pelvis and false. It is formed by the sacral promontory, ala of the sacrum, sacroiliac articulation, iliopectineal line, iliopubic eminence, pectineal line of the pubis, pubic tubercle, pubic crest and symphysis pubis. The plane of the brim is at an angle of 55–60 degree to the horizontal and it is called the angle of inclination. Sacralisation of 5th lumbar vertebra increases angle of inclination and it is called high assimilation pelvis.

The brim is oval in shape. Four diameters at the brim are anteroposterior, transverse and two oblique diameters and posterior sagittal diameter.

- *Anteroposterior diameter at pelvic inlet:* has three diameters namely anatomical conjugate, obstetric conjugate and diagonal conjugate.
  - *Anatomical conjugate* (true conjugate) of the pelvic inlet—11 cm. It is the distance between the sacral promontory to the inner margin of the upper border of pubic symphysis.
  - *Obstetric conjugate*: is the distance between the sacral promontory and the nearest point on the posterior surface of symphysis pubis and normally it measures 10 cm or more. This cannot be measured directly by clinical examination. This is arrived for clinical purpose, by subtracting 1.5–2 cm (for inclination, thickness and height of the pubic symphysis) from diagonal conjugate.
  - *Diagonal conjugate*: distance between sacral promontory and apex of the pubic arch and can be measured clinically—12.5 cm (Fig. 16.2).
- *Transverse diameter*: is the greatest distance between the widest point apart on the linea terminalis on either side and measures 13.5 cm. Since it is the widest diameter, foetus usually engages in this diameter.
- *Each of the two oblique diameters (right or left)* extends from one of the sacroiliac joint to the opposite side iliopectineal eminence—12.5 cm.
- *Posterior sagittal diameter*: extends posterior to the point of intersection of anteroposterior diameter and the transverse diameter to the middle of the sacral promontory—5 cm.
- *The pelvic cavity extends from the pelvic brim above to the pelvic outlet below.*

The pelvic cavity is in the shape of bent cylinder with the posterior aspect formed by sacrum, which is longer than the anterior formed by the pubic bone. At the level of ischial spines is the smallest diameter of the pelvis and its interspinous diameter usually—10 cm and it is the plane of least pelvic dimensions (Table 16.1).

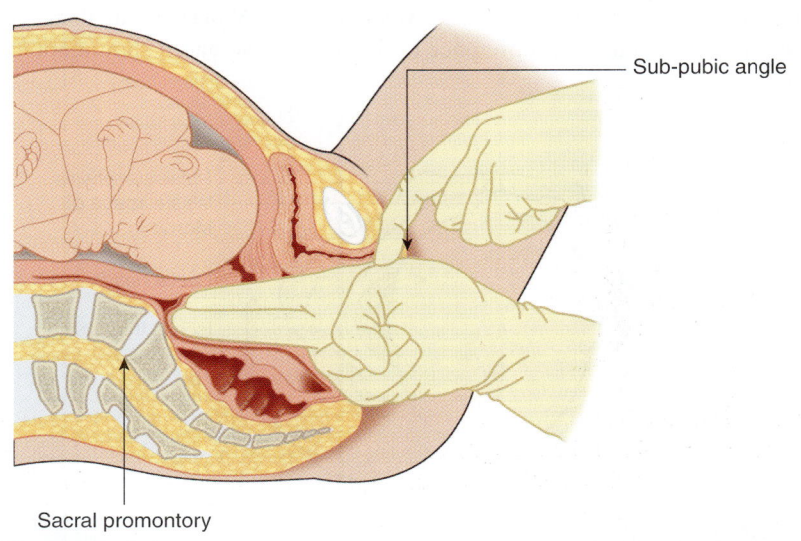

FIGURE 16.2 **Diagonal Conjugate**

174 CASE 16 VIVA VOCE (ORAL EXAM)

Table 16.1 Different Pelvic Plane

Plane of Greatest Pelvic Dimensions	Plane of Least Pelvic Dimensions
It is the mid-point of posterior surface of pubic symphysis to junction of 2nd and 3rd sacral vertebrae and middle of acetabulum called plane of greatest pelvic dimensions	It extends from lower border of the pubic symphysis to the tip of ischial spines and posteriorly to the 4th and 5th sacral vertebra
This part of the cavity is roomy	In this plane engagement and internal rotation occurs
This has no obstetrical significance	It is very important clinically because arrest of foetal descent occurs most frequently in this plane

- *Anteroposterior diameter*: it is from mid-point on the posterior surface of symphysis pubis to junction between 2nd and 3rd sacral vertebra—12 cm.
- *Transverse diameter*: is the distance between the ischial spines—10 cm.
- *Posterior sagittal diameter*: extends posterior to the point of intersection of anteroposterior diameter and the transverse diameter (mid-point of interspinous diameter) to the junction of the 4th and 5th sacral vertebra and it is 6 cm.

THE PELVIC OUTLET

- It is diamond shaped and irregular in outline, consisting of two triangles with common base, that is ischial tuberosities. Pelvic outlet bounded posteriorly by the tip of sacrum; laterally by ischial tuberosities, sacro-sciatic ligaments; anteriorly by the lower border of pubic symphysis and area under the pubic arch.
- Pubic arch is formed by the descending rami of both sides. The sub-pubic angle usually in women is about 90 degrees. Usually sub-pubic arch is rounded, hence when well-flexed head is under the arch, less space is wasted. The **waste space of Morris** is the distance between the pubic symphysis and the circumference of the foetal head and it should not exceed 1 cm (Fig. 16.3).

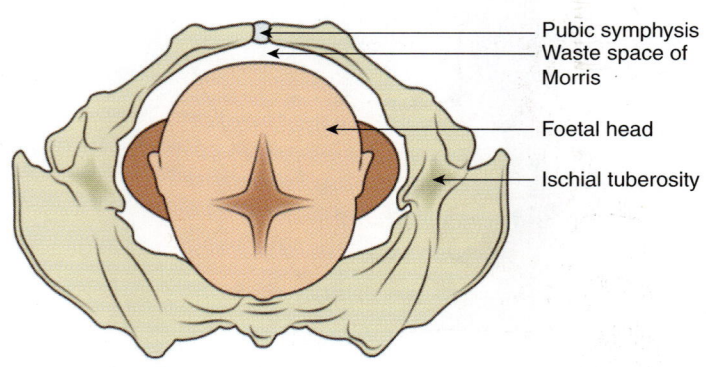

FIGURE 16.3 Waste Space of Morris

BONY PELVIS AND FOETAL SKULL **175**

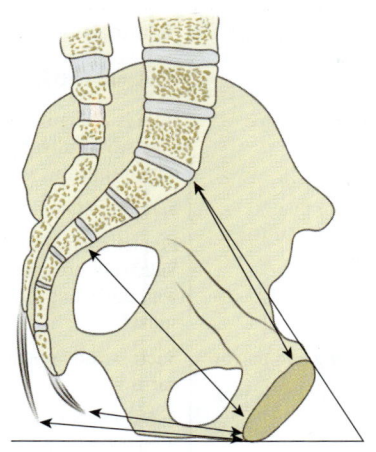

FIGURE 16.4 Line Diagram of Curve of Carus

From Holland & Brews Manual of Obstetrics, fourth ed., Fig 1.14 Classification of pelvic shapes, p. 14.

Diameters
1. Anteroposterior diameter—is between inferior border of the pubic symphysis to the tip of the sacrum: 12.5–13 cm
2. The transverse diameter—is the distance between the inner edges of the ischial tuberosities: 11 cm
3. The posterior sagittal diameter—extends posteriorly to the point of intersection of anteroposterior diameter and the transverse diameter to sacrococcygeal junction: 7.5 cm (Fig. 16.2)

Pelvic axis (curve of Carus): It is **C** shaped. Pelvic axis is formed by joining the mid-point of the anteroposterior diameters at the inlet, cavity and outlet. It is uniformly curved first downwards and backwards up to ischial spines and then abruptly forwards (which is not a uniform curved path) and it is through this, foetus negotiates (Fig. 16.4).

During pregnancy and labour due to the effect of relaxin and progesterone, there is physiological enlargement of pelvic diameters, which return to normal after delivery. Pubic bones may be separate by 2–3 mm.

Type of female pelvis according to Caldwell and Moloy:
This is based on the X-ray studies and it is a morphological classification (Table 16.2).

Diameters of Pelvis in Various Plane			
Diameters	Pelvic Brim (cm)	Cavity (cm)	Outlet (cm)
Anteroposterior	True conjugate—11 Diagonal conjugate—12.5	11.25–12	13
Transverse	12.5–13.5	9.25–10.5	10.5–11
Posterior sagittal	4.25–5	5–6.25	6.25–7

Table 16.2 Description of Different Types of Pelvis and Its Clinical Importance

Gynaecoid Pelvis	Anthropoid Pelvis	Android Pelvis	Platypelloid Pelvis
50% of the pelvis are gynaecoid	Pelvis is that of an ape pelvis	Inlet is triangular or heart-shaped with anterior narrow apex	It is a flat female type, it is rarest—3% of women only
Inlet is slightly oval or round and transverse diameter more than anteroposterior diameter	All anteroposterior diameter more than transverse diameter (oval anteroposteriorly)	Sacrum is flat	All anteroposterior diameters are short
Sacrum is well-curved, wide and concavity and inclination of sacrum is average	Ischial spines mostly prominent	Funnel-shaped cavity Side walls are converging with projecting ischial spines	All transverse diameters are long (oval transverse)
Ischial spines not prominent (transverse diameter is >10 cm)	Sacrum is long and narrow	Sacro-sciatic notch is narrow	Sacro-sciatic notch is narrow
Wide sacro-sciatic notch	Sacro-sciatic notch is wide	Sub-pubic angle is narrow <90 degree	Sub-pubic angle is wide
Pubic arch is wide	Sub-pubic angle is narrow Since posterior segment of pelvis is more, head engages in anteroposterior diameter and face to pubis and delivery occurs	Engagement is delayed; instrumental deliveries are difficult and deep transverse arrest is common	The sacrum usually is well-curved and rotated backward
Most favourable pelvis for vaginal delivery		Android pelvis have poor prognosis for vaginal delivery	Face presentation and asynclitic engagement are encountered in this type of pelvis

Clinically favourable pelvis:
- Sacral promontory should not be felt
- Side walls should be parallel
- Ischial spines should not be prominent
- Sub-pubic arch should admit two fingers and sub-pubic angle should be >90 degree
- Intertuberous diameter should admit four knuckles on pelvic examination

Significant clinical points:
- Intermediate-type pelvis and mixed types are much more frequent than pure types
- Obstetric conjugate can be measured only radiologically
- Diagonal conjugate can be estimated clinically
- Ischial spines can be felt by vaginal examination
- Narrowing of mid-pelvis or pelvic outlet will cause obstructed labour
    Pelvic inadequacy may be due to the following:
    - big baby
    - contracted pelvis
    - abnormal position
        - High inclination of pelvis can cause delay in engagement, favours occipito-posterior position and interferes with internal rotation
        - Best test of pelvic adequacy is progress of labour ending in vaginal delivery of an average-sized live foetus

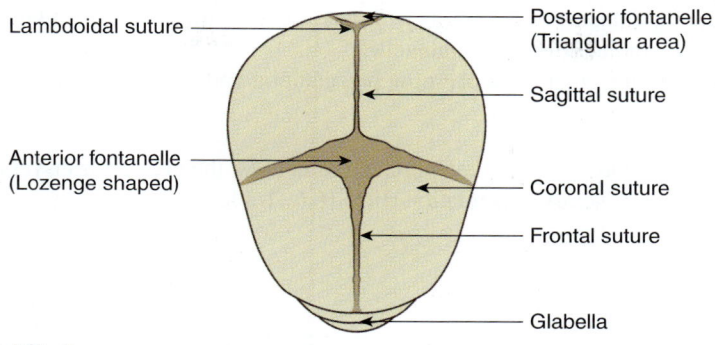

FIGURE 16.5 Foetal Skull

FOETAL SKULL

The skull is formed of the face, the vault and the base. The bones that form the skull are: two frontal bones, two parietal bones, two temporal bones, wings of the sphenoid and occipital bone.

The bones of the face and base are heavy and fused (Fig. 16.5).

The bones of the vault are two frontal, two parietal bones and one occipital bone.

Foetal skull, sutures and fontanelles

Areas of skull and foetal sutures are given in Table 16.3.

Suture: bones of the vault of the skull are not firmly united and they are joined by thin piece of membrane called suture.

Fontanelle: more than one sutures meet at an irregular space, which is enclosed by a membrane called fontanelle.

Anterior fontanelle: diamond-shaped space between coronal and sagittal suture bounded by two parietal bone on either side posteriorly and in front two frontal bones and ossifies at 18th month. It is felt easily when head is deflexed or extended.

Table 16.3 Areas of Skull and Foetal Sutures

Areas of Skull	Foetal Skull Sutures
Vertex—is a diamond-shaped area between anterior and posterior fontanelles and parietal eminences	Frontal suture—lies between two frontal bones
Face—lies between root of the nose and sub-orbital ridges and chin	Sagittal suture—lies between two parietal bones
Brow—lies between anterior fontanelle to orbital ridges	Coronal suture—lies between parietal and frontal bones
Bregma—anterior fontanelle Lambda—posterior fontanelle	Lambdoid suture—lies between parietal and occipital bones
Occiput—is the bony prominence behind and below post-fontanelle	Temporal suture—lies between inferior margin of the parietal and upper margin of temporal bone of the same side

Posterior fontanelle (lambda): triangle-shaped space between sagittal and lambdoid suture bounded by three sutures, which radiate from the fontanelle.

It gives an important information concerning presentation and position of the foetus.

Foetal skull diameters

Bi-parietal diameter, 9.5 cm—it is between parietal eminences; the greatest transverse diameter which is the engaging diameter in vertex presentation (Fig. 16.6; Table 16.4).

Sub-occipito-bregmatic 9.5 cm
Sub-mento-bregmatic 9.5 cm
Mento-vertical 13.5 cm
Occipito frontal 11.5 cm

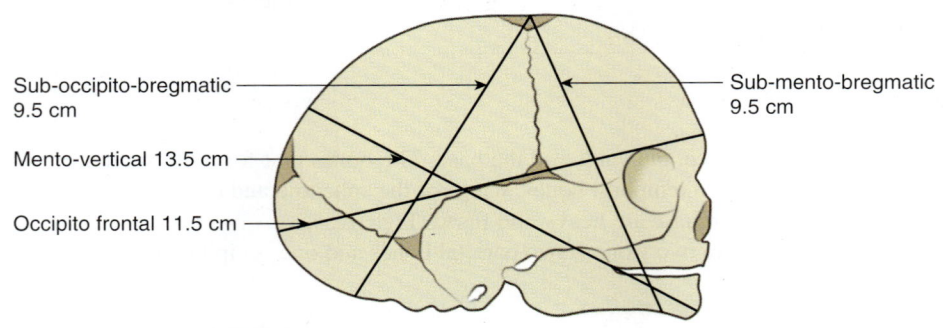

FIGURE 16.6 Line Diagram of Diameters

Table 16.4 Foetal Diameters, Measurements and Presentation

Foetal Diameters	Measurements (cm)	Bones Which Forms the Landmark in Various Presentation	Presentation
Sub-occipito-bregmatic diameter—middle of the bregma to just below occipital prominence—occurs in well-flexed head in labour	9.5	Occipital bone is the landmark in vertex presentation	Vertex
Occipito frontal—root of the nose to the most prominent point of the occiput—a deflexed head presents with this diameter	11.5	Occipital bone	Vertex
Mento-vertical—chin to most prominent point of the occiput. It is the presenting diameter in brow presentation and the largest diameter of the foetal head	13	Frontal bone is landmark for brow presentation	Brow
Sub-mento-bregmatic—chin to middle of bregma	9.5	Mentum is landmark for face presentation	Face

Moulding of the head

The bones of the vault are not joined and bones slide under each other. This reduces the diameter of the skull during labour and it is known as moulding. Only up to 4 mm of moulding is normal. Alteration in shape of the foetal head disappears within few hours of birth.

It occurs with descent of the foetal head into the pelvis to reduce the head circumference.

Frontal bones slips under the parietal bones.

Parietal bones override each other.

Parietal bones slips under the occipital bone.

Degrees of moulding:

Grade 1: The bones come in approximation but do not overlap

Grade 2: Overlapping of bones, which is easily reducible

Grade 3: Fixed overlapping and not reducible

Caput succedaneum—is localized swelling of the scalp formed by effusion of serum, during labour. It is present at birth and resolves spontaneously within next few days (Figs 16.7 and 16.8).

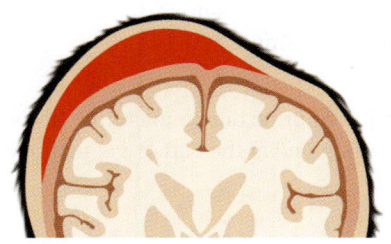

FIGURE 16.7 Line Diagram of Caput Succedaneum

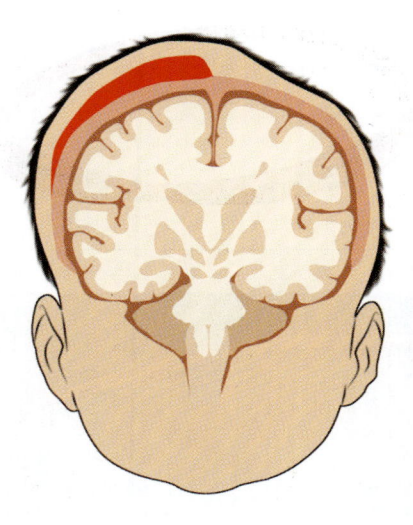

FIGURE 16.8 Cephalhaematoma

Cephalhaematoma—this is caused by sub-periosteal haematoma affecting one or more of the bones of the vault of the skull and it is limited by suture lines.

Significant clinical points of foetal skull:
- During vaginal examination, palpation of posterior fontanelle indicates position of head
- Palpation of anterior fontanelle indicates degree of flexion of head

Condition of the baby can be assessed after birth—if fontanelles are raised, it denotes raised intracranial tension and when depressed, it is due to dehydration.

INSTRUMENTS
RUBBER CATHETER (FIG. 16.9)

Uses in obstetric conditions:
- Used in pregnancy with retention of urine due to retroverted gravid uterus and in retention of urine puerperium
- During labour, when woman is unable to pass urine
- Before application of forceps and vacuum

Uses in gynaec conditions:
- To catheterise bladder in retention of urine due to mass like fibroid, large ovarian tumour impacted in pouch of Douglas; before starting and at the end of vaginal operation

FOLEY'S CATHETER (FIG. 16.10)
- Used for continuous bladder drainage—in conditions like APH, PPH, eclampsia, retention of urine in retroverted gravid uterus, post-operative following LSCS. In second trimester MTP for

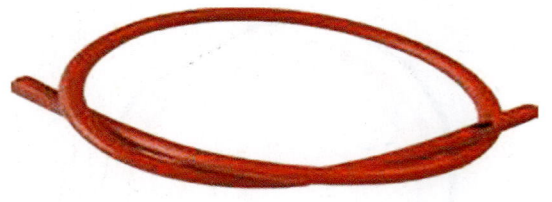

FIGURE 16.9 Rubber Catheter

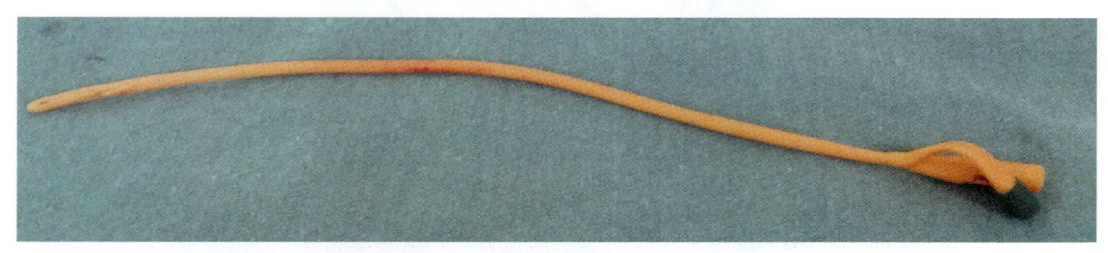

FIGURE 16.10 Foley's Catheter Uses—Self-Retaining Catheter

extra-amniotic instillation of ethacridine. For diagnosis of incompetent cervix in non-gravid uterus, catheter can be introduced without resistance through the internal os.
- Used in sonosalpingography
- Used in mechanical induction of labour and it is placed in endocervical canal and bulb is inflated with 30 mL of normal saline
- Used in amnioinfusion

SIM'S SPECULUM (FIG. 16.11)

In obstetrics:
- To visualise the cervix
- Usually double-bladed speculum is used
- Used in first trimester surgical evacuation and in MTP
- To inspect cervical tear following instrumental delivery, traumatic PPH
- To confirm leakage of amniotic fluid through os in cases of suspected PPROM or PROM
- During encerclage operation and to remove the stitch at the onset of labour or at 38 weeks
- Used to inspect bluish discoloration of cervix in early pregnancy
- To rule out local causes for first trimester bleeding and local cause in APH
- In second trimester MTP during instillation of ethacridine lactate
- To apply intracervial PGE_2 (Dinoprostone gel) for induction of labour

OVUM FORCEPS (FIG. 16.12)

- This instrument does not have a ratchet (something like lock). Tip is spoon-shaped to hold tissue and to avoid perforation.

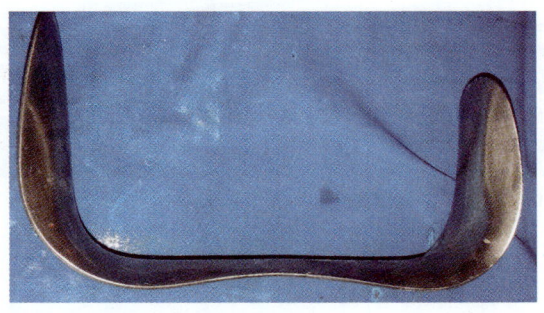

FIGURE 16.11 Sim's Speculum

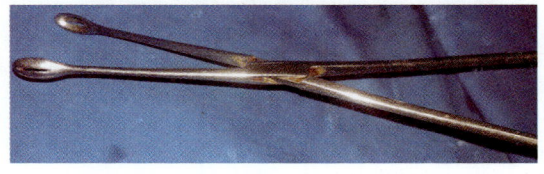

FIGURE 16.12 Ovum Forceps

CASE 16 VIVA VOCE (ORAL EXAM)

Uses:
- To remove products of conception
- To remove remnants of placental bits
- This instrument is used for removing the products of conception in inevitable, incomplete abortion and in MTP procedures

HEGAR'S DILATORS (FIG. 16.13)
- Double-ended dilators are used to dilate cervix in pregnant uterus. Hegar's dilators have no acute angulation. In pregnancy, the ante version and retro version gets corrected and uterus becomes pear-shaped.
- Dilators vary from 1 to 2 mm to 16/16 mm. These dilators are used to dilate the cervix in procedures during pregnancy.
- Used to dilate external os and gradually internal os. Before using this, uterine sound is used to find out length of the uterus. It can cause perforation, if too much force is used. Forcible dilatation can cause cervical incompetence.
- No. 8 Hegar's dilator when passed without difficulty in non-pregnant cervix, confirms incompetent os.

SPONGE HOLDING FORCEPS (FIG. 16.14)
- Tip of the instrument is ring shaped with grooves and has a ratchet, that is lock
- It is used for holding a gauze piece for painting the area before operation

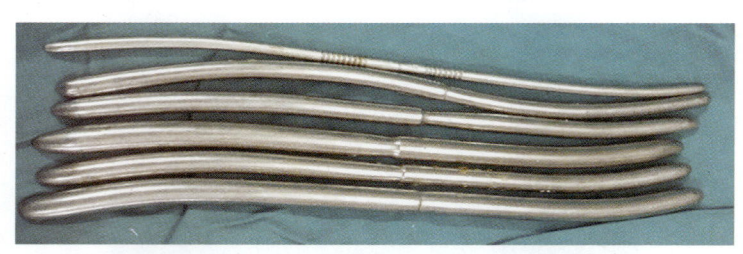

FIGURE 16.13 Hegar's Dilators

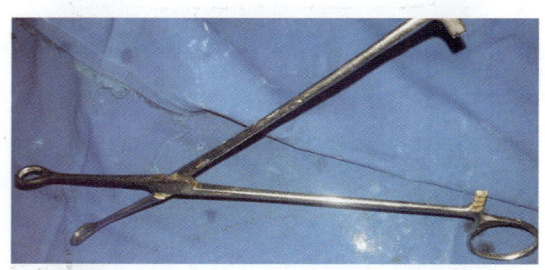

FIGURE 16.14 Sponge Holding Forceps

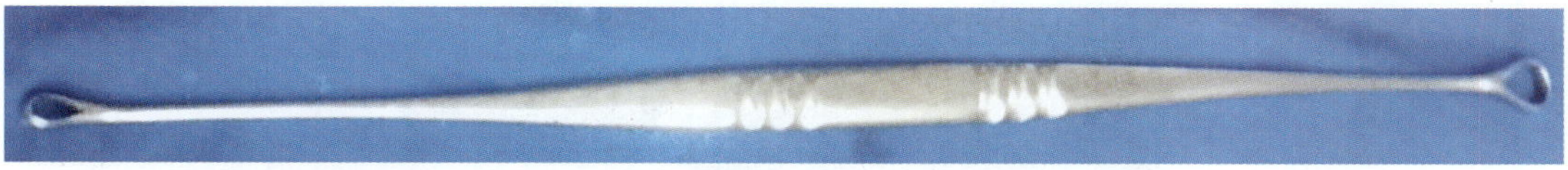

FIGURE 16.15 Uterine Curette

- It is used for holding lips of the pregnant cervix in all surgical procedures because it causes less trauma and bleeding as pregnant cervix is soft and vascular. It is used in os tightening operation and removal of stitch
- In second trimester MTP, to hold the cervix before insertion of Foley's catheter
- In exploring cervix after forceps delivery and to identify and suture the cervical tear (usually four sponge holding forceps are used, minimum three needed to 'walk around' the cervix)

UTERINE CURETTE (FIG. 16.15)

- Diagnostic dilatation and curettage (D&C) is done commonly in conditions like AUB, endometrial carcinoma, infertility, tuberculosis of endometrium. D&C also has therapeutic advantage of reducing the bleeding in menorrhagia apart from being diagnostic
- Complications: immediate—perforation; delayed–infection
- Remote—vigorous curettage especially in post-partum and post-abortal period can lead to Asherman's syndrome

OBSTETRIC FORCEPS

Types:
  Low mid-cavity axis traction forceps and outlet forceps
Pre-requisites for application of forceps:
- Cervix should be fully dilated and effaced
- Membranes should be absent
- Head must be engaged
- Rectum and bladder must be empty
- Presentation should be cephalic with sagittal suture in AP diameter
- No CPD

Contraindications:
- Incomplete dilatation of cervix malpresentation
- Obstructed labour
- Unengaged head

Indications for forceps:
- Foetal distress
- Maternal exhaustion or delay in second stage of labour
- Heart disease, anaemia, eclampsia, VBAC, cord prolapse

184   CASE 16 VIVA VOCE (ORAL EXAM)

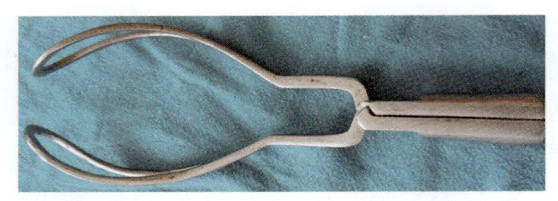

FIGURE 16.16   Outlet Forceps

Prophylactic forceps
When head is on the perineum, outlet forceps is applied to prevent prolonged pressure on perineum causing denervation injury to the muscles and prevent subsequent genital prolapse.

Wrigley's outlet forceps (Fig. 16.16)
Parts of the forceps: blade, shank, handle
- Blade has a gap called fenestra and it has two curves namely cephalic curve and slight pelvic curve. Right and left blades are named according to the relation to the side of maternal pelvis to which it is applied. Cephalic curve fits the foetal head. Pelvic curve enables it to be introduced more or less in axis of parturient canal.
- Shank is very small which connects blade and handle.
- Handle is small.
- Screw is absent which has english lock, socket system; each blade fitting one another.

Outlet forceps
- Promotes only extension of the head
- Applied when foetal head is on the perineum; rotation does not exceed 45 degree (Fig. 16.16)
- Sagittal suture in AP diameter
- Foetal scalp visible at the introitus without separating the labia. It can be used during caesarean section to deliver the head especially when it is mobile head

Axis traction forceps (Fig. 16.17)
- It has got blade, shank, lock, handle with screw and axis traction rod and traction handle.
- Axis traction rod is fitted to the shank.

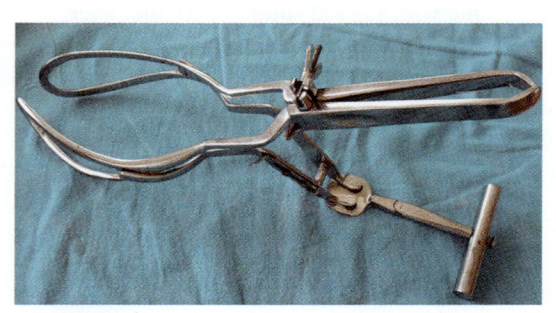

FIGURE 16.17   Axis Traction Forceps

- It has two axis rods. Each rod has a knob, groove and traction handle.
- Fixation screw placed at the end of the handle keeps the blades in proper fitting.

Advantages:
- Traction can be applied in correct direction with minimal force
- Used as low forceps at +2 station
- Used as low mid-cavity forceps whenever vertex is at +1 station
- Sagittal suture in AP diameter
- Rotation of 45 degree or less

Functions of forceps:
- Traction—18 kg for primi, 13 kg for multi
- Protection—acts as protective cage
- Rotation—nowadays not used

Complications:
- *Maternal*: lacerations of the perineum, cervical tear, PPH, shock, sepsis, rarely rupture uterus colporrhexis
- *Foetal*: cephalhaematoma, asphyxia, tentorial tear, facial palsy, cerebral palsy

Trial forceps

It should be done in operation theatre after informed consent under double set up with facilities for immediate CS.
- It is attempted in theatre in cases of doubtful mild contraction of the pelvis with a tentative pull and is done to expedite the delivery
- If there is difficulty in application, locking or traction, procedure is abandoned
- In these situations, we have to inform patient and caesarean is to be done

Failed forceps
- Error in judgment of CPD.
- After applying forceps, failure to deliver the foetus.

MR syringe and Karman's cannula (Fig. 16.18A)
- It is a plastic syringe with plastic cannula used for suction evacuation sterilised by immersing in antiseptic lotion.
- Five sizes of cannula are available (4, 6, 8, 10, 12 mm). It is used up to 6 weeks of pregnancy. This syringe is used for menstrual regulation. The capacity is 50 mL.
- The tip has a rubber attachment with valve.
- The piston when withdrawn can be locked. It creates negative pressure.
- Plastic cannula is inserted into the uterine cavity and the valve is released and with negative pressure of 60–80 mmHg, contents of the uterine cavity are sucked out. This should be repeated till the cavity is empty. Complication of the procedure is incomplete evacuation because of limited suction pressure.
- **Advantage**: No electricity is needed, less chance for perforation and haemorrhage. It can be done as office procedure. Manual vacuum aspiration (MVA syringe; Fig. 16.18B) (double valve) are in

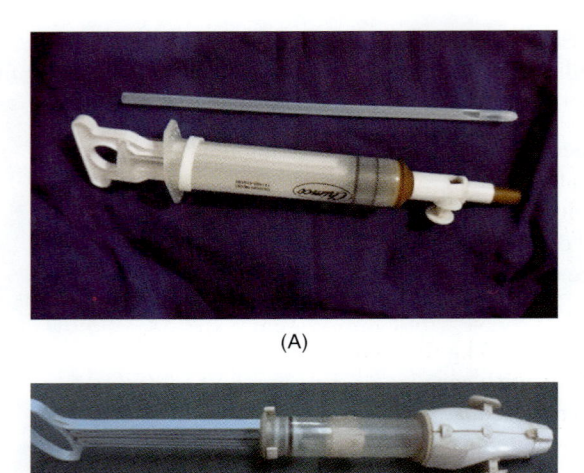

186 CASE 16 VIVA VOCE (ORAL EXAM)

FIGURE 16.18

(A–B) MR syringe and MVA.

use nowadays and can be used up to 12 weeks of pregnancy; 60 cm^3 plastic aspirator with similar principle as Karman's syringe. It is made of silicone and can be autoclaved.

SUCTION CANNULA (FIG. 16.19)

This instrument is used for first trimester MTP, suction of vesicular mole.
- It is numbered as per outer diameter.
- The size of the cannula selected is equal to number of weeks of pregnancy.
- The tip is blunt (to prevent perforation). Below the tip are two sharp openings for suction and curetting the cavity.
- Suction cannula is attached to electric suction apparatus and products of conception are evacuated by creating negative pressure.
- Usually suction force of 60–80 mmHg is applied. Rotational and to and fro movements are done to empty the cavity. Grating sensation and gripping of the cannula indicates that the procedure is complete.
- Complication—incidence of perforation is higher when compared to Karman's cannula.

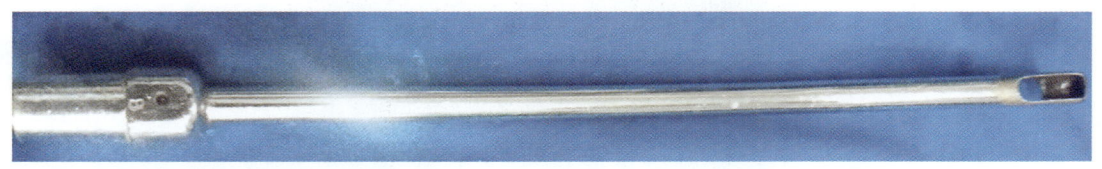

FIGURE 16.19 Suction Cannula

- Questions regarding MTP act and methods will be asked
- MTP act was enacted in 1971 and came into vogue in April 1972
- It allows deliberate termination of pregnancy up to 20 weeks, reasons being medical, social and eugenic
- Up to 12 weeks, a single medical practitioner can certify and after 12 weeks, two medical practitioners should give opinion
- First trimester methods:
  - Medical abortion by mifepristone and misoprostol up to 7 weeks
  - Menstrual regulation by Karman's syringe up to 6 weeks
  - Menstrual vacuum aspirator—MVA till 12 weeks
  - Suction evacuation, D&C till 12 weeks
- Second or mid-trimester methods:
  - Medical methods—misoprostol every 4–6 h, followed by Syntocinon
  - Extra-amniotic ethacridine lactate
  - Surgical—hysterotomy

EPISIOTOMY SCISSORS (FIG. 16.20)
- Used to perform episiotomy
- Blunt end should be introduced inside vagina.

Details: *refer Case 2.*

VENTOUSE (VACUUM EXTRACTOR)
- It was introduced by Malmstrom (Fig. 16.21).

Different parts of the ventouse:

Vacuum bottle, manometer, pump/vacuum generator, metal or silastic cup, traction tubings

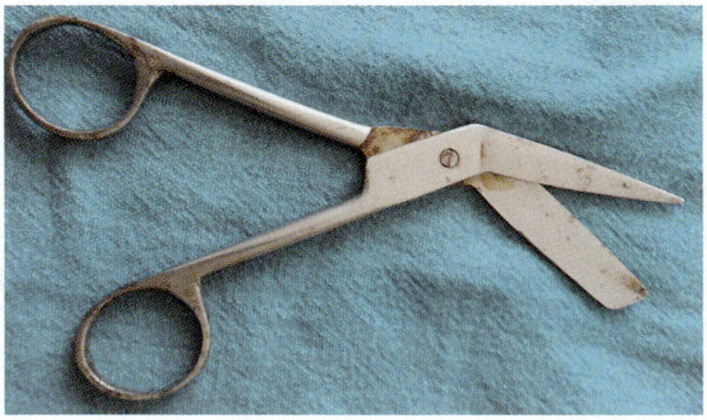

FIGURE 16.20   **Episiotomy Scissors**

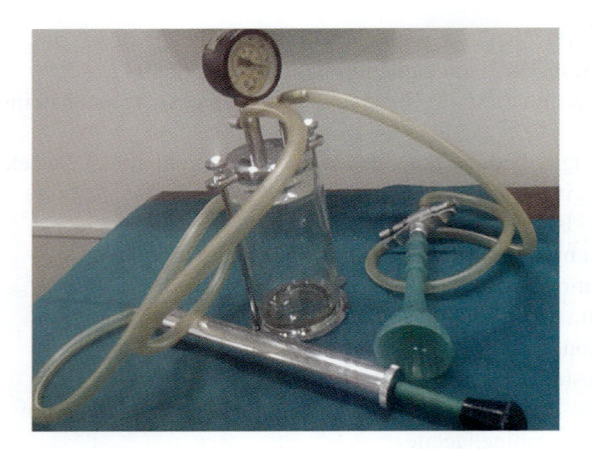

FIGURE 16.21 Ventouse

- There are four different size metal cups/silastic cups (30, 40, 50, 60 mm diameter). The metal cup has knob on the outer surface to indicate the direction of occiput. The cup has traction chain. Vacuum glass suction bottle with rubber cap has connections, one to suction cup, another to the manual or electrical pump and another to manometer.

Pre-requisites for application of ventouse: In modern obstetrics, pre-requisites are similar to that of forceps application
- Cervix should be fully dilated (rim of cervix may be present)

In modern obstetrics:
- Only in full dilatation, application is done. When applied with incomplete dilatation, it may lead to cervical tear and stretch of ligaments and genital prolapse can occur later
- Pre-requisites are similar to that of forceps application. Head should be engaged
- Bladder and rectum should be empty, no CPD

Indications: incomplete rotation/as alternative to forceps

Three basic procedures:
- Application of correct sized cup
- Creating negative pressure and chignon
- Delivery of head by traction

Procedure:
- Largest possible cup according to the dilatation of the cervix is to be selected.
- Cup is placed over the head (make sure it is not over the fontanelle) about 3 cm anterior to posterior fontanelle and the knob of the cup should point towards the occiput—to promote flexion of the head
- Negative pressure is created, which is gradually increased from 0.1 to 0.8 kg/cm^2 or 760 mmHg, over a period of 8–10 min
- The vacuum created between scalp and cup results in artificial caput called chignon
- After this, traction is given during contraction and along with maternal pushing efforts foetal head is delivered

Contraindications:
- Foetal distress where immediate delivery is needed, premature baby
- Face presentation
- After-coming head in breech presentation

Advantages over forceps:
- It can be applied even when rim of cervix is present
- Maternal and foetal injury is less
- It aids in rotation
- It does not require extra space for application

Complications:

Maternal:
- Usually is less
- Maternal tissue can get entrapped between cup and scalp and cause avulsion injury

   Foetal: intracranial haemorrhage, cephalhaematoma

DISPOSABLE CORD CLAMP

Cord is usually clamped only after cessation of the pulsation and it is cut in between two clamps. This allows 80–100 mL of blood to the baby (Fig. 16.22).

Indications of early cord clamping:
- Rh isoimmunisation
- Pre-term and LBW babies
- Baby born to HIV mother, asphyxiated baby

Conditions where long cord is left:
- Baby born to Rh negative mother, pre-term baby
- Asphyxiated baby

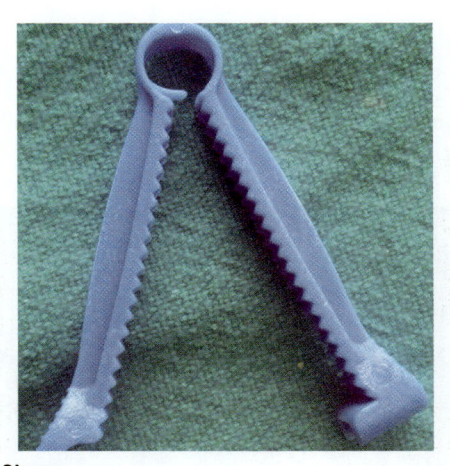

FIGURE 16.22 **Disposable Cord Clamp**

190   CASE 16 VIVA VOCE (ORAL EXAM)

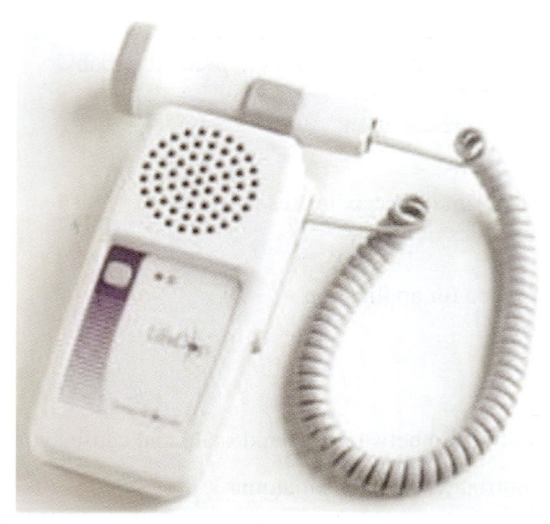

FIGURE 16.23   Hand Doppler

HAND DOPPLER (FIG. 16.23)

- Cardiac activity can be detected by TVS by 6 weeks
- Foetal heart can be heard with stethoscope or Pinard's foetoscope
- Hand Doppler can pickup foetal heart rate (FHR) by 10–12 weeks
- Normal FHR: range—120–160 min^{-1}
- Mild tachycardia: 160–180 min^{-1}
- Severe tachycardia: more than 180 min^{-1}
- Mild bradycardia: 100–120 min^{-1}
- Moderate: 80–100 min^{-1}
- Severe: less than 80 min^{-1}

PINARD'S FOETOSCOPE

- This is used for auscultation of foetal heart. The tapering rim is applied to ear and the other side to the mother's abdomen (Fig. 16.24).

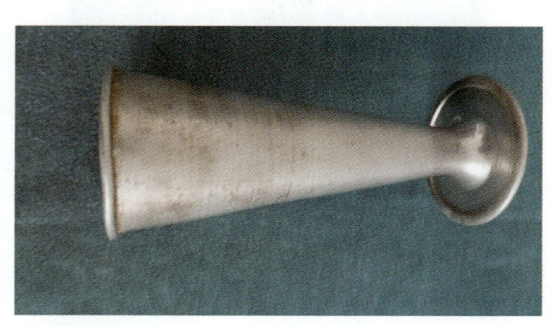

FIGURE 16.24   Pinard's Foetoscope

- In cephalic presentation, foetal heart is heard on the spinoumbilical line on the same side as the back.
- In breech presentation, foetal heart is heard above the umbilicus.
- In transverse lie, foetal heart is heard at the level of umbilicus.

UMBILICAL CORD CUTTING SCISSORS (FIG. 16.25)
DISPOSAL MANUAL MUCUS SUCKER

- It is used to suck out the secretions from the naso–oropharynx following the delivery of the head of the baby (Fig. 16.26)
- Useful in normal delivery and also in meconium aspiration

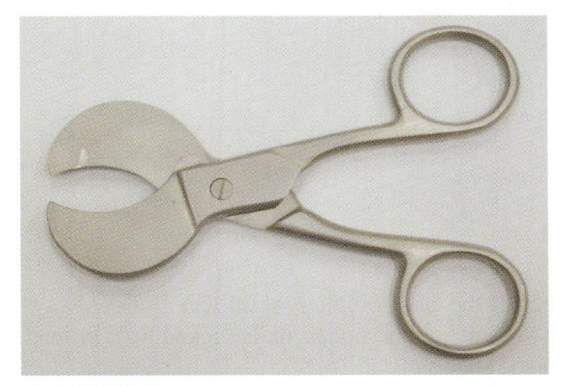

FIGURE 16.25 Umbilical Cord Cutting Scissors

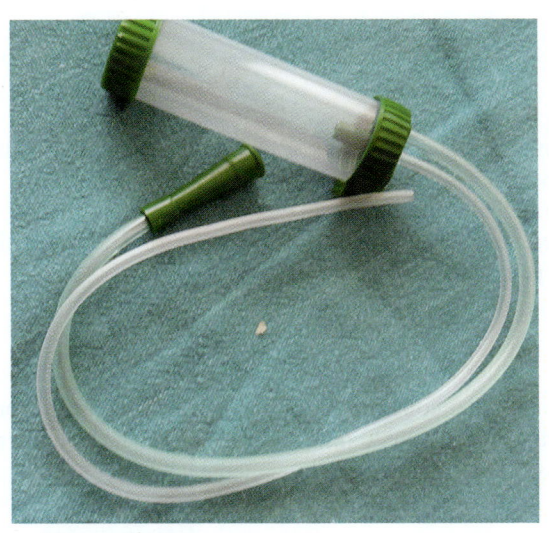

FIGURE 16.26 Disposal Manual Mucus Sucker

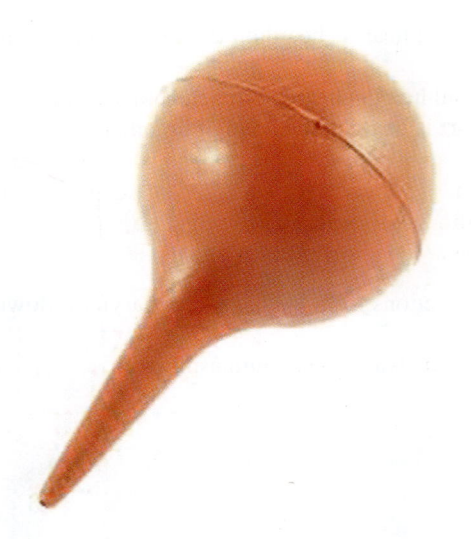

FIGURE 16.27 Bulb Sucker

BULB SUCKER

This can also be used in clearing the naso–oropharyngeal secretions. Always suck oropharynx, then nasopharynx. If meconium is present, and nasopharynx is sucked first, instead of oropharynx, meconium aspiration can occur due to stimulation (Fig. 16.27).

MEDICINES
INJ. CARBOPROST

It is PGF_2 alpha and is used in atonic PPH.

One millilitre contains 250 µg and always it should be given intramuscularly at an interval of 16 min, maximum of eight doses.

Contraindication: bronchial asthma
Complications: nausea, vomiting, diarrhoea, chills, shivering, exaggeration of bronchial asthma
Prophylactic dose in prevention of PPH: 125 µg

INJ. OXYTOCIN

It is oxytocic, which stimulates the contractions of uterus. It is used in IM route and IV in drip.

Half-life 3–4 min, duration of action 20 min, onset of action 2.5 min after IM.
Each ampoule contains: 1 mL = 5 units.

Used for induction and augmentation of labour—5 units in primi, and 2.5 units in multi in 500 mL of RL solution as infusion.

Used in incomplete abortion, inevitable abortion and vesicular mole—to control bleeding.

For active management of third stage of labour—10 units IM given within 1 min of delivery of the baby. It is first line of management in atonic PPH, up to 20–40 units in 500 mL of saline can be used.

Complications of oxytocin: when used for induction or augmentation of labour
Maternal: uterine hyper-stimulation, constriction ring, rupture uterus, water intoxication (high dose)
Foetal: foetal hypoxia, foetal distress and death; neonatal hyperbilirubinaemia

INJ. METHYLERGOMETRINE

It is and alkaloid of ergot given in oral, intramuscular and intravenous route.

One ampoule contains 1 mL, which contains 0.2 mg.

Onset of action: IV—within 1.5 min, IM—7 min, oral after 10–12 min.

Uses: after or during evacuation, in cases of abortion and vesicular mole and in atonic PPH to control bleeding. It is given intravenously.

Prophylactic methergin—given at the delivery of the anterior shoulder in conditions like anaemia, IUD, abruption, polyhydramnios, multiple pregnancy.

Nowadays not used routinely due to its side-effects.

Contraindications: heart disease, pre-eclampsia, eclampsia, following delivery of first child in multiple gestation

Side-effects: nausea, vomiting, rise of blood pressure, myocardial infarction and can interfere with lactation

TAB. MISOPROSTOL

It is methyl ester of PGE_1.

It can be used orally, vaginally and rectally.

It causes uterine contractions, cervical softening and dilatation.

It is used in medical abortion, missed abortion, incomplete abortion, second trimester abortion, atonic PPH.

It is used before instrumentation for cervical dilatation.

Dose: Tab 100 μg, 200 μg

For medical abortion: Day 1—mifepristone 200 mg followed 48 h later vaginally or orally; misoprostol 600–800 μg

In atonic PPH, it can be given up to 1000 μg per rectum

Side-effects: nausea, vomiting, diarrhoea, chills, shivering, headache

TAB. MIFEPRISTONE—RU486

It is a derivative of norethindrone. It has anti-progestational action.

Each tablet—200 mg.

It binds to progesterone receptor at endometrium or decidua.

It is used in medical abortion, emergency contraception and in fibroid uterus.

DINOPROSTONE GEL—PGE$_2$O

It is an intracervical gel used for ripening the cervix; 500 µg, in induction of labour when Bishops score less than 6. It can be repeated after 6 h. Maximum dose: 3 doses.

Oxytocin can be given only 6 h after the last dose of PGE$_2$.

Side-effects: diarrhoea, vomiting, uterine hypertonus. It should be used with caution in hepatic, renal disorder and asthma

INJ. MAGNESIUM SULPHATE

Refer Case 4.

LSCS PROCEDURE

Under suitable anaesthesia (spinal/epidural/general, based on the patient's condition) abdomen is opened either by midline, paramedian or suprapubic transverse incision (Pfannenstiel). Rectus sheath is opened, rectus muscle retracted and general peritoneum is opened.

Doyen's retractor is introduced and loose fold of peritoneum (uterovesical fold of peritoneum) over the lower segment (Fig. 16.28) is cut transversely and lower flap of the peritoneum is pushed down.

Small incision on the lower segment is made by scalpel until the membranes are exposed. Then both index fingers are introduced (Fig. 16.29) and muscles of the lower segment are split transversely (or) incision is extended on either sides using scissors to make it a curved (curvilinear) one about 10 cm in length, with concavity directed upwards; membranes are ruptured.

Head is delivered by introducing the palm of the hand (Fig. 16.30) and fingers to lever out the head while assistant gives fundal pressure. After delivery of the trunk (Fig. 16.31), 10 units oxytocin IM to be given by the anaesthesiologist, rest of the body is delivered slowly.

As soon as the head is delivered, the mucus from mouth, pharynx and nostrils are sucked out using rubber catheter (Fig. 16.32). Cord is cut in between clamps (Fig. 16.33) and the baby is handed over to the paediatrician. Removal of the placenta is done after spontaneous separation of placenta (Fig. 16.34) and membranes are removed in toto (Fig. 16.35).

Suture of uterine wound: the margins of the wound are picked up by Allis tissue forceps. Suturing is done in two layers with catgut—one chromic or vicryl with round body needle (Fig. 16.36). A continuous running suture of deeper muscles excluding the decidua is taken and second layer is also sutured by continuous sutures—inverted Lemberts sutures—burying the first layer (Fig. 16.37). Tubes and ovaries are to be examined. After complete haemostasis, abdomen should be closed in layers.

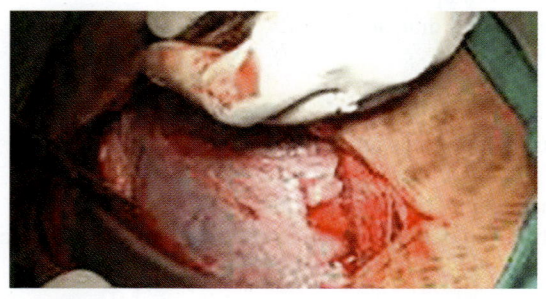

FIGURE 16.28 UV Fold of Peritoneum

LSCS PROCEDURE 195

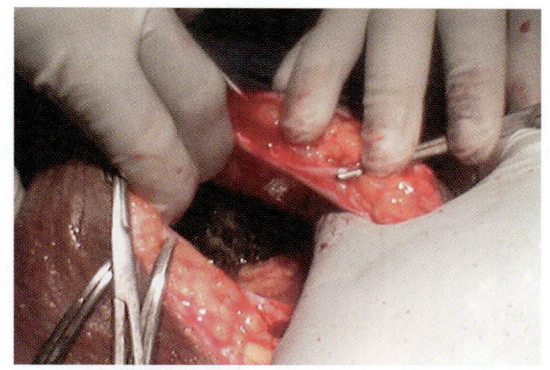

FIGURE 16.29 Lower Uterine Incision Extended

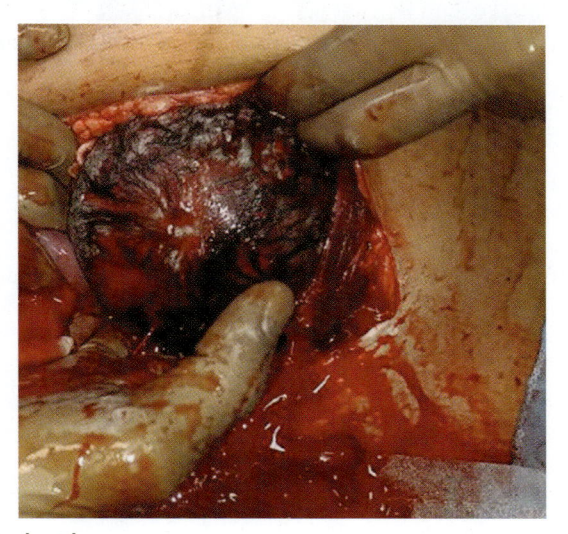

FIGURE 16.30 Hand is Introduced

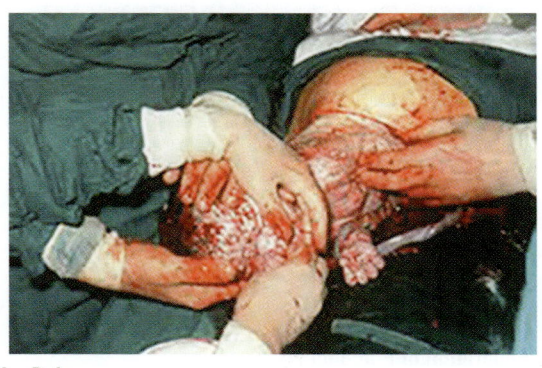

FIGURE 16.31 Delivery of the Baby

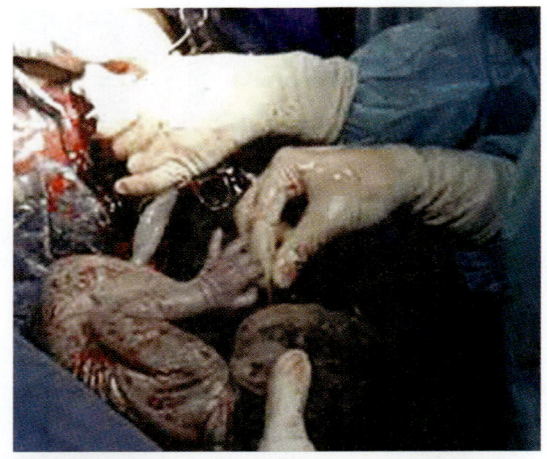

FIGURE 16.32 Mucus From Mouth, Pharynx and Nostrils are Sucked Out Using Rubber Catheter

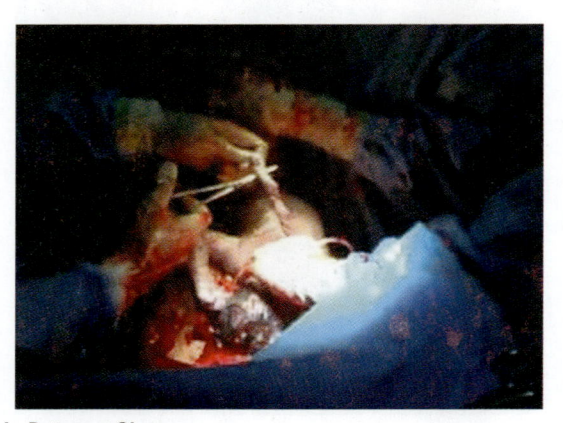

FIGURE 16.33 Cord is Cut In Between Clamps

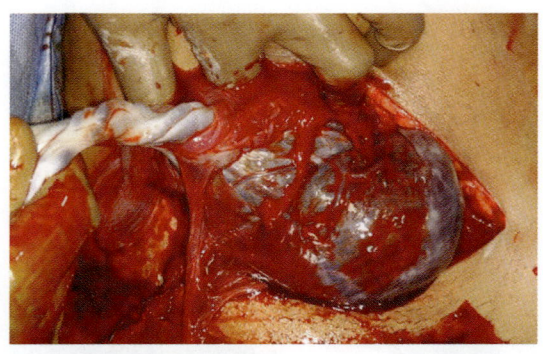

FIGURE 16.34 Spontaneous Separation of Placenta

LSCS PROCEDURE

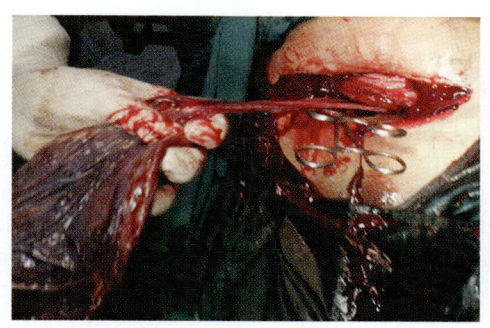

FIGURE 16.35   Membranes are Removed

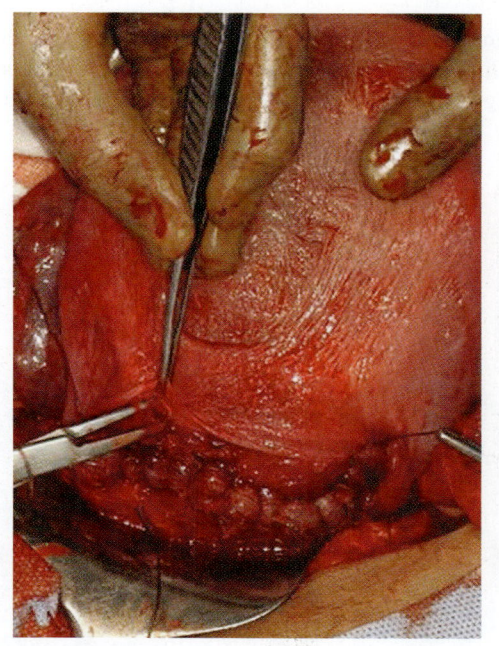

FIGURE 16.36   Suture of Uterine Wound

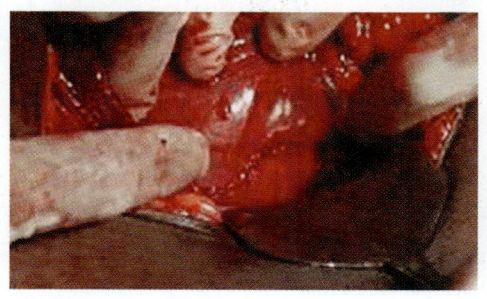

FIGURE 16.37   Inverted Lemberts Sutures

SPECIMENS

SPECIMEN OF ANENCEPHALUS BABY FOETUS (FIG. 16.38)

It is the specimen where vault is absent and facial portion is normal and has 'frog's eye appearance'. By USG, diagnosis can be made at 11–14 weeks. Maternal alpha foetoprotein is increased. Polyhydramnios can occur. It is a lethal anomaly and a type of open neural tube defect; 70% cases occur in female foetuses. MTP is advised before 20 weeks. One of the causes for it is folic acid deficiency, which can be prevented by administration of 400 μg of folic acid 12 weeks before pregnancy and continued till the end of first trimester.

SPECIMEN OF HYDROCEPHALUS FOETUS

When undiagnosed till term, it can go for post-dated pregnancy due to absent foetal hypothalamo pituitary adrenal axis and shoulder dystocia can happen in labour. In this specimen, head is enlarged and its circumference is bigger and hence it is hydrocephalus (Fig. 16.39). This is due to accumulation

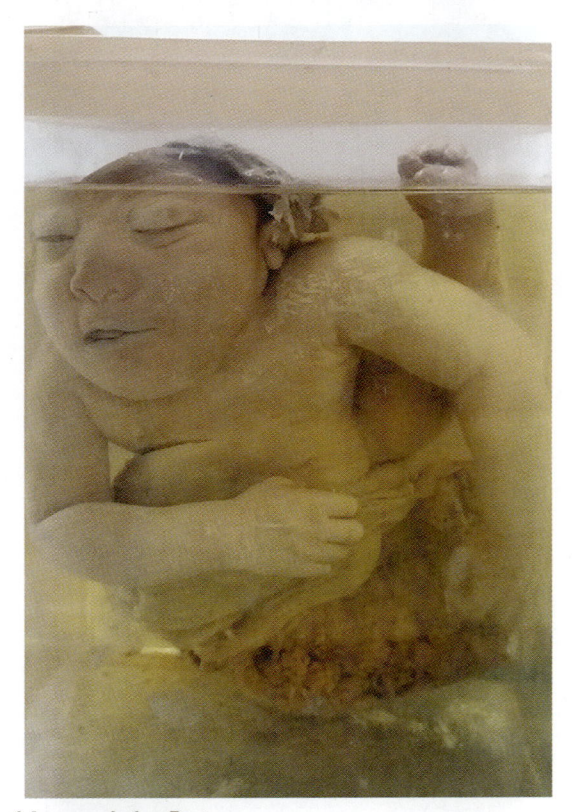

FIGURE 16.38 Specimen of Anencephalus Foetus

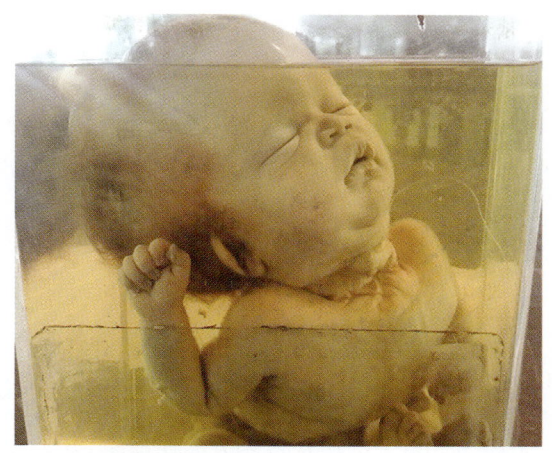

FIGURE 16.39 Specimen of Hydrocephalus Baby

of excessive amount of CSF in the ventricles resulting in separation of sutures. It can be diagnosed by USG (ventriculomegaly).

It can cause breech presentation. If undiagnosed till term, it can cause CPD/obstructed labour.

In severe form where thinning of the cerebral cortex due to ventriculomegaly is diagnosed, early termination of pregnancy is advised. In minor degree, after delivery, baby can be treated by ventriculoperitoneal shunt.

If diagnosed in labour, tapping of CSF can be done under USG guidance either per abdomen or through dilated cervix and delivery done after the head circumference decreases.

SPECIMEN OF ENCEPHALOCOELE (FIG. 16.40)

This is a specimen of anomalous foetus with a swelling in the occipital region, most probably encephalocoele.

FAQ: What are the common causes for anomalous foetus? How will you terminate if it is lethal and foetus is 20 weeks?

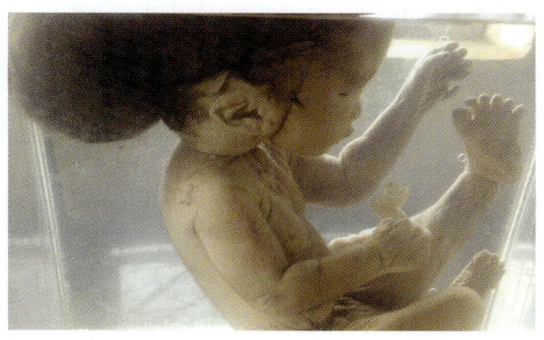

FIGURE 16.40 Specimen of Encephalocoele

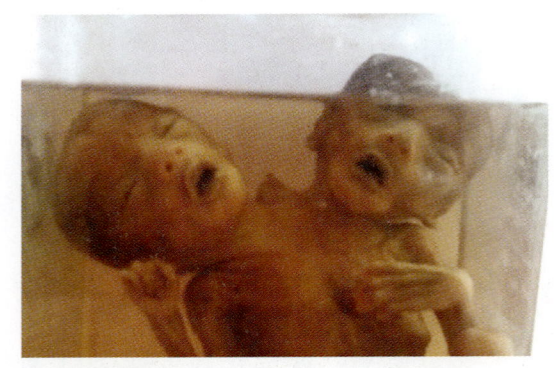

FIGURE 16.41   Conjoint Twins—Thoracopagus

Causes for foetal anomaly are multi factorial: genetic, maternal diabetes, folic acid deficiency, use of anti-convulsants, certain viral infections, teratogenic drugs, drug abuse, foetal alcohol syndrome.

Termination of mid-trimester pregnancy in lethal anomaly is undertaken after counselling and high-risk consent. Two medical practitioners should give opinion.

MTP is done by medical methods or Tab. misoprostol.

Other methods are extra-amniotic ethacridine.

CONJOINT TWINS—THORACOPAGUS (FIG. 16.41)

Conjoint twin is extremely rare. When division occurs after 2 weeks of the development of embryonic disc, conjoint twin is formed.

Four common types—craniopagus (cephalic), thoracopagus (upper thorax fused—most common type), pygopagus (posterior fusion) and ischiopagus (caudal fusion).

Antenatal diagnosis helps to plan method of delivery and paediatric team can be alerted. Management depends on extent and site of union. When diagnosed late—may require classical caesarean section.

SPECIMEN OF VESICULAR MOLE (FIG. 16.42)

This specimen has various sized grape-like structures called vesicles and it is the vesicular mole specimen.

It is an abnormal pregnancy, with hydropic degeneration of chorionic villi, trophoblastic proliferation, and obliteration of vessels in the villi.

In complete mole, karyotype is 46xx where both chromosomes are of paternal origin.

Complications:

Pre-eclampsia, haemorrhage, invasive mole with intra-peritoneal haemorrhage, persistent gestational trophoblastic neoplasia with metastasis in 16%–20%.

Antenatal diagnosis:

Uterine size > period of gestation, with continuous or intermittent uterine bleeding, absent foetal parts. It is diagnosed by high beta-hCG level and USG appearance of 'snow storm'.

Management: vesicular mole once diagnosed, needs surgical evacuation.

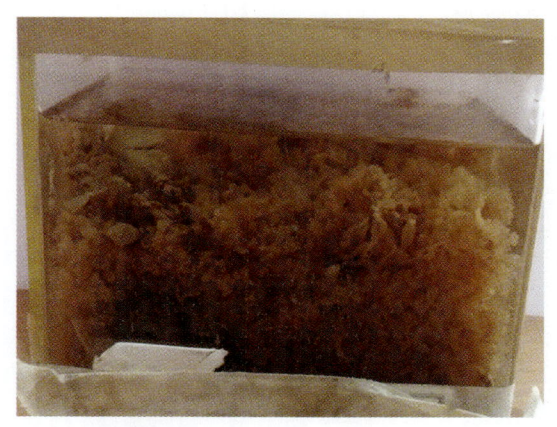

FIGURE 16.42 Specimen of Vesicular Mole

Preliminary X-ray of chest, thyroid function test, blood grouping and cross-matching are done and blood is kept ready.

Regardless of the size of uterus, suction evacuation is to be done with adequate blood along with 10 units of oxytocin drip to promote uterine contraction and prevent haemorrhage due to atonicity; material is sent for HPE.

Follow up: β-hCG to be done weekly till three negative values; then monthly for 3 months and if negative, 6 monthly in 1st and 2nd year. In every visit, detailed history and gynaec examination is to be done to rule out abnormal bleeding PV/sub-urethral nodules/lung metastasis and presence of theca lutein ovarian cysts.

FAQ: What is hydatiform mole, its clinical features, diagnosis, management, complications and follow up?

SPECIMEN OF RUPTURE UTERUS (FIG. 16.43)

Specimen of gravid uterus with rent from lower segment extending to upper segment, without cervix so it is a subtotal hysterectomy specimen.

FAQ: What are the causes for threatened rupture and rupture, signs and symptoms, diagnosis and management?

Obstructed labour may be due to CPD, transverse lie, tumours in lower uterine segment, conjoint twins, lead to threatened rupture and if not identified and treated end in rupture uterus.

In threatened rupture: H/O prolonged labour, maternal exhaustion, tachycardia, foetal distress, stretched lower uterine segment with Bandtl's ring per abdomen, with hot dry vagina with excessive caput and moulding of head are present.

In rupture uterus: maternal shock will be present; foetal parts felt superficially, uterine contour is lost, loss of FH, and receding of foetal presenting part per pelvic examination, with fresh bleeding PV and occasional haematuria may be present.

Management:

Immediate delivery in obstructed labour by caesarean and laparotomy and repair of rent or hysterectomy in rupture uterus.

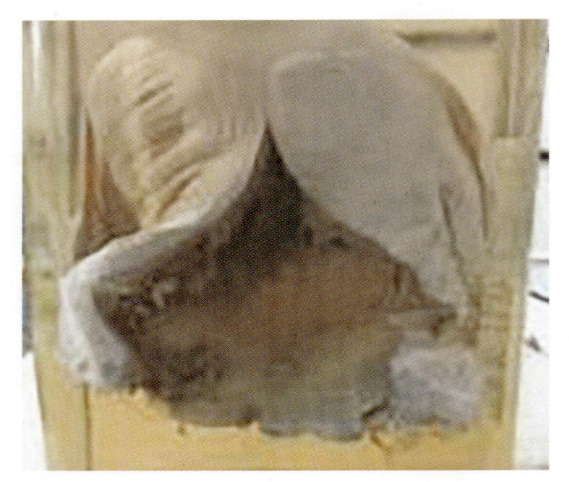

FIGURE 16.43 Rupture Uterus

SPECIMEN OF COUVELAIRE UTERUS WITHOUT CERVIX (FIG. 16.44)

Specimen of gravid uterus without cervix, ecchymosis in the lower uterine region, so it is a subtotal hysterectomy specimen probably due to Couvelaire uterus.

FAQ: Clinical features of abruptio placentae, pathophysiology of Couvelaire uterus, investigations complications and management—refer Case 4—Abruptio placenta.

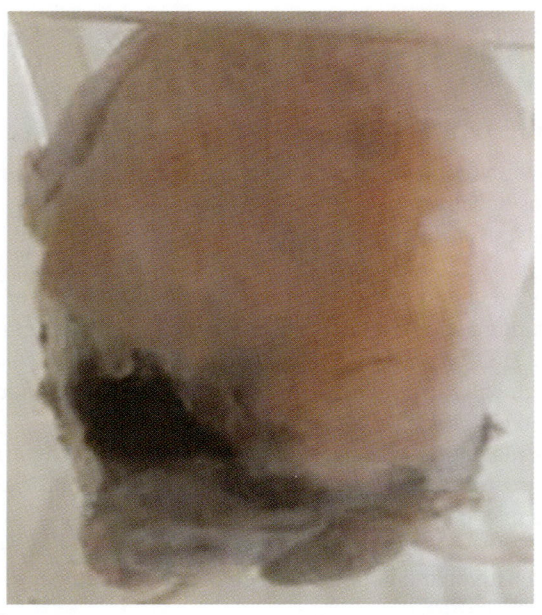

FIGURE 16.44 Couvelaire Uterus

NST AND CTG

NST done in antenatal period, which shows FHR acceleration with foetal movement and no uterine contraction (Fig. 16.45).

Interpretation of a CTG tracing requires description of the following:
Baseline FHR
Beat-to-beat FHR variability
Presence of accelerations
Periodic or episodic decelerations
Changes or trends of FHR patterns over time
Uterine activity (contractions)

Normal pattern trace (Fig. 16.46):
Baseline rate 110–160 beats/min, with normal beat-to-beat variability of 5–16 beats/min, two or more accelerations of 16 beats/min lasting for 16 s in response to a foetal movement over a period of 20 min

Absence of late or variable decelerations

Variable deceleration: deceleration is independent of uterine contraction, it may be due to cord compression and may relieved by change in position.

Early deceleration (Fig. 16.47): deceleration coincides with uterine contraction and FHR returns to normal when contraction passes off. It can be due to head compression during labour.

Late deceleration—beat to beat variability present and late deceleration present beyond uterine contraction (Fig. 16.48).

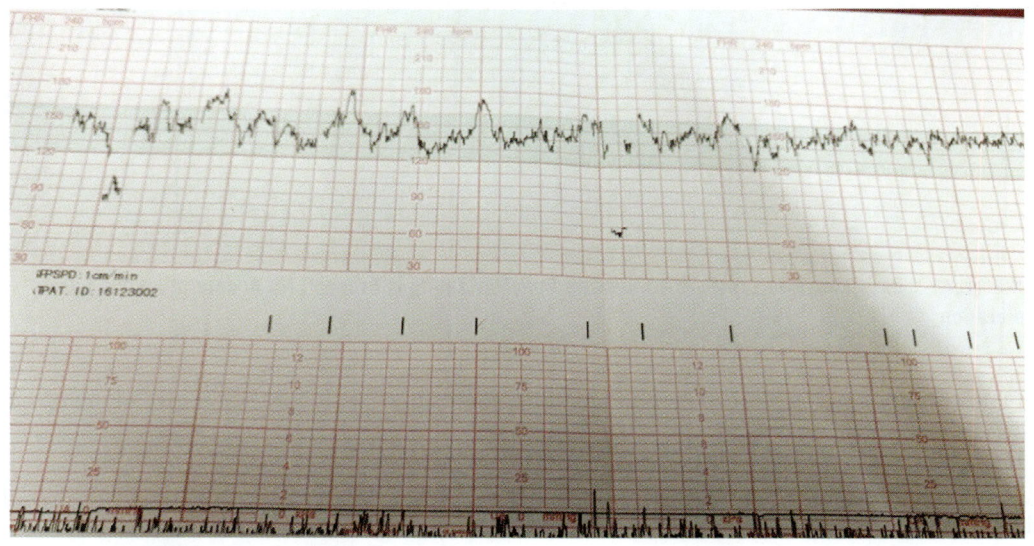

FIGURE 16.45 Antenatal Tracing-NST

204 CASE 16 VIVA VOCE (ORAL EXAM)

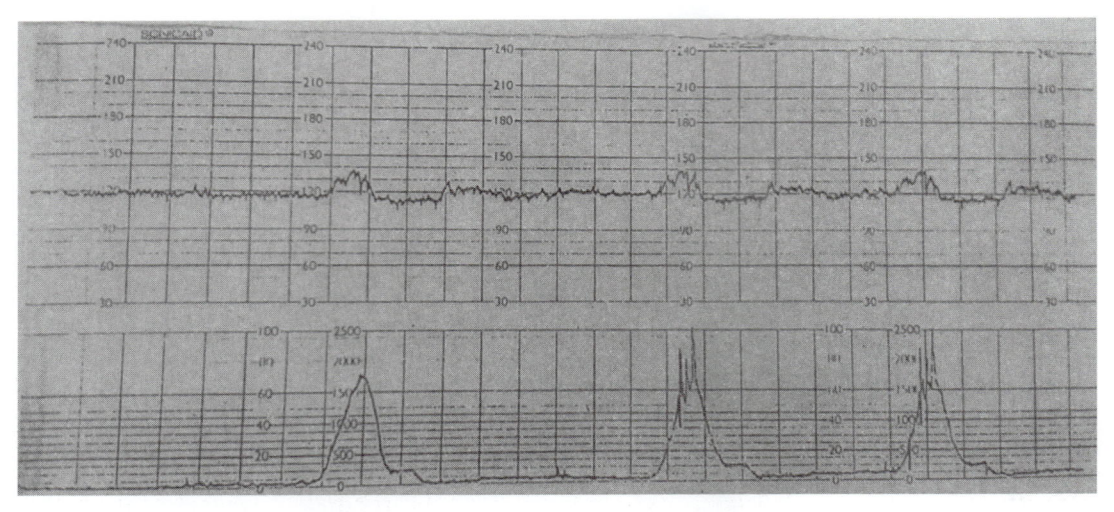

FIGURE 16.46 Normal Pattern

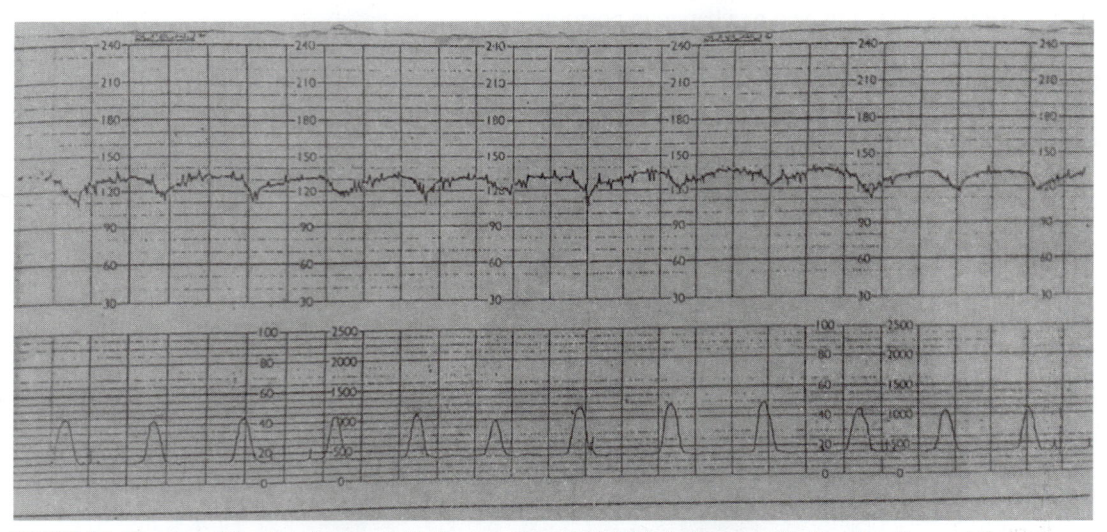

FIGURE 16.47 Base Line Heart rate—140, Beat-to-Beat Variability is Present, No Acceleration and Early Deceleration

FHR does not return to normal even after uterine contraction passes off. Suggestive of uteroplacental insufficiency and foetal hypoxia.

What are the causes for foetal distress?

Chronic causes for foetal distress are placental insufficiency due to anaemia, PIH, GDM, renal disorders and other medical illness and prolonged pregnancy.

Acute causes for foetal distress are cord, compression during labour, cord prolapse, tachysystole, hyper-stimulation of uterus, prolonged labour, APH—abruptio, vasa praevia and placenta previa.

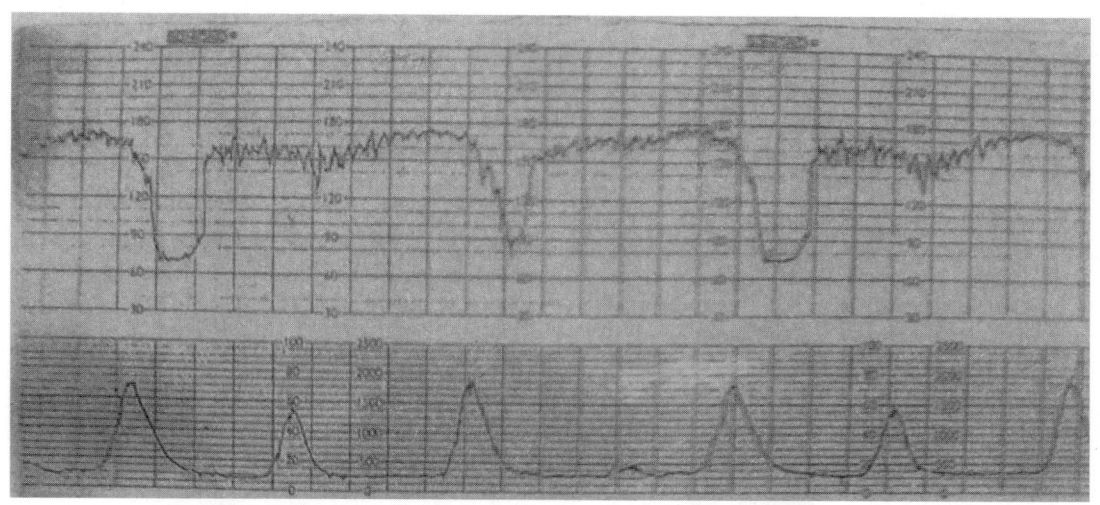

FIGURE 16.48 Late Deceleration

What are the signs of foetal distress?

- In labour, findings of meconium-stained liquor, big caput and excessive moulding of head denotes foetal distress.
- Abnormal CTG tracing in labour:

Foetal tachycardia, foetal bradycardia, loss of beat-to-beat FHR variability and persistent late deceleration indicate foetal distress.

- During pregnancy:

Decreased or absent foetal movements, non-reactive NST, severe oligohydramnios with abnormal Doppler study of umbilical and middle cerebral artery indicate foetal distress.

What are the tests for antepartum foetal surveillance?
DFMC, NST, AFI, foetal Doppler study.

What is the significance of early and late deceleration?
Early deceleration is due to vagal stimulation because of head compression during labour and late deceleration is due to placental insufficiency.

What measures will you take when there is foetal distress?
Stop the oxytocin drip, start IV crystalloids, put patient in left lateral position, administer nasal O_2. Administer tocolytics, if uterine hyper-stimulation is present.

What will you do when liquor is meconium stained?
If CTG is normal and delivery is imminent, allow natural vaginal delivery or instrumental delivery.
If CTG is abnormal, caesarean is done.
In thick meconium-stained liquor, amnioinfusion is given while awaiting for delivery, which is imminent or taking up for LSCS. It decreases meconium aspiration syndrome.

What is modified biophysical profile?
Refer Case 5

USG PICTURES

Gestational Sac shows gestational sac (Fig 16.49), which can be detected at 4 weeks by transvaginal USG, when β-hCG is 1000–1200 IU/L.

By TAS, when β-hCG is 6000 IU/L, which is the discriminatory level, GS will be 1–3 mm in diameter and grows at the rate of 1 mm/day and appears on one side of the cavity line, not in the middle of it.

GESTATIONAL SAC WITH YOLK SAC

Gestational Sac with yolk sac (Fig. 16.50). Yolk sac can be seen at 5 weeks in transvaginal USG.

Yolk sac appearance is a definite sign of intra-uterine pregnancy.

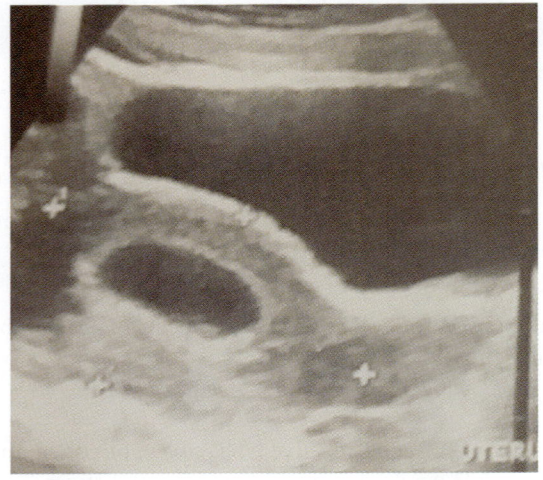

FIGURE 16.49 Gestational Sac

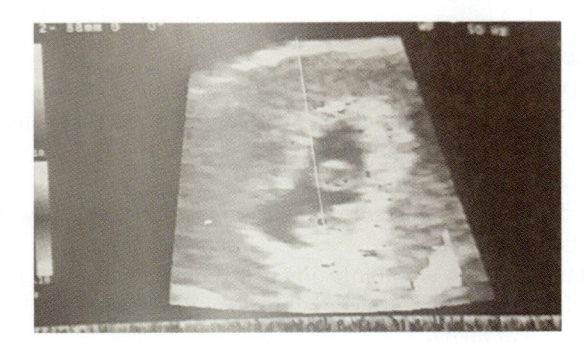

FIGURE 16.50 Yolk Sac

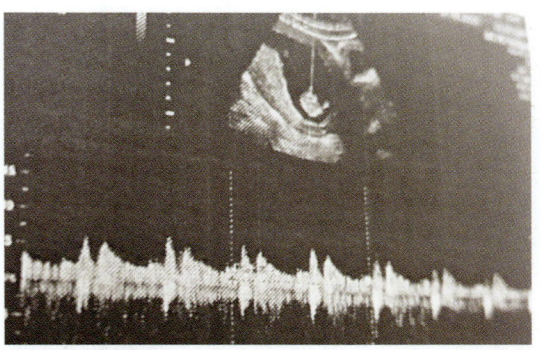

FIGURE 16.51 Foetal Cardiac Activity

FOETAL CARDIAC ACTIVITY

Foetal cardiac activity (Fig. 16.51). With transvaginal USG, foetal cardiac activity can be picked up by 6 weeks in M-mode. Foetal cardiac activity may be seen even before a foetal cell mass can be identified. The foetal cardiac activity is one of the earliest signs that the pregnancy is viable.

CROWN–RUMP LENGTH (CRL) (FIG. 16.53)

CRL (Fig. 16.52) is the measurement of the length of human embryo and foetus from the top of the head (crown) to the bottom of the buttocks (rump). It can be used to estimate gestational age. From 7 to 12 weeks, crown–rump length is predictive of gestational age ±4 days.

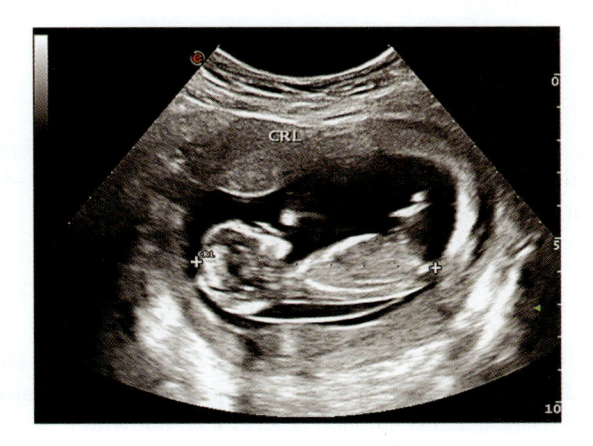

USG FINDINGS OF MISSED ABORTION (FIG. 16.53)

USG shows large gestational sac without visual evidence of a yolk sac. Hence, it can be blighted ovum.
Absence of growth of the gestational sac or foetal pole over a 5-day period of observation; absence of a visible foetal heartbeat when the CRL is greater than 5 mm; gestational sac larger than 8 mm mean

FIGURE 16.52 CRL

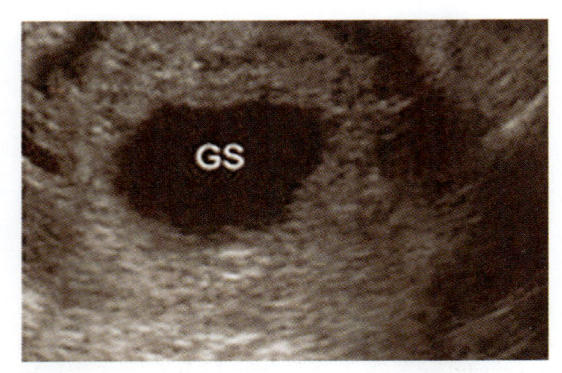

FIGURE 16.53 Missed Abortion

diameter without visual evidence of a yolk sac; foetal pole more than 4 mm diameter, without cardiac activity; yolk sac that is abnormally shaped or echogenic (sono dense rather than the normal sono lucent); loss of foetal cardiac activity that was previously seen.

Management: sometimes expulsion of products of conception occurs spontaneously.

When pregnancy is less than 10 weeks, instead of surgical methods, medical methods are useful in expulsion of the products followed by curettage, if medical method fails.

Products are to be sent for HPE.

When products are retained for more than 5–6 weeks, risk of DIVC develops.

Question regarding diagnosis, DIVC and other complications, management of missed abortion can be asked.

USG FOR NT (FIG. 16.54)

USG for NT is done at 11–13.6 weeks. It is a translucent nuchal space (anechoic space) at the posterior part of foetal neck. It is a soft marker for trisomy 21, 13, 18, Turner's syndrome and other chromosomal defects. When NT is >3 mm, it is a strong marker for chromosomal anomaly.

USG OF VESICULAR MOLE

USG of vesicular mole is a sonographic appearance of a complete hydatidiform mole. The classic sonographic appearance is that of a collection of blood with numerous small (3–10 mm) anechoic spaces (snowstorm or granular appearance) (Fig. 16.55).

Questions related to gestational trophoblastic tumours can be asked.

TWIN PEAK SIGN

The twin peak sign (Fig. 16.56) (also known as the lambda twin peak sign) is an ultrasound finding that is helpful in determining the chorionicity of a multi-foetal pregnancy especially in early pregnancy up to 14–16 weeks. Placental tissue extends into and tapers to a point within twin membranes.

Dichorionic twins present with a 'lambda sign' but its absence does not exclude it.

USG PICTURES   209

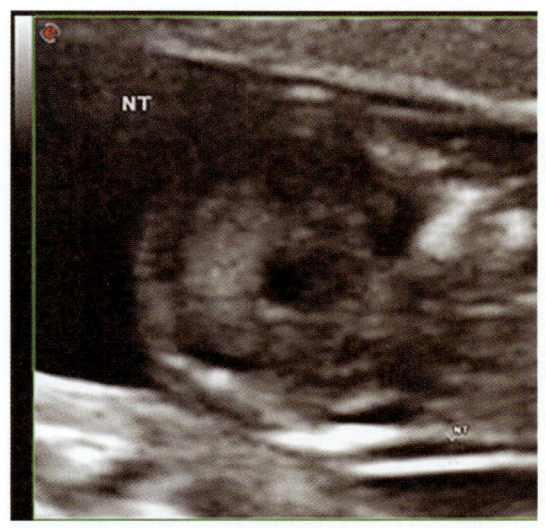

FIGURE 16.54   Nuchal Translucency

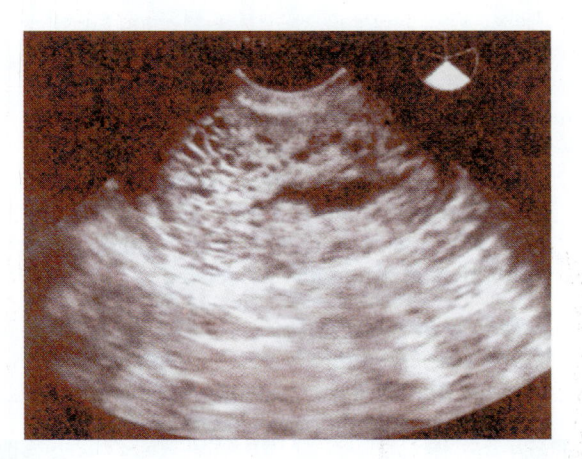

FIGURE 16.55   Vesicular Mole

From Manuel of Obstetrics, fourth ed., Shirish p. 252 Fig. 38.4.

T SIGN (FIG. 16.57)
T sign is an USG finding in monochorionic diamniotic pregnancy. The presence of a 'T-sign' at the inter-twin membrane–placental junction is indicative of monochorionic-diamniotic twin (the junction between the inter-twin membrane and the external rim forms a right angle).

PLACENTA PREVIA
USG show entire placenta covering the internal os (Fig. 16.58).

210 CASE 16 VIVA VOCE (ORAL EXAM)

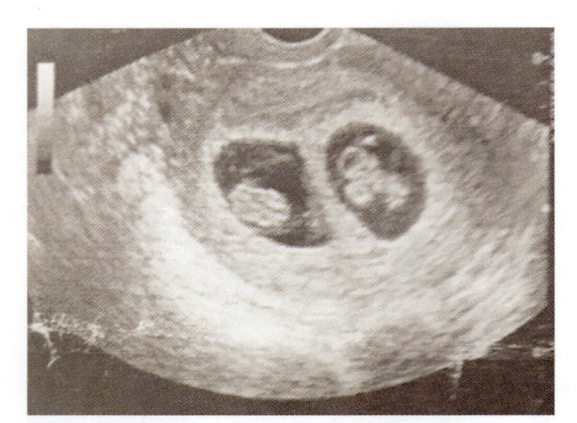

FIGURE 16.56 Twin Peak Sign

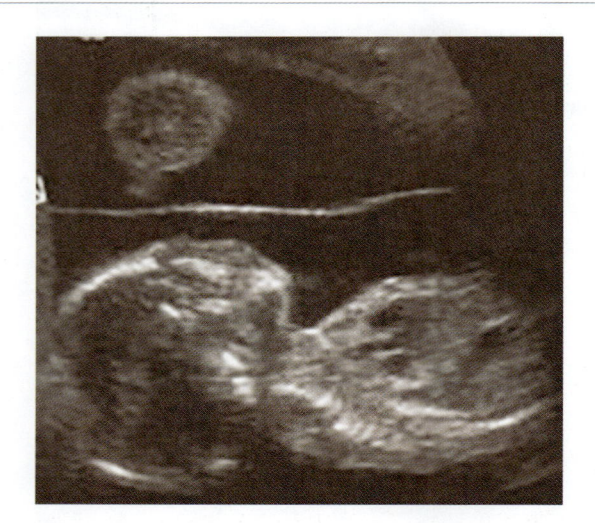

FIGURE 16.57 T Sign

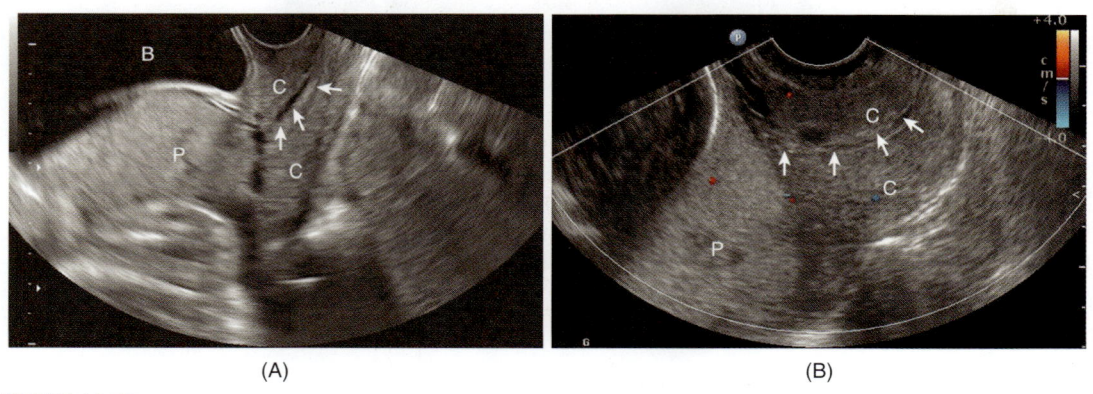

(A) (B)

FIGURE 16.58

(A) Partial Placenta Previa (B) Total Placenta Previa

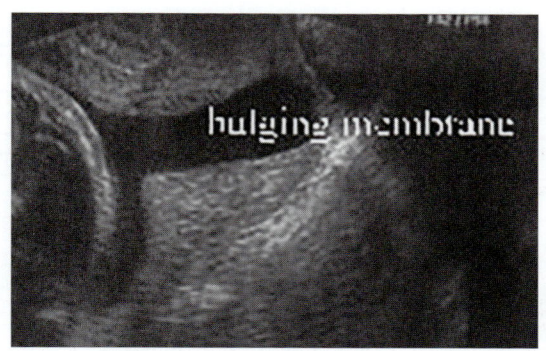

FIGURE 16.59 Incompetent os

Main symptom of placenta previa is painless bleeding usually at the end of second and third trimester.

Management: expectant or McAfee regime followed when GA < 37 weeks, patient is stable, not in labour.

Active line—when GA > 37 weeks, bleeding is profuse, foetus is dead, patient in labour.

For total placenta previa—LSCS.

Question about placenta previa, differential diagnosis and management can be asked.

USG PICTURE OF INCOMPETENT OS

USG picture shows a short (about 2–3 cm) cervix with dilated internal os with bulging membrane (Fig. 16.59).

In cervical incompetence, there will be painless spontaneous dilatation of the cervix. It is a common cause of second trimester pregnancy loss. Treatment is encerclage. Refer RPL Case 13.

Any questions related to abortion, gestational sac in the adenexa with vascularity (ring of fire) its treatment and causes for recurrent pregnancy loss can be asked.

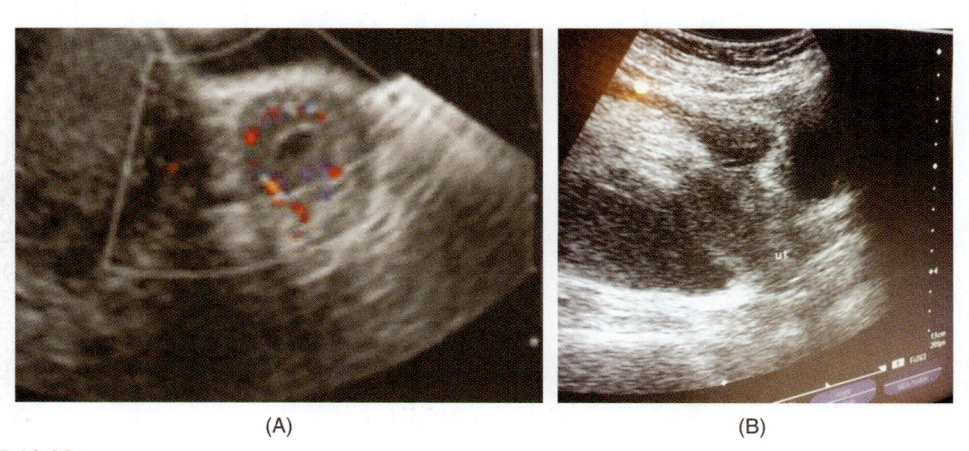

FIGURE 16.60

(A) Gestational sac in adenexa, (B) USG empty uterus with fluid in POD.

From Manual of Obstetrics, fourth ed., Shirish p. 232 Fig. 33.2.

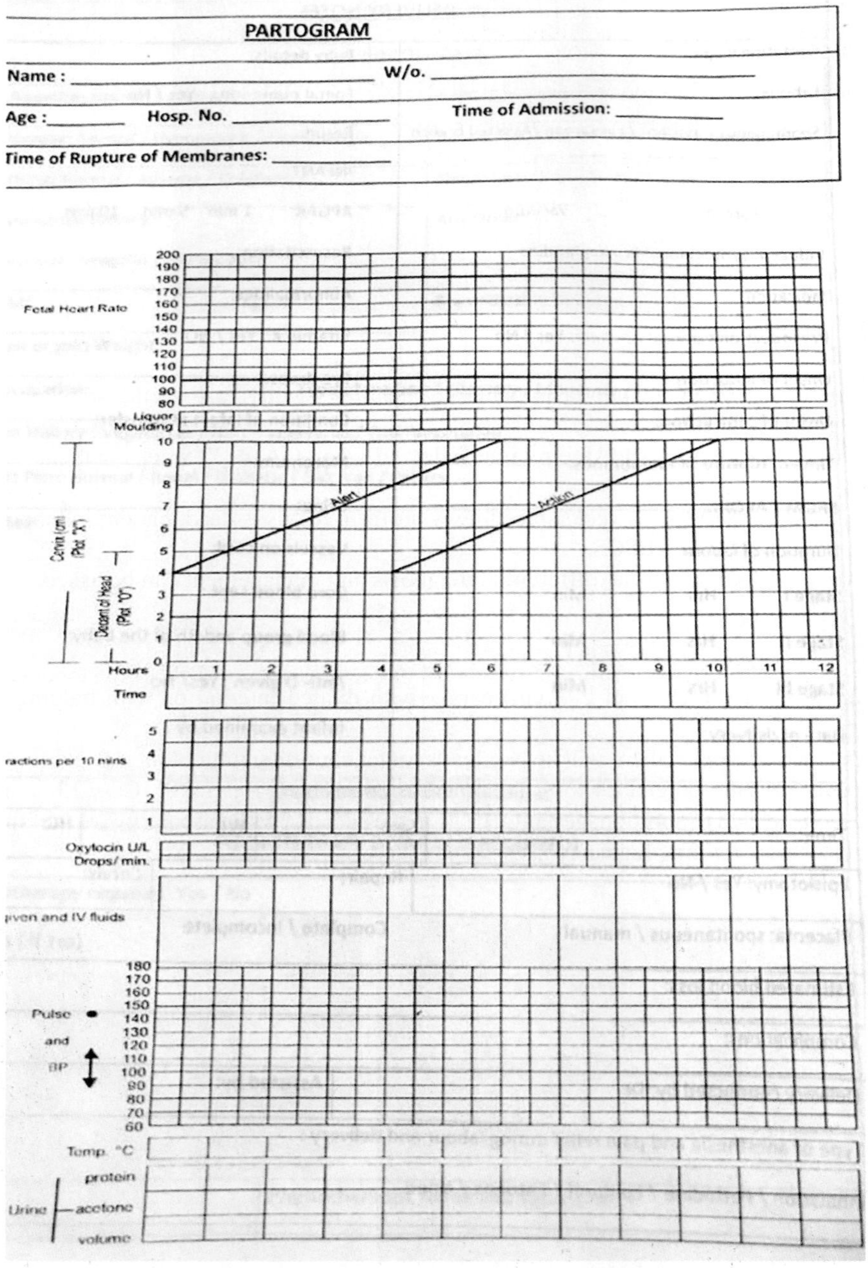

FIGURE 16.61 Partogram

USG SHOWS ECTOPIC GESTATION

Fig. 16.60A–B shows empty uterus with adnexal cyst with internal echo like foetal pole—unruptured ectopic gestation.

Fig. 16.60B shows fluid collection in the pouch of Douglas and empty uterus—may be ruptured ectopic gestation.

Questions related to ectopic gestation can be asked.

PARTOGRAM (FIG. 16.61)

Partogram is graphical representation of all the events in labour.

Partogram has three components namely foetal records, maternal records and progress of labour and it is marked in nine compartments.

In the partogram, rate of cervical dilatation and descent of head is plotted in *Y*-axis, against time in *X*-axis.

Rate of cervical dilatation in multi is 1.5 and 1 cm/h in primi. Progress of labour is assessed by descent of head and dilatation of cervix.

Alert line is drawn from 4 to 10 cm dilatation of cervix and it indicates rate of dilatation and therefore if line of cervical dilatation moves towards right of the Alert line it indicates slow or delay in progress.

Action line is drawn 4 h towards right of Alert Line.

When cervical dilatation crosses this line definite decision for appropriate management is to be taken.

Questions regarding Friedman curve, progress of labour, causes for dystocia in labour can be asked.

PART 2

GYNAECOLOGICAL CASES

1. GYNAEC CASE SHEET WRITING 217
2. A CASE OF VAGINAL DISCHARGE 233
3. A CASE OF ABNORMAL UTERINE BLEEDING 241
4. A CASE OF GENITAL PROLAPSE 255
5. A CASE OF FIBROID UTERUS 265
6. A CASE OF CANCER CERVIX 275
7. A CASE OF INFERTILITY 289
8. A CASE OF PRIMARY AMENORRHOEA 299
9. A CASE OF SECONDARY AMENORRHOEA 307
10. A CASE OF OVARIAN TUMOUR 315
11. A CASE OF POST-MENOPAUSAL BLEEDING PV 325
12. A CASE OF URINARY INCONTINENCE 333
13. VIVA VOCE EXAMINATION IN GYNAECOLOGY 339

CASE 1

GYNAEC CASE SHEET WRITING

GYNAECOLOGICAL HISTORY TAKING AND PHYSICAL EXAMINATION

To present the gynaec case in an organized way one should know the outline of history taking. History should be taken in a systematic way so that important facts are not missed which will give a clue to the diagnosis. If there is a detailed history of the patient taken and good physical examination done, it will lead to probable diagnosis and relevant investigations to be done and gives an idea about risk factors and prognostic indicators.

Introduce yourself and be polite and gentle towards the patient.

PATIENT'S DETAILS AND HISTORY

Name………………………....... Age…………. Address……………….. Occupation…………………..
Socioeconomic class……………............ Parity……………......... Present complaints……………..............
Menstrual history……………………......... Marital history……… Obstetric history………………..........…..
Contraception history ………….. Past medical history…………… Past surgical history……………
Past treatment history……………………. Family history…………….. Personal history ……………..

IMPORTANCE OF AGE (TABLE 1.1)

Table 1.1 Common Gynaecological Problems, Which Can Occur in Various Age Groups

Children	Adolescent Age	Reproductive Age	Older Age
Vaginal discharge, bleeding, foreign body in the vagina, sexual abuse	Pain abdomen, mass abdomen, menstrual problems, vaginal discharge, cyclical abdominal pain, urinary symptoms like retention of urine, not attained menarche, precocious puberty	Symptoms of pregnancy-related complications like incomplete abortion, missed abortion, septic abortion, vesicular mole, ectopic gestation, inability to conceive, pain abdomen, menstrual problems, mass abdomen, vaginal discharge, mass descending from vagina, urinary symptoms like burning micturition, retention and frequency of micturition, urge incontinence, stress incontinence.	Problems associated with menopause, pain abdomen, mass abdomen, post-menopausal bleeding PV, vaginal discharge, urinary symptoms like frequency, urge incontinence, stress incontinence and retention of urine

OCCUPATION

Occupation of woman and her husband gives an idea about the socioeconomic status.
Working in stressful work environment can give rise to menstrual problems.
In case of infertility—husband's occupation is important like night shift, working in hot environment, frequent traveller to be elicited.

IMPORTANCE OF SOCIOECONOMIC CLASS

Lower socioeconomic class prone for cancer cervix, tuberculosis, reproductive tract infection
Higher socioeconomic class prone for endometriosis, obesity leading to anovulation, endometrial carcinoma

IMPORTANCE OF PARITY

Multi-incidence of cancer cervix and genital prolapse are more common.
Nulliparous—fibroid, endometriosis, endometrial carcinoma. Ovarian tumours are more common.

PRESENT COMPLAINTS

Following basic complaints for which a woman can approach gynaecologist:
- Menstrual problems
- Pain abdomen
- Vaginal discharge
- Mass abdomen
- Mass descending P/V
- Problems related to coitus

MENSTRUAL PROBLEMS

- *Heavy menstrual bleeding* (HMB) (menorrhagia—cyclical menstrual bleeding which is excessive in amount, duration or both) more than 7 days or more than 80 mL
- Frequent cycles (*polymenorrhoea or epimenorrhoea*) less than 21 days
- Frequent cycles with HMB (*polymenorrhagia*)
- Infrequent cycles (*oligomenorrhoea*) more than 35 days
- Scanty periods with normal cycle (*hypomenorrhoea*)
- Painful periods—*dysmenorrhoea*
- Absence of periods—*amenorrhoea*
- Irregular inter-menstrual bleeding—*metrorrhagia*

When there is HMB, elicit following history:
- How many pads she uses per day?
- Whether it is fully soaked, partly soaked, or only spotting.
- Association with clots.

- Whether it affects her routine work.
- Normal menstrual blood loss is 50–80 mL and menstrual blood does not clot because of the fibrinolytic activity. When there is excessive menstrual bleeding normal fibrinolytic activity is not enough to lyse the clots present and clots may be passed.

Causes of menorrhagia
- AUB
- *Pelvic causes*: fibroid, adenomyosis, pelvic inflammatory disease (PID), endometriosis, early TB endometritis, IUCD, feminising ovarian tumour
- *Endocrine causes*: hypothyroidism and hyperthyroidism in initial stages
- *Blood dyscrasias*: idiopathic thrombocytopenic purpura (ITP), leukaemia, bleeding and coagulation disorders like Von Willebrand's disease
- *Systemic causes*: liver disorder (inability to conjugate oestrogens)
- *Functional*: emotional upset

Causes of hypomenorrhoea
- Asherman's syndrome, later stages of TB endometritis, OCP use, thyroid dysfunction

Causes of oligomenorrhoea
- PCOD, obesity, hyperprolactinemia, hyperthyroidism, strenuous exercise

Causes for polymenorrhoea
- Usually due to accelerated follicular phase

Causes for metrorrhagia
- Cervical polyp, cancer cervix, tuberculous ulcer of cervix, endometrial/fibroid polyp, prolapse of uterus with decubitus ulcer

Dysmenorrhoea
- It can be primary or secondary
  - *Primary*—spasmodic dysmenorrhoea—pain starts with menstruation or starts with menstruation in the absence of pelvic pathology and gradually intensity of pain lessens with onset of flow by 2nd day. It is usually associated with constitutional symptoms like vomiting and sweating. Pain is spasmodic, suprapubic, radiates to back and thigh
    - It is mostly seen in nulliparous individuals in ovulatory cycle. Women with anxiety and stress are more prone for this disorder
  - *Secondary dysmenorrhoea*—secondary to pelvic pathology
    - Occurs few years after menarche. Pain starts a few days before menstruation and increases with onset of menstruation

Spasmodic dysmenorrhoea
- Cramping pain secondary to underlying organic disease of the pelvic organs like submucus fibroid, endometrial polyp, IUCD

Congestive dysmenorrhoea
- Pain will be present preceding and during periods and may indicate—fibroid, endometriosis, PID, adenomyosis, IUCD in situ

Triple dysmenorrhoea
- Pain before, during and after periods (typical of endometriosis and adenomyosis)

Membranous dysmenorrhoea
- It is actually a type of spasmodic dysmenorrhoea characterized by the passage of an endometrial cast

Amenorrhoea
- It may be physiological or pathological
    - Physiological—occurs before menarche, during pregnancy, lactation and after menopause.
    - Pathological—primary amenorrhoea or secondary amenorrhoea

Primary amenorrhoea—failure of onset of menstruation before the age of 16 years regardless of the development of secondary sexual characters. Presently the upper age limit is reduced to 15 years due to decrease in mean age of menarche.

Primary amenorrhoea is defined as absence of menses by 13 years of age when there is no development of secondary sexual characters or absence of menses by 15 years of age when there is development of secondary sexual characters

Common causes—chromosomal, dysfunction in hypothalamo pituitary axis (HPO) axis, genital tract developmental defects

Secondary amenorrhoea—Absence or failure of occurrence of menstruation for 6 months or a length of period 3 times the previous menstrual cycles in women who have previously menstruated

Common causes—HPO axis dysfunction, PCOD, stress and emotional upset, premature ovarian failure, thyroid dysfunction, hyperprolactinemia, TB endometritis

PAIN ABDOMEN

Following points to be elicited:
- Site/duration/nature/radiation/aggravating and relieving factors/relation to menstrual cycle
- Period of amenorrhoea/cyclical pain (due to cryptomenorrhoea—occurrence of menstruation without external bleeding, due to imperforate hymen or transverse vaginal septum/cervical atresia) (Table 1.2)

Table 1.2 Different Causes of Pain

Lower Abdominal Acute Pain	Period of Amenorrhoea With Pain Abdomen	Chronic Dull Aching Lower Abdominal Pain
May be due to PID	During pregnancy or with use of OCP—red degeneration of fibroid	PID
Torsion of ovarian cyst, torsion of pedunculated-fibroid	Pregnancy related causes like, any type of abortion, ectopic gestation—(TRIAD of symptoms—amenorrhoea, pain abdomen, bleeding PV)	Non-gynaec conditions
Rule out other surgical conditions—appendicitis, ureteric colic		
UTI		

PID, Pelvic inflammatory disease.

VAGINAL DISCHARGE

Following features are noted:
- Colour/amount/odour/itching/relationship to menstrual cycle/nature of the discharge
- Curdy white—*moniliasis or candidiasis*
- Profuse, slightly greenish/creamy, frothy—*trichomoniasis*
- Greenish white, homogenous, malodorous discharge—*bacterial vaginosis*
- Associated with itching—*moniliasis and trichomoniasis*
- Pruritus in relationship to menstrual cycle—premenstrual pH of vagina is acidic and hence pruritus due to moniliasis gets improved after periods and pruritus due to trichomoniasis get worsened after periods (due to alkaline pH)
- Blood stained discharge—cervical lesions like polyp, erosion, cervicitis, cancer cervix
- Presence of systemic disease—diabetes, long-term illness, patient on broad-spectrum antibiotics and immunocompromised state can cause vaginal Moniliasis. Oral pill usage increases chances of monilial infection.

MASS ABDOMEN

Following points to be noted:
- Duration/site/whether associated with pain and vomiting/constitutional symptoms
- Pressure symptoms/association with menstrual problems
- Acute pain with mass—one has to rule out torsion of subserous fibroid and torsion of ovarian mass
- Mass abdomen with menstrual problems may be due to *fibroid/endometriosis/adenomyosis ovarian tumour—sex cord-stromal tumours (feminizing or functioning ovarian tumour)—granulosa/theca cell tumour*

MASS DESCENDING P/V

- Common causes—prolapse uterus, infravaginal elongation of cervix, fibroid polyp, cervical polyp inversion of uterus
- History in uterine prolapse—following history should be asked for:
  - Duration, presence of precipitating factors like chronic cough, ascites, constipation, details about child birth like duration of labour, place of birth, weight of the baby and spacing of child birth
  - Urinary symptoms like frequency and burning micturition (due to cystitis)
  - Difficulty in initiating act of micturition—mass has to be reduced before micturition because intra-abdominal pressure is raised during straining and urine is pushed into cystocele below the level of internal meatus
  - Incomplete emptying of bladder and stasis leads to cystitis
  - Stress urinary incontinence may be present due to descent of bladder neck and internal urinary meatus below the level of pelvic floor muscles and lack of support to urethral sphincter
  - Associated low back pain due to stretching of uterosacral ligament
  - Vaginal discharge due to decubitus ulcer
  - Associated bowel disturbances, constipation and sense of incomplete emptying in rectocele, incontinence of flatus or stools (due to complete perineal tear)

PROBLEMS RELATED TO COITUS

- Painful coitus (dyspareunia)
- Superficial dyspareunia—due to vulvovaginitis, pain during penetration
- Deep dyspareunia—deep seated pelvic pain during or after intercourse due to endometriosis, PID

HISTORY
MENSTRUAL HISTORY

- Should include present and past menstrual cycle
- Age of menarche—onset of first menstruation
- Cycle length—from first day of periods to next periods
- Normal 28 days ± 7 days
- Duration of flow—Normal 3–5 days
- Amount of flow—how many pads she soaks per day—whether fully soaked, partly soaked or spotting, passage of clots (indicates HMB)
- Painless periods may indicate anovulation
- Whether associated with pain or not—if so whether it is present before, during or after periods
- Regularity of the cycle—whether it occurs at regular intervals

For example:

1. Cycle can be expressed as 4/28 days regular, moderate, painless, LMP
2. 6–10/35–45 days, irregular, profuse with clots, painful, LMP

Age of menarche (mean age 10–16 years, peak 12–13 years)
Precocious puberty: development of progressive isosexual secondary sexual characteristics before the age of 8 years and menarche before 9 years
Delayed puberty: absence of secondary sexual characters by 13 years and menarche by 15 years
Primary amenorrhoea: absence of menarche by 15 years, regardless of the development of secondary sexual characters

MARITAL HISTORY

- Duration of marriage
- In case of infertility—whether she is living with her husband. H/O consanguineous marriage

OBSTETRIC HISTORY

- H/o abortion, parity, number of children and mode of delivery, number of live babies, last child birth, birth weight of the babies in prolapse of uterus

CONTRACEPTION HISTORY

- Temporary or permanent method. Combined pill or low dose pill or emergency pill, barrier method, natural method, intra-uterine contraceptive device—duration of usage

- Permanent: puerperal sterilisation or interval sterilisation, either by conventional method or by laparoscopy

PAST MEDICAL HISTORY
- Diabetes, hypertension, tuberculosis, thyroid problems, asthma, allergy, epilepsy H/O radiation H/O chemo therapy

PAST SURGICAL HISTORY
- H/O previous gynaec surgeries like diagnostic/operative laparoscopy for fibroid, endometriosis, Fothergill's operation, myomectomy, vaginal or abdominal hysterectomy, surgery for vault prolapse

TREATMENT HISTORY AND SCREENING TEST
- History of previous treatment for present complaints. Past or present medications, for example, treatment for infertility
- Screening test—previous Pap smear and it's report if available

FAMILY HISTORY
- Fibroid uterus, ovarian, uterine, breast malignancy and any other malignancy, tuberculosis, diabetes, hypertension

PERSONAL AND SOCIAL HISTORY
- Smoking, alcohol, drug abuse, H/O multiple sexual partners and diet.

EXAMINATION
PHYSICAL EXAMINATION
Proper general examination and systemic examination is mandatory in every patient. This should be followed by thorough gynaec examination. She should be explained about the speculum and pelvic examination and procedure is to be carried out after getting permission. A lady attendant should be present during examination by a male doctor

GENERAL EXAMINATION
- *Build*: thin—hyperthyroid, (menstrual problem, infertility), obese—PCOD, infertility, endometrial carcinoma, hypothyroidism
- *Nourishment*: moderately nourished/poorly nourished—anorexia nervosa, tuberculosis, malignancy

224 CASE 1 GYNAEC CASE SHEET WRITING

- *Stature*:
  - Short stature—may be due to constitution/Turner's syndrome
  - Tall may be due to androgen insensitivity syndrome
- *Anaemia*: can occur in AUB, fibroid, other causes of abnormal uterine bleeding, malignancy
- *Pedal oedema* may be due to pressure symptoms in cases of huge fibroid, malignant ovarian tumour or huge benign ovarian tumour, anaemia with CCF due to menorrhagia
- *Jaundice*
- *Lymphadenopathy*: superficial lymph nodes and left supra clavicular node—Virchow's node (indicates secondaries from ovarian malignancy)
- *Thyroid*: menstrual problems may be due to hypo- or hyperthyroidism
- *Breast*: discharge—serous/blood stained/, milky discharge (galactorrhoea), lump
- *Vitals*: pulse, BP
- *Temperature*: febrile in acute PID
- *Respiratory and cardio vascular system* to be examined

ABDOMINAL EXAMINATION

This is like any other abdominal examination, which includes fundamentally inspection, palpation, percussion and auscultation

- *Inspection*: look for distension, mass, engorged veins, swelling in the hernial orifices, any surgical scar
- *Palpation*: bladder should be empty before examining the patient (Fig. 1.1)
  - If mass is present following points to be noted:
    - Situation—which quadrant it occupies
    - Size
    - Borders—lower pole is not felt in uterine swelling except in subserous fibroid, whereas lower pole is felt in ovarian mass

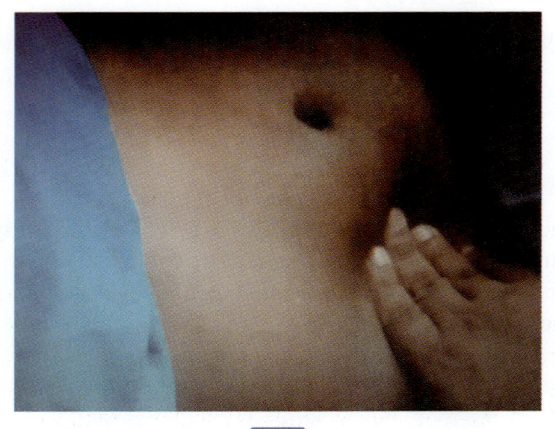

FIGURE 1.1 Palpating the Mass

Scan to play Examination of mass abdomen

- Consistency—soft or cystic—benign ovarian mass, solid–fibroid, ovarian malignancy/hard and variable—malignant ovarian tumour
- Tenderness—(torsion ovarian tumour or subserous fibroid, PID) or non-gynaec causes like appendicitis, ureteric colic, cystitis, diverticulitis
- Mobility—mesenteric cyst—oblique mobility, across right hypochondrium to left iliac fossa (perpendicular to the attachment of the mesentery), ovarian cyst—side to side and if with long pedicle upwards and downwards mobility may be present
- Rigidity—indicates peritonitis
- Hepatomegaly and splenomegaly to be ruled out in all cases
- *Percussion*: shifting dullness and fluid thrill should be tested when ascites or ovarian tumour is suspected
  - In ascites: flanks will be dull on percussion. Shifting dullness will be present
  - In the presence of mass: mass will be dull on percussion with resonance in flanks
- *Auscultation*: in big uterine fibroid, uterine souffle will be heard

GYNAEC EXAMINATION

This examination is very essential and challenging part. It is very sensitive to the woman and hence done in privacy and should be done gently and patient should be covered up to below knee and one should make the woman comfortable

Gynaec examination includes inspection of the vulva, labia majora, minora and clitoris. Inspection of vagina and cervix done with speculum. Per vaginal examination is a bimanual examination. Sometimes one has to do per rectal examination

Inspection:
- Inspect—mons pubis, pubic hair type
- Labia majora and minora—if any ulcer is present one should describe it. Redness/scratch marks—present in case of vulvovaginitis
- Vulva—swelling, growth or ulcer to be noted
- Enlargement of clitoris (clitoromegaly)—may be present in primary amenorrhoea or virilising tumours of the ovary
- Urethral meatus—sub-urethral nodule (chorio carcinoma)/urethral caruncle
- Presence of cystocele, rectocele, descent of cervix—if present to be noted.
  - *Various positions for gynaec examination*:
    - Dorsal position: patient's legs flexed at the hip and knee with feet resting on the examination couch (Fig. 1.2).
    - Sim's lateral position: woman will be on left lateral position with left knee extended and right knee flexed and she can be asked to hold the right thigh. This position is used in cases of prolapse uterus to look for enterocele and rectocele (Fig. 1.3).
    - Lithotomy position: flexion at hip, thighs are abducted and knees are partly flexed and feet are placed in lithotomy rods. This position is usually used in vaginal surgeries (Fig. 1.4).
- *Procedure for Sim's speculum examination*:
  - It is usually done in dorsal position and can be done in Sim's position also. Labia minora is separated with index finger and thumb of left hand to visualise introitus and gently with right hand, Sim's bivalve speculum which is pre sterilised is introduced.

226 CASE 1 GYNAEC CASE SHEET WRITING

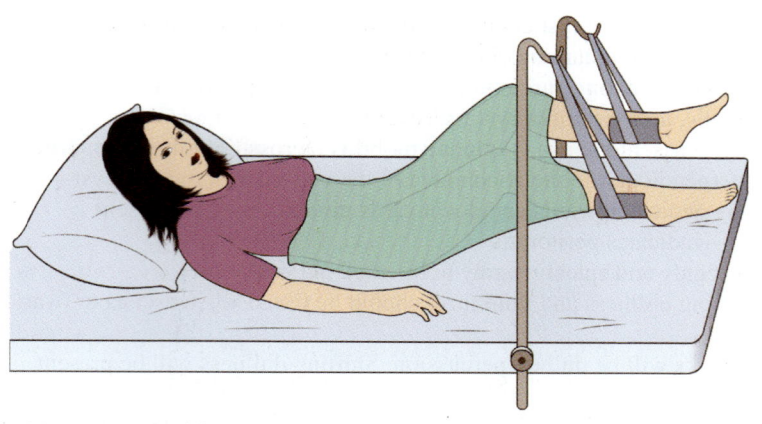

FIGURE 1.2 Dorsal Recumbent Position

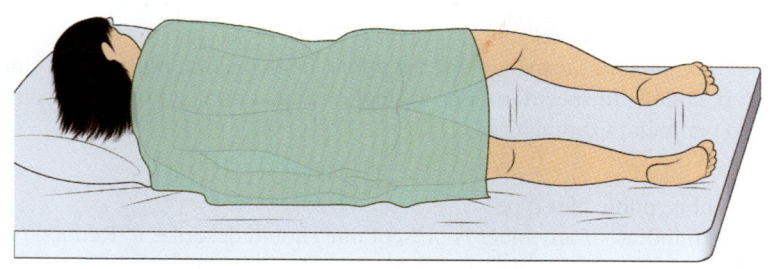

FIGURE 1.3 Sim's Left Lateral Position

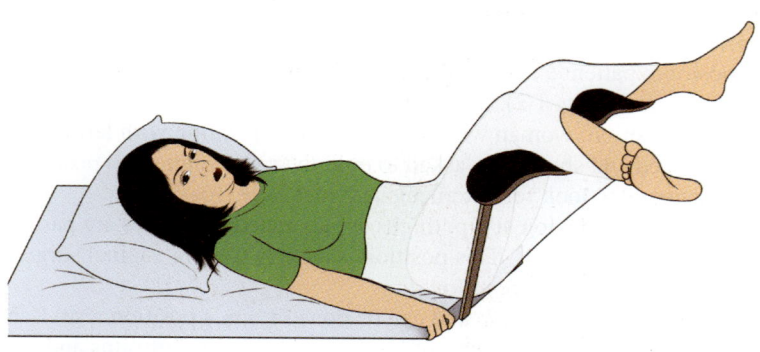

FIGURE 1.4 Lithotomy Position

- One blade of the speculum is held in the palm and the other blade gently introduced into the introitus with blade parallel to the introitus and gently advanced anteriorly or posteriorly to visualise the cervix and the vagina.
- Care should be taken during removal also and should be done gently.
  - Sim's speculum is used for visualisation of vagina and cervix (ulcer, polyp and erosion of cervix, vaginal or cervical discharge) (Figs 1.5–1.6 ▶)
  - Cusco's bivalve self-retaining speculum can be used to visualise the cervix and not the vagina. No need for assistant to hold the speculum (Figs 1.7 ▶ and 1.8)

Pelvic examination is always bimanual (to be avoided in virgins with intact hymen)

- *Procedure for pelvic examination:*
This is done in dorsal position with empty bladder. Middle and index fingers of the right hand with palmar aspect facing upwards, is gently inserted into the vagina and left hand is kept over the lower abdomen and bimanual examination is done.

In bimanual examination, middle and index fingers of the right hand are introduced into the vagina to palpate the cervix and fingers of the left hand are kept over the suprapubic region to find

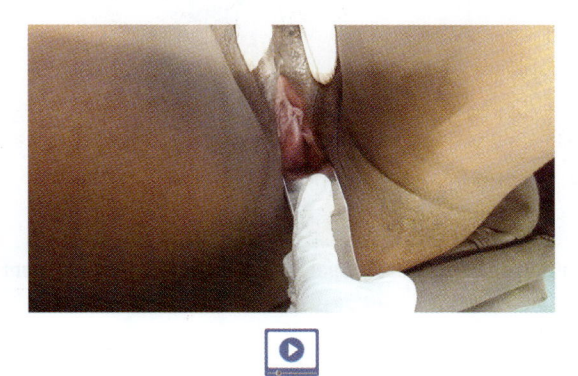

FIGURE 1.5 Visualisation of Anterior Vaginal Wall Using Sim's Speculum

▶ Scan to play How to use Sim's speculum

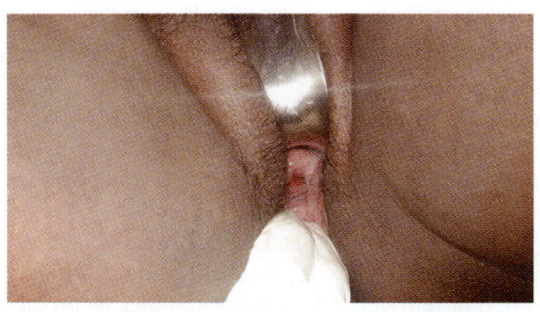

FIGURE 1.6 Visualisation of Cervix and Posterior Vaginal Wall Using Sim's Speculum

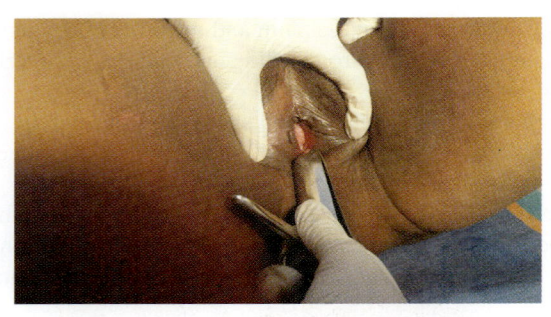

FIGURE 1.7 Introducing the Cusco's Speculum

Scan to play How to use Cusco's speculum

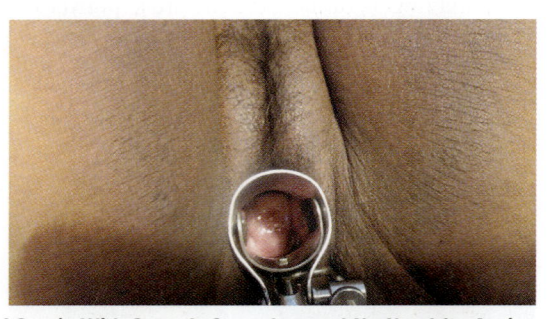

FIGURE 1.8 Visualisation of Cervis With Cusco's Speculum and No Need for Assistant

out the size of the uterus. Then the fingers in the vagina are gently moved towards one fornix and fingers on the abdomen to the iliac fossa of the same side to find out if there is mass in the fornix and then moved to the other fornix (Figs 1.9–1.11).
- *During bimanual pelvic examination following points are noted*:
  - Cervix
    - Position of cervix—cervix points forwards in retroverted uterus and backwards in anteverted uterus
    - Tenderness on cervical movement—ectopic gestation, PID
    - Movement of cervix—when movement of cervix is transmitted to the mass felt per abdomen, it is uterine swelling. If it does not move, it may be ovarian mass
  - Uterus
    - *Size*—enlarged in fibroid, adenomyosis, endometrial carcinoma, pyometra, haematometra, may be irregularly enlarged in fibroid. Uniformly enlarged in adenomyosis
    - *Position*—anteverted or retroverted (retroverted in uterine prolapse). Fixed retroversion occurs in PID and endometriosis

EXAMINATION   229

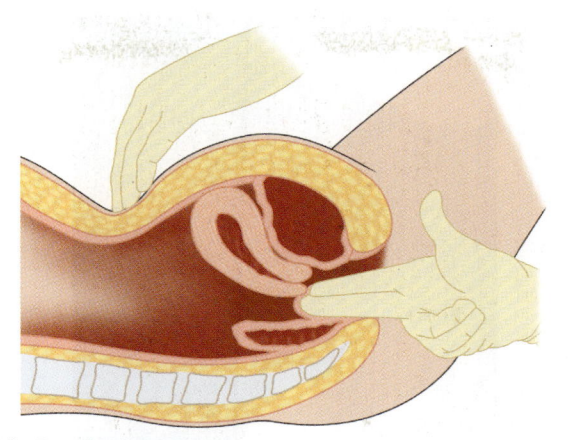

FIGURE 1.9   Bimanual Pelvic Examination Procedure

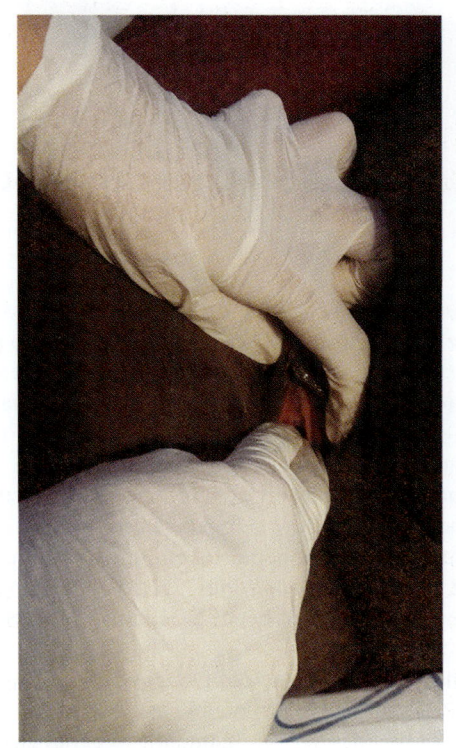

FIGURE 1.10   Gentle Insertion of Middle and Index Finger

230 CASE 1 GYNAEC CASE SHEET WRITING

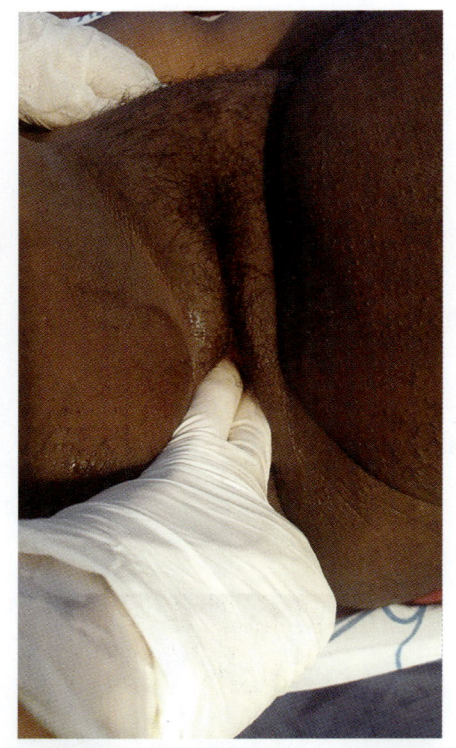

FIGURE 1.11 Fingers in the Vagina Will Palpate Cervix Left Hand is Kept Over Lower Abdomen to Asses Size of Uterus

- *Consistency*—soft in pregnancy, pyometra, haematometra, firm in fibroid and adenomyosis
- *Mobility*—fixed in endometriosis, PID cancer cervix—due to parametrial infiltration
- *Forniceal palpation*: feel for mass—its size and shape (retort shaped in hydrosalpinx)
  1. Tenderness—ectopic gestation, tubo-ovarian mass (TO mass)
  2. Adnexal mass—consistency—tense and cystic in benign ovarian mass firm in endometriosis and firm to hard or variable in malignancy
  3. When ovarian mass is very closely adherent to uterus the movement of cervix will be transmitted to the mass, and may be mistaken for uterine swelling
  4. Pedunculated uterine mass can be mistaken for ovarian mass

Per rectal examination (P/R): *In following conditions, P/R is done.*
- *In unmarried women*—hymen is intact and hence P/V cannot be done and hence P/R has to be done.
- *Endometriosis*—nodules may be felt in pouch of Douglas.
- *Ovarian malignancy*—nodules may be felt in pouch of Douglas.
- *Cancer cervix*—infiltration of the uterosacral ligament and parametrial involvement to stage the disease.

- To rule out the involvement of rectal mucosa in cancer cervix.
- *Uterine prolapse*—to diagnose rectocele.

SUMMARY
- The detailed history and physical examination done properly will help to make differential diagnosis or provisional diagnosis and helps to decide about investigations to be done.
- All points must be presented briefly, with regard to gynaec history, obstetric history, past medical or surgical history, physical examination and diagnosis must be made.

DIAGNOSIS
For example, mention about degree of prolapse with or without cystocele/rectocele/enterocele with or without decubitus ulcer.

CASE 2

A CASE OF VAGINAL DISCHARGE

PATIENT'S DETAILS

Name.. Age................. Address.......................... Occupation.............
Socioeconomic Class......................... Para........................

PRESENT COMPLAINTS

- C/O vaginal discharge:
    - Duration
    - Consistency—sticky—candidiasis
    - Colour—curdy white—candidiasis, yellowish—Trichomonas infection
    - Odour—fishy (*Gardnerella vaginalis*), foul smelling—cancer cervix
    - Blood stained—cancer cervix, polyp, erosion cervix
    - Intermittent profuse watery discharge (hydrops tubae profluens)
    - Associated with itching—Trichomonas infection and candidal infection
    - H/O local drug application, vaginal douche, deodorants and H/O allergy or contact dermatitis
- *Pruritis in relation to menstrual cycle*: premenstrual pH of vagina is acidic and hence pruritus due to moniliasis improves after periods. Pruritus due to trichomoniasis worsens after periods (due to alkaline pH)
- *In addition to aforementioned following details to be elicited*: diabetes and hepatitis, chronic illness on long-term antibiotics, immunosuppressive drugs, steroids, HIV, pediculosis or scabies, use of intrauterine contraceptive device/oral pill, foreign body insertion in children, recurrent reproductive tract infection, pigmentation or depigmentation—(vulval dystrophy)

• History suggestive of UTI (dysuria) • H/O painful coitus (dyspareunia) • H/O pain lower abdomen and low back pain	All these symptoms indicate pelvic inflammatory disease (PID)

HISTORY

MENSTRUAL/MARITAL/PAST OBSTETRIC HISTORY/CONTRACEPTIVE HISTORY/MEDICAL/SURGICAL/FAMILY HISTORY/PERSONAL HISTORY

- Refer Case 1

To view the lecture notes log in to your account on www.MedEnact.com

PAST MEDICAL HISTORY
- Previous H/O abnormal discharge may indicate reproductive tract infection. H/O abortion/recent child birth—PID
- H/O tuberculosis/diabetes/exposure to STI

EXAMINATION
GENERAL EXAMINATION
- As in Case 1

LOCAL EXAMINATION
- *Vulva*—following points are to be noted—redness, scratch marks, excoriation, signs of inflammation, curdy white discharge, lesions like tinea, scabies, ulcer, cancerous lesion, pigmentation or depigmentation
- *Speculum examination*: to visualise vagina and cervix
- *Vagina*—the following points are to be noted:
  - Yellowish frothy discharge and inflamed vagina, strawberry spots indicate—*Trichomonas infection.*
  - Curdy white discharge, which tends to stick to vagina and inflamed vagina indicates—*moniliasis or candidiasis.*
  - Profuse non-itchy discharge—suggest bacterial vaginosis, *ulcer or growth in vagina.*
  - Intermittent profuse watery discharge occurs in *tubal carcinoma known as hydrops tubae profluens.*
- *Blood stained discharge*: cervical—erosion, polyp, ulcer, cancerous growth, ulcer or growth in vagina

BIMANUAL PELVIC EXAMINATION
- Examination is done to assess uterine size, tenderness, mobility and adnexal swellings to rule out associated problems like PID, rarely tubal disease

SUMMARY
Name.......................... years old.......................... parous woman.......................... having excessive discharge PV.................... duration.................. describe nature of discharge................... any systemic illness.......................... any h/o previous medication

DIAGNOSIS
Vaginal discharge for evaluation

INVESTIGATIONS
ROUTINE AND SPECIFIC INVESTIGATIONS
SPECIFIC INVESTIGATIONS
- *Vaginal discharge*:
  - *Wet film* preparation in saline—motile flagellate organism—*Trichomonas vaginalis*
  - *Wet film*—clue cells (presence of epithelial cells with bacteria)—*bacterial vaginosis*
  - *Wet film* in KOH—hyphae seen in *candidiasis*
- *Whiff test*—fishy odour when KOH is added—*bacterial vaginosis*
- *Gram stain* of vaginal discharge and urethral swab for *gonococci*
- *Vaginal discharge* for culture and sensitivity—Saboraud's medium—*candidiasis*
  - Feinberg Whittington medium—*Trichomonas* Vaginalis
  - Blood agar or Thayer Martin medium—*Gonococcus*
- *Pap smear*—refer cancer cervix Case 6
- *VIA*, visual inspection with acetic acid; *VILI*, visual inspection with Lugol's iodine—refer cancer cervix Case 6
- *Biopsy cervix*—when ulcer is present biopsy is to be taken at edge of ulcer including the normal tissue. Biopsy is also to be taken whenever there is a growth in the cervix
- *Colposcopy*—in indicated cases
- *When tuberculous ulcer is* suspected as aetiology—other tests for tuberculosis and biopsy from lesion is to be taken
- *Urine sugar and blood sugar* to rule out diabetes in cases of candidiasis
- *Urine bile salts and serum bilirubin to rule out acute or chronic liver disease* which may cause pruritus vulva

CASE DISCUSSION
VAGINAL DISCHARGE
- *Definition of leucorrhoea*: excessive normal vaginal discharge which is non-purulent macroscopically and microscopically and non-offensive, non-irritant, and never causes pruritus
- *Physiological causes for leucorrhoea*:
  - *During puberty*—due to increased levels of oestrogen
  - *Around ovulation*—peak rise of oestrogen
  - *Pre-menstrual phase*
  - *During sexual intercourse*
  - *Pregnancy*—hyperoestrogenism with increased vascularity
- *Normal vaginal pH*:
  - 5.7 in newborn
  - 6–8 in children
  - 4 at puberty
  - 4.5 in reproductive age group
  - 4 in pregnancy
  - 7 in menopause

CASE 2 A CASE OF VAGINAL DISCHARGE

- *Normal defence mechanism of genital tract*:
  - *Vulva:* Apposition of the labia protects entry of organisms. Apocrine glands secretion is rich in undecylenic acid, which is fungicidal.
  - *Vagina*: Apposition of anterior and posterior vaginal walls.
    Mature well developed stratified squamous epithelium.
    Vaginal pH is normally acidic, lower than 4.5 and it is maintained by lactic acid produced from glycogen in epithelial cells by Doderlein's lactobacilli.
    It is dependent on the presence of oestrogen. Whenever acidity is reduced, the pathogenic organisms will be able to survive.
  - *Cervix:* Cervical mucus is bacteriolytic.
  - *Uterus:* Endometrium sheds periodically which tend to eliminate any infection, which may try to gain access.
  - *Tubes:* Tubal ciliary movements towards uterus prevents ascending infection.

Types of Abnormal Vaginal Discharge, Their Probable Cause and Management

Type of Discharge	Probable Diagnosis	Morphology	Clinical Features	Treatment
Profuse, thin creamy or slightly green in colour, irritating and frothy	Trichomoniasis	Protozoa, actively motile, have anterior flagella central axostyle, moves along the mucous membrane	Discharge causes pruritus, strawberry-vagina (Fig. 2.1). Can have urinary problems, dysuria, dyspareunia	Metronidazole 200 mg t.d.s. × 7 days. For both partners or 2 g metronidazole single dose
Thick, curdy or flaky discharge	Candidiasis (moniliasis)	Commonest organism—*Candida albicans*, Gram-positive, grows in acid medium	Vaginal irritation pruritus, vaginal wall congested, discharge visible at the vulva (Fig. 2.2), mucocutaneous junction and in posterior fornix	Anti-fungal agents like imidazole, miconazole, clotrimazole-creams × 3–6 days; clotrimazole-vag tab 100 mg × 7 days oral; single dose of fluconazole 150 mg, ideally both partners to be treated
White, milky, non-viscous discharge adherent to vaginal wall, non-itchy, may be foul smelling pH (5–7)	Bacterial vaginosis (termed vaginosis because it is associated with alteration in normal vaginal flora and not due to any specific infection)	Polymicrobial condition caused by *Haemophilus vaginalis, Gardnerella/Mobiluncus/Mycoplasma hominis. Mobiluncus* is a Gram-positive curved rod with cork-screw spinning anaerobe	Women will have minimal vulval irritation, congestion of vaginal walls (Fig. 2.3)	Metronidazole 500 mg twice daily × 7 days, ampicillin 500 mg or cephalosporin 500 mg b.i.d. × 7 days, clindamycin locally or orally 300 mg × 7 days
Purulent vaginal discharge	Gonococcal vulvovaginitis	Gram-negative intracellular diplococcus-*Neisseria gonorrhoea*	Discharge, vaginal inflammation, vulval, irritation, pruritus, dysuria, rectal discomfort	Inj. cefoxitin 2 g IM plus probenecid 1 g orally × 14 days. Followed by doxycycline 100 mg b.i.d or oral tetracycline 250 mg q.i.d. × 14 days. Treat male partner

CASE DISCUSSION **237**

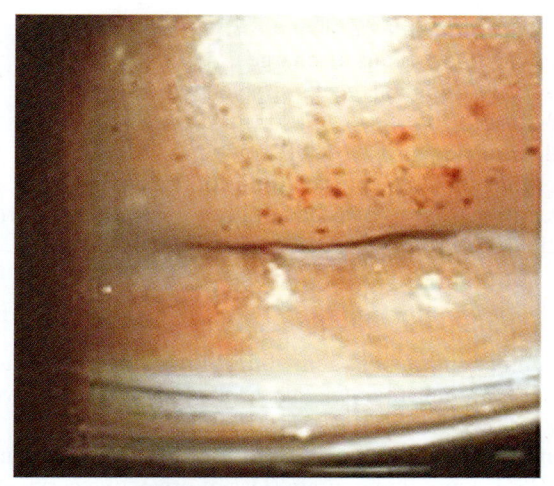

FIGURE 2.1 Trichomoniasis Strawberry-Appearance of Cervix

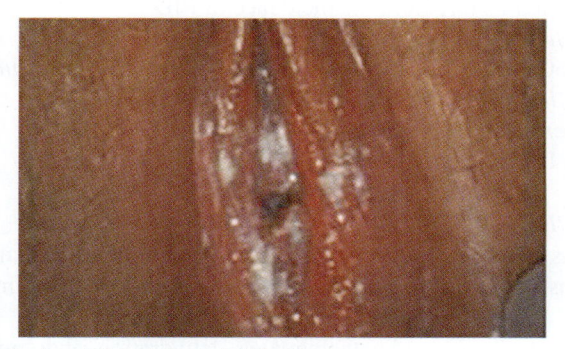

FIGURE 2.2 Moniliasis Vaginal and Vulval-Curdy White Discharge

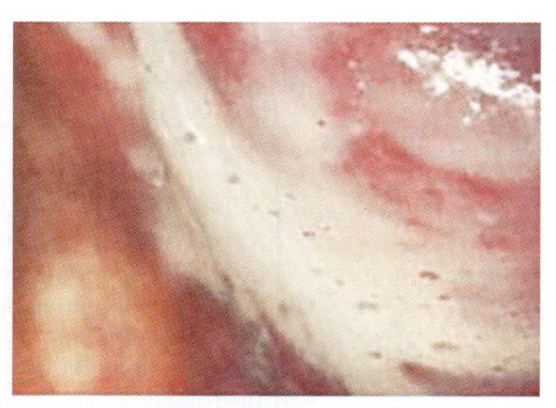

FIGURE 2.3 Bacterial Vaginosis Milky, Non-Viscous, Non-Itchy Discharge

- *Amsel's criteria for diagnosis of bacterial vaginosis*:
  - Thin, white or yellow, homogeneous discharge
  - Clue cells on microscopy—epithelial cells stippled with bacteria
  - pH of vaginal fluid > 4.5
  - Release of fishy odour on adding 10% KOH solution
  - At least three out of four should be present for a confirmed diagnosis

  The modified Amsel's criteria says two instead of three out of the four criteria to be present to diagnose bacterial vaginosis

PELVIC INFLAMMATORY DISEASE CAUSES VAGINAL DISCHARGE

- *Definition of PID*: inflammation of upper genital tract involving uterus, tubes and ovaries
- *PID is result of polymicrobial infection due to ascending infection from vagina and endocervix and it can occur in the following events*:
  - Menstruation, abortion, delivery, manual removal of placenta (raw surface prone for infection)—D&C, HSG, sonosalpingogram (loss of protective cervical mucus resulting in ascending infection)
  - IUCD insertion increases threefold the incidence of PID
- *Organisms responsible in PID*:
  - STI accounts for 60%–70% of cases—*Gonococcus, Trichomonas, Chlamydia*
  - Pyogenic—*Staphylococcus, Streptococcus, Escherichia coli*
  - Anaerobes—*Bacteroides, Peptococcus*
  - *Actinomyces* with IUCD
  - Tuberculosis
- *Symptoms of acute PID*:
  - General symptoms and signs: pelvic pain, fever, mucopurulent vaginal discharge, painful coitus, heavy menstrual bleeding, painful periods, dysuria, urinary symptoms (Tables 2.1 and 2.2).
  - Patient may be febrile. Tachycardia, tachypnoea, dehydration, abdominal tenderness, rigidity, distension may be present.
  - S/E purulent vaginal discharge may be present.
  - P/V cervical motion tenderness.
  - Uterine tenderness, forniceal tenderness, tender TO mass, pelvic abscess may be present.

Table 2.1 Stages of Acute PID (Gainesville Classification)

Stage	Clinical Presentation
Stage I	Acute salpingitis without peritonitis—no adhesion
Stage II	Acute salpingitis with peritonitis—purulent discharge
Stage III	Acute salpingitis with superimposed tubal occlusion or tubo ovarian complex
Stage IV	Ruptured tubo ovarian abscess
Stage V	Tubercular salpingitis

PID, Pelvic inflammatory disease.

Table 2.2 Symptoms and Signs of Chronic PID

Symptoms	Signs
Lower abdominal pain, painful coitus	Tenderness in lower abdomen
Menstrual abnormalities like menorrhagia, dysmenorrhoea, polymenorrhoea, polymenorrhagia	Discharge from vagina, cervix
	Fixed retroverted, tender, uterus
Low back ache	Hydro salpinx, TO mass
Infertility	
Discharge PV	

- *Following are the investigations for PID*:
    - *Total count, differential count*—leucocytosis, raised ESR
    - *C-reactive protein*—elevated
    - *High vaginal swab* for culture and sensitivity
    - *Endo cervical smear* for gonorrhoea (diplococci) and chlamydia
    - *USG*—tubo ovarian mass, abscess
    - *Laparoscopy* is done in doubtful cases, to rule out other causes of acute abdomen like ectopic, appendicitis, torsion or rupture of ovarian cyst and endometriosis and it is also useful to stage the severity of PID
- *Treatment*

> The aim of the therapy is to cure the disease and prevent future infertility and chronic sequelae.

- *In mild cases*: ambulatory management can be advocated and admission is required if woman is not responding to treatment in 48 h.
- *Acutely ill patients and complicated cases with TO mass*: need hospitalisation and parenteral antibiotics
- *Medical*: cefoxitin 2 g IV 6th hourly and doxycyline 100 mg IV route followed by oral route or clindamycin 900 mg 1V 8th hourly + gentamycin 2 mg/kg every $\times$ 8 h for at least 48 h followed by doxycycline 100 mg b.i.d. $\times$ 14 days
- *Indications for surgery*:
    - Drainage of pelvic abscess—by laparotomy/laparoscopy/colpotomy
    - Not responding to medical treatment or worsening of the clinical condition
    - Removal of septic focus as in septic abortion
    - Laparotomy for suspected perforation, intestinal injury

KEY POINTS

- Leucorrhoea is an excessive normal vaginal discharge, which is not itchy and is non-purulent, non-offensive.
- Leucorrhoea can be physiological which occurs during ovulation, premenstrual, puberty, pregnancy and during sexual excitement.

CASE 2 A CASE OF VAGINAL DISCHARGE

- Pathological vaginal discharge is mainly infective and commonest infective conditions are trichomonas vaginitis, moniliasis and bacterial vaginosis.
- Amsel's criteria are used for diagnosing bacterial vaginosis.
- There are several defence mechanisms, which protect the women from infection.
- Evaluation of women with vaginal discharge is done by taking history about nature of discharge, physical examination, wet film examination, Gram staining and Pap smear.
- Partner must be evaluated and treated.
- Acute PID should be differentiated from acute appendicitis and ruptured ectopic.
- PID can be treated with antibiotics either as out patient or inpatient and in some instances women require surgical management.
- Infertility, tubal damage, ectopic pregnancy are late sequelae of PID.

FREQUENTLY ASKED QUESTIONS

1. What is leucorrhoea?
2. What are the common causes of vaginal discharge?
3. What are the causes of pruritus vulva?
4. How will you diagnose Trichomonas vaginitis and treat it?
5. How will you diagnose moniliasis and it's treatment?
6. What are Amsel's criteria for diagnosing bacterial vaginosis?
7. How will you diagnose bacterial vaginosis and treat it?
8. What are the normal defence mechanisms of genital tract?
9. What are the causative organisms for PID?
10. What are the stages of PID?
11. What are the symptoms of acute and chronic PID?
12. Cancer cervix questions—refer cancer cervix Case 6.

CASE 3

ABNORMAL UTERINE BLEEDING

PATIENT'S DETAILS
Name.. Age.................. Address........................... Occupation.............
Socioeconomic Class.......................... Para........................

PRESENT COMPLAINTS (MAY BE)
- Heavy menstrual bleeding during periods (menorrhagia)
- Frequent periods (polymenorrhoea)
- Frequent and profuse periods (polymenorrhagia)
  Previously mentioned complaints may be due to dysfunctional uterine bleeding (DUB), fibroid, adenomyosis, PID, endometriosis, IUCD usage, thyroid dysfunction, coagulation and bleeding disorder
- In case of intermenstrual bleeding (metrorrhagia), cervical polyp, submucous fibroid, fibroid polyp, cancer cervix, erosion cervix, TB cervix has to be ruled out
- Period of amenorrhoea followed by bleeding PV in reproductive age—pregnancy-related causes like abortion, ectopic gestation, vesicular mole has to be rule out, it can be due to metropathia haemorrhagica [anovulatory abnormal uterine bleeding (AUB), polycystic ovarian disease]
- Post-coital bleeding—cancer cervix, erosion cervix, cervical polyp, TB cervix has to be ruled out
- Pre- or post-menstrual spotting—may be due to irregular ripening and irregular shedding, respectively, which occurs in ovarian dysfunction
  Due to deficient corpus luteum and inadequate support of progesterone, irregular ripening of endometrium and break through bleeding occurs
  Patient will present with pre-menstrual spotting in irregular ripening
  Patient will present with post-menstrual spotting: in irregular shedding of endometrium that occurs due to persistent corpus luteum
- Irregular bleeding may be due to irregular intake of OCP, progesterone only pill

To view the lecture notes log in to your account on www.MedEnact.com

HISTORY

HISTORY OF PRESENT ILLNESS

After elaborating the present complaints, following history has to be elicited:

- If c/o heavy menstrual flow:
  - Duration of flow
  - Amount of flow—how many pads she soaks per day—whether fully soaked, partly soaked or spotting, history of passage of clots (indicates menorrhagia)
  - Clots are present because normal fibrinolytic activity in the uterus is not enough to take care of excessive bleeding
- Painless periods—may indicate anovulation (metropathia haemorrhagica)
- Painful menstruation—if present, whether pain is present before, during or after periods (causes may be fibroid, adenomyosis, endometriosis, PID, bleeding due to IUCD usage)
- Bleeding from other sites may be due to coagulation disorder
- History suggestive of anaemia like fatigue, palpitation, swelling of legs, chest pain
- Mass abdomen—to rule out fibroid, functioning ovarian tumour
- Increase in weight—to rule out myxoedema, PCOD
- Weight loss—rule out tuberculosis, malignancy, hyperthyroidism
- Recent change in physical activity or mental status, prolonged illness, drug intake
- Similar episodes in the past; if present, whether prior investigations or treatment for the same was undertaken by the patient

PREVIOUS MENSTRUAL HISTORY

- Age of menarche/regularity of menstrual cycles
- Flow—scanty/moderate/heavy
- Painful/painless—painful may mean ovulatory cycle, secondary dysmenorrhoea due to fibroid, endometriosis, adenomyosis; painless—anovulatory cycle
- LMP

PAST OBSTETRIC HISTORY

- If there is H/O abortion whether spontaneous or induced, period of amenorrhoea/when abortion occurred/medical abortion or surgical abortion/post-abortal period
- H/O vesicular mole, H/O IUCD insertion, number of deliveries and mode of delivery, H/O contraception—temporary or permanent method

CONTRACEPTIVE HISTORY

- Irregular intake of oral combined contraceptive pill, IUCD usage, and sterilisation can cause menstrual disturbances
- Since DUB is AUB in the absence of pelvic pathology and other systemic and endocrine disorder, proper history should be elicited to rule out other causes for AUB before arriving at a diagnosis of DUB

PAST MEDICAL HISTORY
- H/O bleeding disorder/coagulation disorder/H/O taking anti-coagulants/prolonged illness and drug intake (H/O hormonal treatment taken for the present complaint)
- H/O hypo or hyperthyroidism/H/O diabetes/hypertension/tuberculosis

PAST SURGICAL HISTORY
- H/O dilatation and curettage or hysteroscopy for AUB in the past

FAMILY HISTORY
- Diabetes, PCOD, familial cancer (to decide about conservation of ovaries, if hysterectomy is contemplated, detailed family history should be taken—prophylactic removal of ovaries is advisable in woman with H/O familial cancer of ovary or breast in her relatives)

EXAMINATION
GENERAL EXAMINATION (REFER CASE 1)
Special attention to be paid for the following details:
- *Build*
    - Obese—PCOD, hypothyroidism
    - Lean—hyperthyroidism
- *Pallor*—indicates severity of bleeding
- *Vitals* to be checked
- *Breast and thyroid* to be examined
- *CVS and RS* to be examined

ABDOMINAL EXAMINATION
If mass is present—it could be fibroid Case 5 or ovarian tumour Case 10.

SPECULUM EXAMINATION
To rule out cervical lesion—erosion, growth, ulcer, polyp and to find out if bleeding is through the os and the amount of bleeding

BIMANUAL PELVIC EXAMINATION
- To find out the following:
    - *Uterine size*—if enlarged may be due to fibroid, adenomyosis
    - *Mobility and tenderness*—uterus may be fixed and tender in PID and endometriosis
    - *Adnexal mass*—present in cases of TO mass, endometriosis, ovarian mass
    - *In case of ovarian mass*—movement of cervix is not transmitted to the mass felt per abdomen; groove sign will be present
    - *In case of fibroid*—movement of cervix is transmitted to mass; groove sign will be absent

PER RECTAL EXAMINATION
- In case of cancer cervix, to stage the disease
- Ovarian tumour—nodules in POD
- Endometriosis—multiple small nodules (cobble stone feel of uterosacral ligament)

SUMMARY
- Name... Age................ Socioeconomic Class........................
  Parous/Nulliparous........................ c/o........................ in chronological order..............................
- Mention about general examination positive findings.................... abdominal examination findings

DIAGNOSIS
- Give only differential diagnosis in AUB—based on history and findings
- For example: if no positive findings are present in general examination, no history pointing to endocrine and systemic disease and if per abdominal findings and PV findings if known are—normal—probable diagnosis is AUB-O

INVESTIGATIONS
- *Haematological test*
  - Haemoglobin, PCV—to rule out anaemia
  - Platelets—to rule out idiopathic thrombocytopenic purpura (ITP)
  - Total count (rarely leukaemia may be the cause for AUB)
  - Bleeding time, clotting time
  - Coagulation profile—if bleeding diathesis or coagulation disorder is suspected or patient is on anti-coagulant therapy
- *Thyroid function test*
- *Pap smear—VIA, VILI, colposcopy/biopsy cervix*—when cervical pathology is suspected, biopsy cervix
- *USG—TAS/TVS*—following details are noted:
  - *Uterine size*—may be increased in the presence of fibroid/adenomyosis
  - *Endometrial thickness* (more than 12 mm in any phase in menstruating woman and more than 4 mm in post-menopausal woman is abnormal)
  - *Endometrial cavity*—presence of polyp, submucous fibroid may be present
  - *Adnexal mass* (TO mass/ovarian mass)
  - *Fluid in pouch of Douglas*
  - *In case of fibroid*—pressure effects on the ureter and kidney to be looked for
- *To rule out endometrial pathology, any one of the following tests can be done*:
  - Endometrial aspiration
  - Dilatation and curettage
  - Fractional curettage (above 40 years of age)
  - Hysteroscopy and directed biopsy

- *CT and MRI, when you suspect ovarian mass*
  - PET scan and FDG PET in cases of cancer cervix

CASE DISCUSSION
AUB

- AUB is defined as any bleeding from the genital tract, which is a deviation from normal in frequency, cyclicity or quantity
  - AUB includes organic causes and systemic causes
  - DUB is AUB without any demonstrable pelvic pathology or systemic and endocrine disorders

NORMAL MECHANISM TO CONTROL BLEEDING IN MENSTRUATION

- Platelet plug and clot formation causes haemostasis
- Vasoconstriction mediated by prostaglandins—PGF2 alpha and thromboxane
- Tissue repair

TYPES OF DUB: OVULATORY—20%; ANOVULATORY—80%

- Ovulatory—irregular ripening, irregular shedding, IUCD insertion, tubal sterilisation
- Anovulatory—threshold bleeding, puberty menorrhagia, metropathia haemorrhagica, pre-menopausal DUB

CAUSES OF AUB IN PUBERTAL/ADOLESCENCE AGE GROUP (AVOID PV/DILATATION AND CURETTAGE/PER RECTAL EXAMINATION CAN BE DONE IN RARE INSTANCES)

- It may be due to immature hypothalamo pituitary ovarian axis
- Bleeding and coagulation disorder—like Von Willebrand's disease, ITP
- PCOS
- Tuberculosis—early stage
- Thyroid disorders
- Feminising ovarian tumour

CAUSES OF AUB IN REPRODUCTIVE AGE GROUP

- DUB
- Thyroid disorder
- PCOS
- Pregnancy-related complications
- Problems related to contraception—temporary and permanent
- Fibroid, adenomyosis, ovarian tumour, PID
- Blood dyskaryosis—ITP/leukaemia—rare cause

CAUSES OF AUB IN PERIMENOPAUSAL AGE GROUP

- Anovulatory bleeding due to depletion of ovarian follicles
- Pre-malignant and malignant condition of uterus, cervix, ovary

- Other conditions like thyroid disorders
- Fibroid, adenomyosis, endometriosis, PID

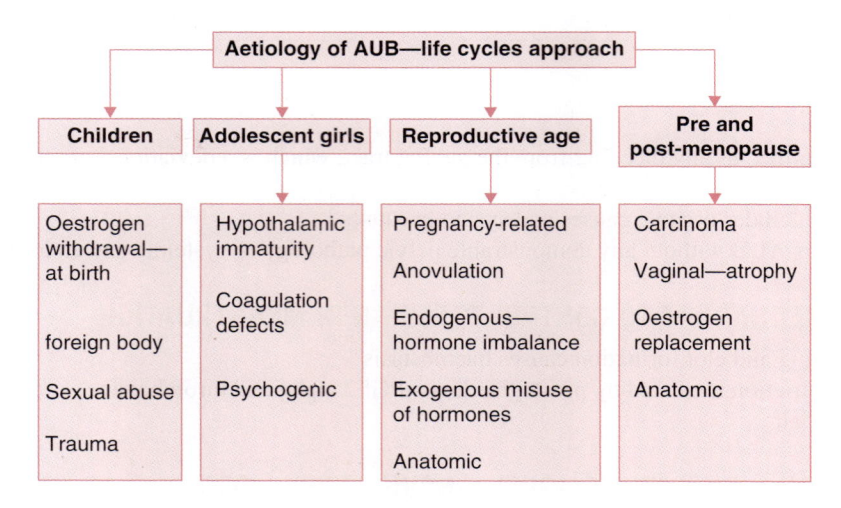

Aetiology of AUB—life cycles approach

Children	Adolescent girls	Reproductive age	Pre and post-menopause
Oestrogen withdrawal—at birth	Hypothalamic immaturity	Pregnancy-related	Carcinoma
	Coagulation defects	Anovulation	Vaginal—atrophy
foreign body		Endogenous—hormone imbalance	Oestrogen replacement
Sexual abuse	Psychogenic	Exogenous misuse of hormones	Anatomic
Trauma		Anatomic	

- FIGO classification system (PALM-COEIN) for causes of AUB in non-gravid women of reproductive age
  - **PALM structural causes** (Fig. 3.1A):
    – P—Polyp (AUB-P)
    – A—Adenomyosis (AUB-A)
    – L—Leiomyoma (AUB-L); sub-classification—SM-1–3, O-4–8
    – M—Malignancy and hyperplasia (AUB-M)

Polyp	
Adenomyosis	
Leiomyoma	→ Submucosal
Malignancy and hyperplasia	Other

| Coagulopathy |
| Ovulatory dysfunction |
| Endometrial |
| Iatrogenic |
| Not yet classified |

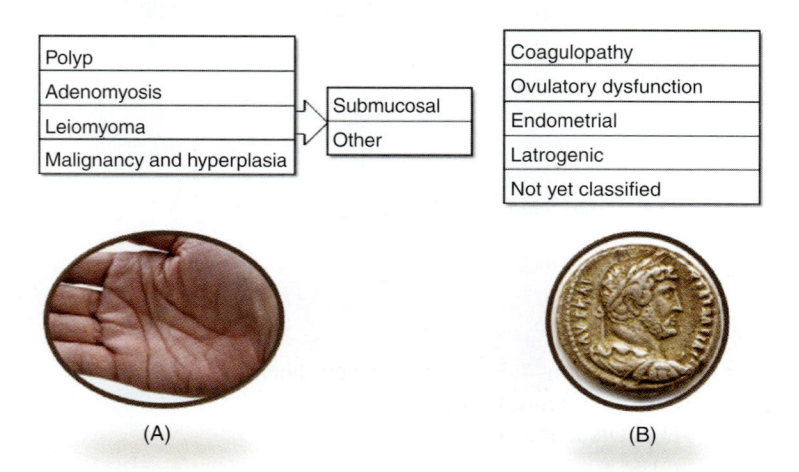

(A) (B)

FIGURE 3.1

(A) PALM structural causes and (B) COEIN non-structural causes.

From VG Pdubidri, SN Daftary, Shaw's textbook of gynaecology, 16th edition. Elsevier 2015: Fig 24.1. pp. 336.

- *COEIN non-structural causes* (Fig. 3.1B)
    - C—Coagulopathy (AUB-C)
    - O—Ovulatory dysfunction (AUB-O)
    - E—Endometrial (AUB-E)
    - I—Iatrogenic (AUB-I)
    - N—Not yet classified (AUB-N)
- Classification for leiomyoma depending on site of fibroid in relation to endometrium, myometrium and serosa

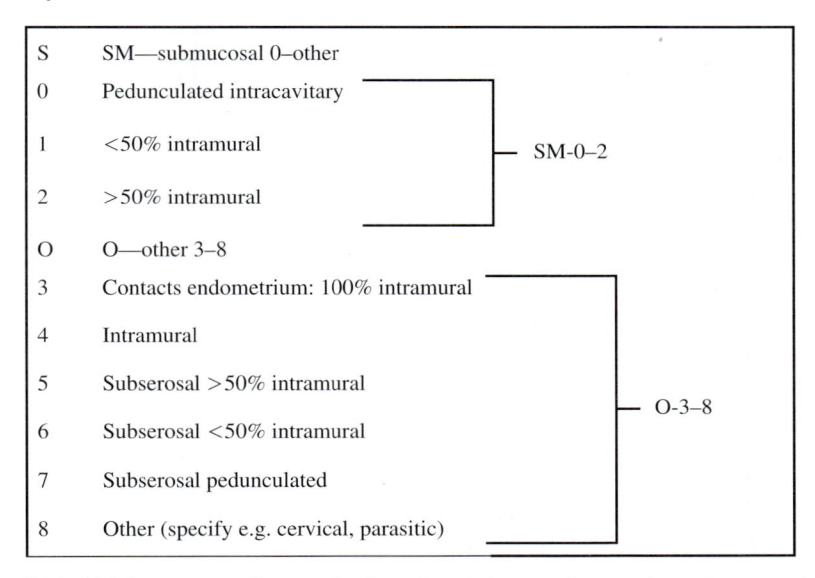

S	SM—submucosal 0–other	
0	Pedunculated intracavitary	
1	<50% intramural	SM-0–2
2	>50% intramural	
O	O—other 3–8	
3	Contacts endometrium: 100% intramural	
4	Intramural	
5	Subserosal >50% intramural	O-3–8
6	Subserosal <50% intramural	
7	Subserosal pedunculated	
8	Other (specify e.g. cervical, parasitic)	

Hybrid leiomyomas (impact both endometrium and serosa)—submucosal and subserosal, each are with less than half the diameter in the endometrial and peritoneal cavities, respectively.

METROPATHIA HAEMORRHAGICA (SCHROEDER'S DISEASE)
- Most commonly seen in perimenopausal women
- Ovarian follicles develop and oestrogen is produced but dominant follicles fail to develop and this leads to failure of LH surge
- There is no ovulation but formation of follicular cyst
- No progesterone is produced and unopposed oestrogen action on the endometrium causes prolonged periods of amenorrhoea
- When endometrium outgrows it's blood supply, bleeding occurs
- Bleeding is profuse and painless as there is lack of progesterone, which results in decreased vasoconstriction and decreased PGF_2 alpha
- The disease is characterised by 2–3 months of amenorrhoea, followed by painless, prolonged profuse bleeding
- Histopathology examination (HPE) of endometrium—Swiss cheese appearance—cystoglandular hyperplasia
- Investigations and management: similar to AUB-O

OVULATORY DUB

- *Irregular shedding*: Incomplete atrophy of corpus luteum due to incomplete withdrawal of LH resulting in persistent secretion of progesterone. Bleeding or spotting continues for variable period after regular periods
- *Irregular ripening*: Poor formation of corpus luteum and inadequate function leads to inadequate production of progesterone, which is inadequate to support the endometrial growth
- Slight bleeding or spotting starts before regular periods

TYPES OF ENDOMETRIAL PATTERN IN AUB

- Normal (60%)—proliferative endometrium or secretory endometrium
- Cystoglandular hyperplasia
- Simple hyperplasia—with or without atypia
- Complex hyperplasia—with or without atypia
- Complex hyperplasia with atypia—chances of malignancy if untreated—30%

CAUSES OF ENDOMETRIAL HYPERPLASIA

- Anovulatory cycles (unopposed oestrogen)
- Metropathia haemorrhagica
- Obese women
- PCOS
- Woman on tamoxifen
- Menopausal woman on HRT without progestogen
- Feminising ovarian tumours

FRACTIONAL CURETTAGE

- Indications:
  - AUB in women above 40 years
  - Post-menopausal bleeding, suspected endometrial carcinoma
- *Procedure*: Patient should be asked to empty the bladder
  - Under suitable anaesthesia, with patient in lithotomy position after cleaning and draping, bimanual examination is performed. Sim's speculum is introduced to retract the posterior vaginal wall and anterior lip of cervix is held with vulsellum.
  - Before introducing the uterine sound and dilating the cervix, endocervical curettings are taken and kept separately.
  - Then uterine sound is introduced to confirm uterine length and position.
  - Cervical canal is dilated with Mathew Duncun dilators and then uterine cavity is curetted by curette, starting from fundus, anterior, posterior and lateral walls of uterus including isthmus.
  - Endocervical and endometrial curettings are sent for HPE.
    Fractional curettage does not include ectocervical biopsy but if lesion is seen on the ectocervix, biopsy should be taken

ENDOMETRIAL ASPIRATION

- It can be done easily with Pipelle or Vabra aspirator without anaesthesia as out-patient procedure. This can be done for post-menopausal women where cervical canal is narrow.
  Adequate sample of endometrium can be obtained.

DILATATION AND CURETTAGE

It is done mainly for diagnostic purpose. It is therapeutic in 30%–40% of cases.
- *Diagnostic*:
  - To study the endometrial pattern
  - To rule out endometrial carcinoma
  - To rule out endometrial tuberculosis

INDICATIONS FOR HYSTEROSCOPY

- If facilities are available, it can be done for all cases of AUB
- It can be diagnostic as well as therapeutic in few cases
- Direct endometrial sampling can be done (advantage is that the exact area of pathology can be visualised and biopsy can be taken from that area)
- *Therapeutic* in the following conditions:
  - Removal of endometrial polyp
  - Removal of submucous fibroid
  - Excision of septum
  - Adhesiolysis in Asherman's syndrome

> Treatment of heavy menstrual bleeding depends on the age, her parity, desire for fertility and associated factors.

MANAGEMENT OF AUB

According to age group:
- *Adolescent age*
  - Treat general cause
  - Treatment is conservative, rule out coagulation disorders
  - Anaemia is corrected and reassurance is given
  - Thyroid dysfunction and coagulation disorders ruled out
  - Treatment is always medical management
  - Initially non-hormonal preparations like non-steroidal anti-inflammatory drug (NSAID), tranexamic acid and ethamsylate are prescribed to decrease blood loss
  - If bleeding is severe, medical curettage using progestogens are advocated to arrest bleeding as it is an anovulatory type
- *Reproductive age 20–40 years*
  - Rule out pregnancy-related problems
  - General—correction of anaemia, diet

- Medical—non-hormonal-NSAID, Tranexamic acid.ethamysylate/hormonal—OCP/Progestogens
- In refractory cases—D&C minimally invasive surgery, surgery—advocated
- *Perimenopausal age*
  - General, medical, surgical
  - Diagnostic curettage is mandatory before any therapy to exclude endometrial malignancy
- General Management: reassurance, diet, anaemia to be corrected

MEDICAL MANAGEMENT FOR AUB
NON-HORMONAL TREATMENT

- NSAID: mefenamic acid, naproxen, ibuprofen can be given during periods
- Anti-fibrinolytics: tranexamic acid, epsilon-aminocaproic acid
- Ethamsylate—prevents capillary fragility

HORMONAL TREATMENT

- To arrest bleeding (when curettage is not done): initial dose of 30 mg of medroxyprogesterone acetate or norethisterone acetate 30 mg is given for 24–48 h till bleeding stops. Dose is gradually reduced to 10 mg twice a day and then 10 mg once a day for a total of 21 days and then stopped. After 2–3 days withdrawal bleeding occurs. This is known as medical curettage
- Maintenance therapy of progesterone: it is usually given for correcting anovulatory cycles. Medroxyprogesterone acetate 10 mg from 15th to 25th day or for 21 days from day 5 for 3–6 cycles
- *MIRENA—LNG IUD: releases 20 µg of levonorgestrel daily and acts locally on the endometrium* It contains 52 mg of levonorgestrel. It causes glandular atrophy and stromal decidualisation. It has dual purpose of providing temporary contraception, as well as curing menorrhagia. Initially it results in scanty periods, later amenorrhoea may result
- OCP: reduces bleeding by 50%. It contains either 20 or 30 µg of ethinyloestradiol with 50–75 µg of levonorgestrel. It is given from 5th to 25th day and can be used for 3–6 cycles; OCP usage leads to better cycle control, controls heavy bleeding flow and corrects anaemia
- Ormeloxifene: SERM—selective oestrogen receptor modulator
Dose 60 mg twice weekly for 12 weeks then once weekly for another 12 weeks
- Danazol: 100–200 mg daily
  - Disadvantage: androgenic side-effects, acne, hirsutism, weight gain, reduced HDL
  - It is not used nowadays
- GnRh analogues:
  - Costly
  - Used when waiting for surgery or in women nearing menopause
  - To prepare endometrium prior to endometrial ablation
  - Injections—3.6 mg IM/monthly (leuprolide)
   When given for more than 6 months, ADD–BACK therapy with low dose oestrogen is to be given, since it causes hot flushes, coronary artery disease, and reduction in bone mineral density

SURGICAL TREATMENT
- Conservative surgery: minimally invasive surgery
- Hysterectomy
- *Concept of endometrial ablation*:
  Ablation causes hypomenorrhoea or amenorrhoea
    - *First generation* techniques: requires hysteroscopy
    - *Second generation*: easy to do and done under mild sedation and does not require hysteroscopy

MINIMALLY INVASIVE SURGERY
- *Indication*:
    - Failed medical therapy
    - Patient wants to conserve uterus
- *Contraindication*:
    - Young woman who wants to preserve fertility
    - Uterus more than 12 weeks
    - Large fibroids
    - Endometrial hyperplasia and carcinoma

ABLATIVE PROCEDURES
- *First generation—requires hysteroscopy*
    - Methods: transcervical resection of endometrium (TCRE), hysteroscope-guided resection
- *Second generation—does not require hysteroscopy and can be done under mild sedation*; it is easy to perform
- Methods:
    - Thermal ablation; microwave ablation
    - Radio-frequency-induced thermal ablation, laser ablation
    - Cavaterm balloon therapy
    - Novasure (impedance-controlled endometrial ablation)

Indications for Hysterectomy and Routes of Hysterectomy

Indications for Hysterectomy	Routes of Hysterectomy
Failed medical therapy	Total abdominal hysterectomy
In older women, endometrial hyperplasia with atypia	Non-descent vaginal hysterectomy
Failed endometrial ablation	LAVH
Associated pelvic pathology like adenomyosis, fibroid	TLH

Normal ovaries are preserved in women <50 years for hormonal function.
In women with H/O familial cancers and in women more than 50 years, ovaries are removed along with uterus.

LAVH, Laparoscopic-assisted vaginal hysterectomy; TLH, total laparoscopic hysterectomy.

STEPS OF ABDOMINAL HYSTERECTOMY
Refer Case 13.

Complications of Abdominaxl Hysterectomy

Immediate	Delayed	Remote
Anaesthesia—complications	Reactionary haemorrhage, abdominal distension paralytic ileus, peritonitis	Adhesion
Haemorrhage	UTI, thrombosis and pulmonary embolism	Incisional hernia
Injury to ureter, bladder, bowel		

- *Other methods of management*:
  Bilateral uterine artery embolisation used for intractable AUB in young woman

KEY POINTS
- AUB can occur at any age and if not treated timely, it can lead to anaemia and treatment depends on the age.
- Abnormal uterine bleeding is bleeding from genital tract, which deviates from normal in frequency, duration and amount.
- Anovulation occurs in adolescent and perimenopausal period and accounts for 80% of AUB.
- The classification of AUB is PALM–COEIN and first four causes namely polyp, adenomyosis, leiomyoma and malignancy will have structural uterine abnormality and are diagnosed by imaging modalities and histopathology.
- In adolescent girls, coagulatory disorders, thyroid dysfunction to be ruled out first and in perimenopausal and post-menopausal women, malignancy to be ruled out.
- For all age group, medical management with non-hormonal and hormonal treatment will be first line of management.
- LNG-IUS and minimally invasive procedures have almost replaced hysterectomy.
- Hysterectomy is the last resort for AUB.

FREQUENTLY ASKED QUESTIONS
1. Definition of DUB and AUB.
2. What are menorrhagia, polymenorrhoea, polymenorrhagia and metrorrhagia?
3. What is the mechanism of control of bleeding in normal menstruation?
4. What are the types of DUB?
5. What are the causes of puberty menorrhagia?
6. What is metropathia haemorrhagica?
7. What is irregular ripening, irregular shedding?
8. What are the causes for perimenopausal bleeding?

9. What are the causes for post-menopausal bleeding PV? Refer Case 11—post-menopausal bleeding PV.
10. How will you do Pap smear and its interpretation? Refer refer Case 6 on cancer cervix.
11. How to do dilatation and curettage, fractional curettage?
12. What is endometrial aspiration?
13. What are the drugs used in the management of menorrhagia?
14. What is endometrial ablation, what is the concept?
15. What is the minimally invasive procedure for AUB? What are first-generation and second-generation procedures?
16. Any questions from cancer cervix, fibroid, adenomyosis, endometriosis, ovarian tumour, endometrial cancer can be asked.

CASE 4

A CASE OF GENITAL PROLAPSE

PATIENT'S DETAILS
Name……………………..………. Age……..... Address…………………… Occupation………………
Socioeconomic Class……………………. Para………………….

PRESENT COMPLAINTS
Mass descending per vaginum—*following history is to be elicited*:
- *Duration*: whether mass is reducible or not (irreducible when oedematous, congested or inspissated with impacted faeces in rectocoele)
- *Micturition problems*: difficulty in initiating act of micturition—mass has to be reduced before micturition, because intra-abdominal pressure is raised during straining and urine is pushed into cystocoele, which is below the level of urethral meatus
  - Stress incontinence
  - Frequency, burning and painful micturition—due to incomplete emptying of bladder and stasis, which leads to infection and cystitis
  - Rarely urinary retention
- *Constipation*, sense of incomplete emptying due to rectocoele
- *Chronic cough*/lifting heavy weights/abdominal mass or distension of abdomen (ascites) which increases intra-abdominal pressure, which can lead to prolapse uterus
- *Vaginal discharge*/inter-menstrual bleeding/post-coital bleeding/post-menopausal bleeding—may indicate congestion/decubitus ulcer or cancer cervix
- *Usage of pessary*
- *Low backache* due to stretching of nerve fibres in uterosacral ligament

HISTORY
MENSTRUAL HISTORY, MARITAL HISTORY, OBSTETRIC HISTORY, CONTRACEPTIVE HISTORY, PAST MEDICAL AND SURGICAL HISORY, FAMILY HISTORY, PERSONAL HISTORY
Refer Case 1.

To view the lecture notes log in to your account on www.MedEnact.com

PAST OBSTETRIC HISTORY
Following history is to be taken in detail:
- Number of pregnancies
- Spacing between pregnancies
- Home delivery, unattended delivery, delivery conducted by untrained dhais
- Prolonged labour with head on the perineum for long time
- H/O episiotomy or H/O perineal tear
- Birth of big baby
- Forceps or vacuum delivery
- Early ambulation in puerperium

CONTRACEPTIVE HISTORY
Refer Case 1.

PAST MEDICAL & SURGICAL HISTORY
- Neurological disease—in cases of nulliparous woman (spina bifida etc.)
- Previous surgery for prolapse in case of recurrence of prolapse
- Hysterectomy in case of vault prolapse
- Previous abdominopelvic resection of rectum, radical vulvectomy leads to weakness of pelvic floor

PERSONAL HISTORY
Refer Case 1.

EXAMINATION
GENERAL EXAMINATION
As in Case 1
Special attention to be paid for the following details:
- *Respiratory system* to be examined to rule out chronic respiratory infection
- *Spine and neurological* examination to be done in case of nulliparous prolapse to find out spina bifida occulta

ABDOMINAL EXAMINATION
- Liver and spleen are palpated to rule out visceroptosis. Palpation is done to rule out mass in the abdomen/ascites

GYNAEC EXAMINATION
- *Inspection*:
    - *External genitalia*—normal or atrophic (atrophic in post-menopausal woman)
    - *Pubic hair*—normal or sparse
    - *Look for descent of cervix*—whether it is at the level of introitus or outside introitus

It should be described as pinkish globular mass lying outside the vulval outlet, it's size (cervix is made out by external os) or as cervix is seen lying outside the vulval introitus
- *Vagina*—rugosity is lost in post-menopausal woman; whether vagina is dry and scaly (post-menopausal woman); presence of ulcer and pigmentation of vagina to be noted
- *Cervix*—look for hypertrophy, erosion, keratinisation, oedema, congestion, pigmentation, ulcer
  If ulcer is present, it is to be described in detail—size, site, formation of slough, bleeding from it (ulcer can be due to decubitus ulcer produced by circulatory changes, congestion, stasis, denudation and ulceration or rarely due to malignancy Fig. 4.1 ▶)
- Look for the following:
  - Cystocoele—prolapse of the upper two-third of anterior vaginal wall
  - Uretherocoele—prolapse of lower one-third of anterior vaginal wall
  - Enterocoele—prolapse of upper one-third of posterior vaginal wall [herniation of pouch of Douglas (POD)]
  - Rectocoele—prolapse of lower two-third of posterior vaginal wall
  - Look for old perineal tear
- *Palpation*:
  - Whether mass is reducible or not
  - Whether you can get above the fundus of uterus

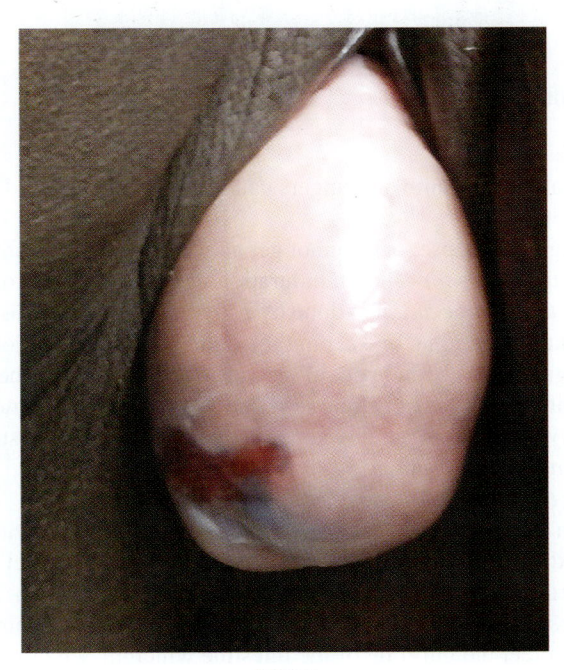

FIGURE 4.1 Third Degree Prolapse With Decubitus Ulcer

▶ Scan to play Examination of uterine prolapse

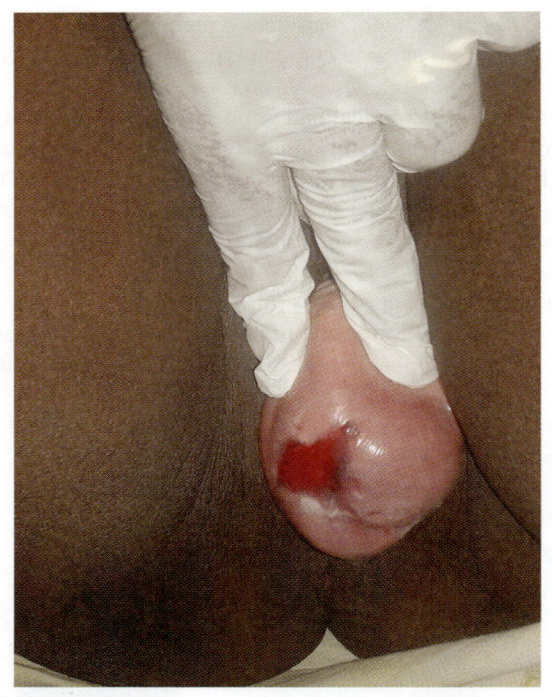

FIGURE 4.2 Third Degree Uterine Prolapse

- In case of procidentia, the thumb and fingers can be approximated and hence one can get above the fundus of uterus
- In case of third degree prolapse, one cannot get above the fundus of uterus Fig. 4.2
- *In case ulcer is present palpate for*—fixity, induration, whether it bleeds on touch
- *Assessment of tone of the levator ani*: it is done by palpating pubovaginalis fibres in the lateral wall of the lower one-third of the vagina, by keeping the thumb over labia majora and two fingers over lower one-third of vagina laterally and patient may be asked to contract the muscle as if trying to hold the act of micturition, and thus the tone of pubovaginalis part of levator ani is assessed
- *Perineal body integrity*: can be palpated by keeping two fingers in the posterior vaginal wall and thumb in the perineum above the anus
- *Differentiating points between enterocoele and rectocoele*:
  - Patient is placed in Sim's position and posterior lip of cervix is held with vulsellum and prolapse is reduced. Sim's speculum is introduced posteriorly to retract posterior vaginal wall. The patient is asked to strain and slowly Sim's speculum is withdrawn. If there is a bulge in the upper one-third posteriorly, it is enterocoele and bulge in lower two-third, then it is rectocoele.
  - Sometimes one can feel the gurgling of the intestine which may be the contents of enterocoele
  - During pelvic examination, patient is asked to strain. If the bulge hits the tip of the finger it is enterocoele and if it touches the pulp of your finger it is rectocoele
  - During per rectal examination, the patient is asked to strain. The rectal mucosa will slide over the finger. Fingers can also be hooked through rectocoele

BIMANUAL PELVIC EXAMINATION
- Uterine size/its position (retroverted in prolapse) fixity/adnexal pathology, if present are noted

PER RECTAL EXAMINATION
- To diagnose rectocoele

SUMMARY
Name........age........belongs to socio economic class nulliparous/parous...mention about her chief complaints with duration........

Mention about general examination findings........

Mention in local examination about inspection findings........describe about mass protruding from vagina, changes in cervix and if ulcer is present in the cervix describe it

DIAGNOSIS
Uterovaginal prolapse........degree with cystocoele/uretherocoele/rectocoele/enterocoele........with/without decubitus ulcer

DIFFERENTIAL DIAGNOSIS
- *Anterior vaginal wall cyst also called as Gartner's cyst*: which has well-defined margins and it is tense and cystic (Fig. 4.3). It cannot be reduced
- *Cervical polyp*: it will be attached to cervix or protruding through os. It may be a mucus polyp or fibroid polyp (Fig. 4.4) (firm polyp which can arise from cervix or seen protruding through cervix)
- *Chronic inversion*: cervix will not be felt and uterine fundus will be outside. Cervix felt as a rim higher and sound cannot be introduced (Fig. 4.5)
- *Congenital infravaginal elongation of the cervix*: fornices are deep and vaginal portion of cervix is long. Usually it is not associated with cystocoele, enterocoele, rectocoele. In uterovaginal prolapse, there will be supravaginal elongation of cervix
- *Urethral diverticula*
- *Prolapse of rectum*

INVESTIGATIONS
- *Urine analysis*—routine and culture sensitivity
- *Complete haemogram*—haemoglobin, PCV, TC, DC
- *Blood* urea and sugar, serum creatinine
- *X-ray chest*—for pre-operative assessment
- *USG*—abdomen and pelvis—to rule out mass
- *IVP*—in long standing prolapse and huge procidentia—ureter gets kinked which may lead to hydroureteronephrosis
- *Pap smear and cervical biopsy* (biopsy from the edge of the decubitus ulcer, if present)

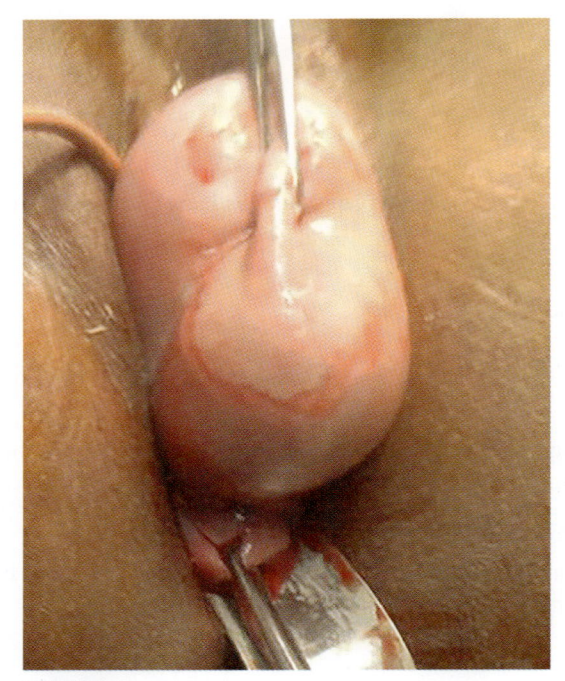

FIGURE 4.3 Anterior Vaginal Wall Cyst

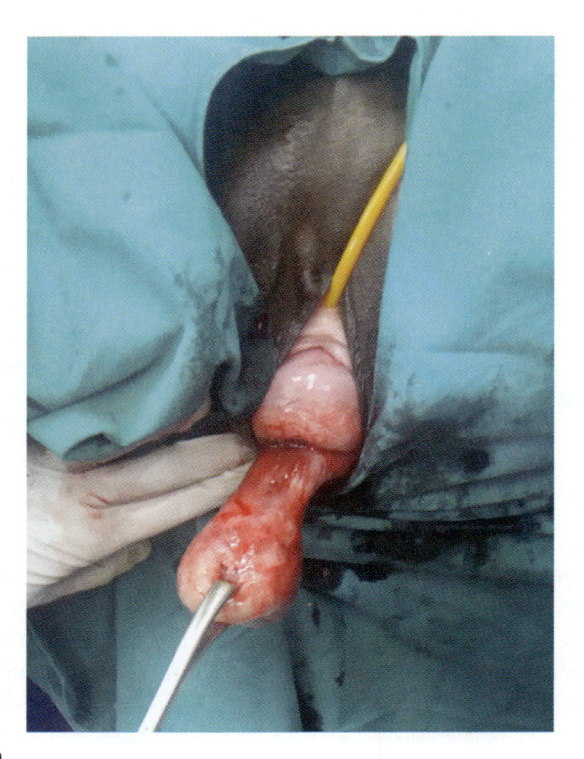

FIGURE 4.4 Fibroid Polyp

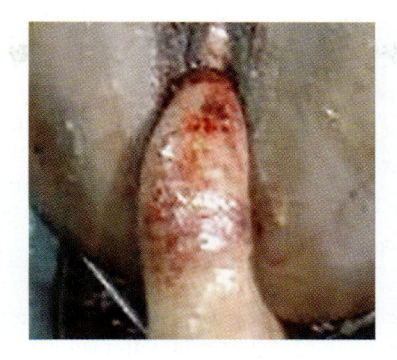

FIGURE 4.5 Chronic Inversion

CASE DISCUSSION

- Supports of the uterus are ligamentary and muscular
- *Following level system was introduced by De Lancey*:
  Level I: ligaments; condensation of the endopelvic fascia pubocervical—anterior; uterosacral—posterior; Mackenrodt's ligament—lateral
  Level II: pelvic fascia and paracolpos connects vagina laterally to white line through arcus tendineus
  Level III: pelvic diaphragm, levator ani muscles namely pubococcygeus part of levator ani—pubouretheralis, pubovaginalis, puborectalis, perineal body
- Anatomical classification of prolapse uterus:

Normal	Cervix at the level of ischial spines
First degree	Cervix below the ischial spines but above the introitus
Second degree	Cervix at the level of introitus
Third degree	Cervix outside the introitus
Procidentia	Uterine fundus outside the introitus

- Pelvic Organ Prolapse Quantification (POPQ) system of classification of prolapse uterus by International Continence Society—hymen is taken as fixed point and six reference points are measured (Table 4.1)
- *Causes of prolapse uterus in post-menopausal women*: it is due to lack of oestrogen, which causes asthenia and atonicity of supports of uterus. In parous women, frequent childbirth, big baby, prolonged labour, instrumental delivery, denervation injury to the ligaments due to stretching in vaginal delivery causes weakness and predisposes to prolapse uterus. Later loss of hormones in post-menopausal age results in prolapse

Table 4.1 Stages of POPQ

Stage 0	No descent of pelvic organs
Stage 1	Lowest point of prolapse does not descend below 1 cm from hymen
Stage 2	Lowest point of prolapse within 1 cm from hymen
Stage 3	Lowest point >1 cm below hymen
Stage 4	Complete prolapse

- *Treatment for decubitus ulcer*: reducing the prolapse relieves congestion and ulcer will be healed. Hence after reducing prolapse, packing the vagina with pack soaked in betadine solution aids in healing. Alternatively pessary can be used to keep the uterus in position which aids in healing the decubitus ulcer
- *Causes for non-healing decubitus ulcer*: diabetes, malignancy
- *Pessary is only palliative for management of prolapse uterus*:
    - Ring pessary made of polyvinyl chloride is used; pessary can be of different sizes

Indications and Disadvantages of Pessary

Indications for Pessary	Disadvantages of Pessary
Early pregnancy up to 12 weeks because after that uterus becomes abdominal organ	Can cause infection and vaginitis
Puerperium	Has to be changed once in 3 months
For healing of decubitus ulcer	Forgotten pessary can lead to ulcer, incarceration, malignancy, VVF
Patient who refuses surgery	Inappropriate sized pessary may not be retained
Patient medically unfit for surgery	

- *Pessary test*: to find out if low backache is due to prolapse of uterus or due to some other reason. It can be used to find out if she will be relieved of her symptoms, if surgery is done

MANAGEMENT

Management of prolapse uterus depends on the following:
- Age
- Degree of prolapse uterus
- Desire for conserving menstrual and reproductive function
- Associated complications
- Desire for menstrual conservation after finishing child-bearing function

Surgery for prolapse uterus:
- In older women and post-menopausal women—Ward Mayo's vaginal hysterectomy with pelvic floor repair (PFR) is done
- In younger and parous women—Fothergill's with PFR or Manchester operation is done
- Nulliparous women—abdominal sling operation

- Very old and unfit for surgery—Lefort's surgery
- *Steps of vaginal hysterectomy*:
  - Refer Case 13
- *PFR*:
  - Includes anterior colporrhaphy and posterior colpoperineorrhaphy
  - For cystocoele—anterior colporrhaphy is done
  - For enterocoele—obliteration of POD, approximation of uterosacral ligament, McCall culdoplasty is done
  - For rectocoele—posterior colpoperineorrhaphy is done

Complications of Vaginal Hysterectomy

Per-Operative	Post-Operative	Remote
Anaesthesia complications, primary haemorrhage	Reactionary haemorrhage, infection of wound	Dyspareunia
Injury to bladder, urethra, ureter, small bowel, rectum	Pelvic abscess, UTI, retention of urine	Vault prolapse
	Thrombosis and pulmonary embolism	

- *Fothergill's operation*: *refer Case 13*; Figs. 13.35 to 13.40
  Indications:
  - Young patient
  - Women who want to conserve menstrual or reproductive function

Steps:
- Preliminary dilatation and curettage (done to prevent post-operative haematometra, to rule out endometrial pathology and for easy formation of cervical lip)
- Amputation of the cervix
- Shortening or plication of the Mackenrodt's ligament
- Fothergill's stitch—it is taken from vaginal wall and Mackenrodt's ligament on one side, anterior surface of cervix, other Mackenrodt's ligament and vaginal wall on opposite side. The stitch is tied at the end after cervical lip formation
- Anterior colporrhaphy and posterior colpoperineorrhaphy
- *Shirodkar's modification of Fothergill's operation*:
  - Amputation of cervix reduces subsequent fertility and future pregnancy complications are increased
  - Hence amputation of the cervix is not done. POD is opened and uterosacral ligaments are divided close to cervix and stumps are crossed and stitched in front of cervix. High closure of POD is done
- *Surgeries for nulliparous prolapse uterus*:
  - Nulliparous prolapse uterus—sling surgery
  - *Purandare's abdomino cervicopexy*—strips of rectus sheath are brought between leaves of broad ligament and stitched in front of uterine isthmus
  - *Shirodkar's sling surgery*—strips of Mersilene tape are attached to cervix posteriorly and brought via retro peritoneum posteriorly and fixed to longitudinal ligament on anterior surface of sacral promontory
  - *Khanna's sling surgery*—sling is attached to cervix and anterior superior iliac spine

- *Surgery for vault prolapse*:
  - Repair of enterocoele with PFR
  - Sacrospinous colpopexy—vaginal approach
  - Sacrocolpopexy—abdominal approach
  - Colpocleisis

KEY POINTS
- Genital prolapse is the common complaint of elderly women and can occur in young women too.
- Aetiology of genital prolapse in post-menopausal women is atonicity and asthenia of muscles and ligaments that support the uterus due to lack of oestrogen. Another cause is injury occurring during repeated childbirth.
- In POPQ system, hymen is the fixed point.
- Symptoms of prolapse, in addition to mass descending PV, are urinary symptoms, backache, vaginal discharge, bowel symptoms.
- Pessary test—to find out if low backache is due to prolapse of uterus or due to some other reason.
- Conservative management is pelvic floor exercise—Kegel's and pessary but pessary does not restore anatomy.
- Management of prolapse depends on age, degree of prolapse, desire for future fertility, associated pathology.
- Vault prolapse can be managed vaginally, abdominally and laparoscopically.

FREQUENTLY ASKED QUESTIONS
1. What are the supports of uterus?
2. What are aetiological factors for prolapse uterus?
3. What are the degrees of uterine prolapse?
4. What are the precipitating and aggravating factors for uterine prolapse?
5. What is the cause of prolapse uterus in post-menopausal age group?
6. How will you differentiate third degree and fourth degree uterine prolapse?
7. What are the urinary symptoms in uterine prolapse?
8. What is the cause for decubitus ulcer and what will you do to heal the ulcer?
9. What are the causes for non-healing ulcer?
10. What are the indications for pessary in uterine prolapse?
11. What is the differential diagnosis of uterine prolapse?
12. What is the type of pessary used in prolapse uterus?
13. How will you decide about the type of surgery?
14. When will you do Fothergill's surgery (Manchester's repair)?
15. What is Shirodkar's modification of Fothergill's repair?
16. What are the steps of Fothergill's surgery?
17. When will you do vaginal hysterectomy with PFR?
18. What are the steps of vaginal hysterectomy with PFR?
19. What are the immediate and remote complications of vaginal hysterectomy with PFR?
20. What is PFR?
21. What are the surgeries done for nulliparous prolapse?

CASE 5

A CASE OF FIBROID UTERUS

PATIENT'S DETAILS
Name.. Age.................. Address........................... Occupation..............
Socioeconomic Class......................... Para.........................

PRESENT COMPLAINTS
Woman may come with the following complaints:
- Menstrual problems like profuse bleeding, pain during menstruation, frequent periods, intermenstrual bleeding
- Mass in the abdomen
- Pain in abdomen, pelvic pain and discomfort
- Heaviness in lower abdomen
- Infertility
- Pressure symptoms—due to huge fibroid—oedema, varicosity in lower limbs
- Urinary symptoms—frequency, retention of urine (anterior and cervical fibroid)
- Rectal symptoms—constipation, feeling of incomplete evacuation due to posterior wall fibroid and posterior cervical fibroid
- Vaginal discharge may be due to fibroid polyp
- Symptoms of anaemia like lethargy, palpitation, chest pain, dyspnoea may be present due to menorrhagia
- 30%–50% of fibroids are asymptomatic and found incidentally

HISTORY
MENSTRUAL HISTORY
Following should be taken in detail:
- Cycle length/number of days of bleeding/number of pads soaked per day/passage of clots/pain during periods
- In fibroid, bleeding can be abnormal/profuse/intermenstrual/frequent

MARITAL HISTORY
Refer Case 1

To view the lecture notes log in to your account on www.MedEnact.com

PAST OBSTETRIC HISTORY
- H/O pregnancy complications in the past like abortion, pre-term labour

CONTRACEPTIVE HISTORY
Refer Case 1

PAST HISTORY
- History of investigations/intake of drugs/surgery done (myomectomy, myolysis—laparoscopy or laparotomy) for fibroid

FAMILY HISTORY
- Fibroid in siblings and mother
- H/O familial ovarian, breast carcinoma, endometrial, colonic cancer (when present prophylactic oophorectomy can be performed with hysterectomy)

PERSONAL HISTORY
Refer Case 1

EXAMINATION
GENERAL EXAMINATION
Refer Case 1

Specific attention for the following details to be made:
- Anaemia, oedema and varicosity of lower limbs
- When fibroid is associated with acute conditions like torsion or red degeneration, pulse may be increased

ABDOMINAL EXAMINATION
- Inspection, palpation, percussion and auscultation to be done as usual
- *If mass is present describe about the following*:
  - Site: the quadrants of abdomen the mass occupies
  - Size: if midline, describe as corresponding to—weeks of pregnant uterus or describe in centimetres
  - Consistency and contour: mostly firm in consistency and may be regular or irregular
  - Lower border felt or not (usually not felt except in pedunculated subserous fibroid)
  - Mobility: side to side may be present
  - Tenderness may be due to torsion, infection, red degeneration

GYNAEC EXAMINATION
(Not to be done by undergraduate but should know what points to be noted)
- Inspection—Ext. genitalia
- Fibroid polyp sometimes can be seen outside the vulval outlet

SPECULUM EXAMINATION
- Cervix is visualised for its displacement or presence of fibroid polyp protruding through the cervix or from cervix

BIMANUAL PELVIC EXAMINATION
- Position of the cervix
- Size of the uterus (uniformly enlarged or irregularly enlarged)
- Whether uterus is felt separately
- Whether movement of cervix is transmitted to the mass felt per abdomen and whether movement of mass is transmitted to the cervix
- Fixity of the mass
- Any other mass in the fornix
- Groove sign is a depression between uterus and mass and it will be absent in fibroid

SUMMARY
- Patient's name………age……nulliparous/parous—c/o……….
- Mention about relevant past history, general examination, abdominal examination findings, local findings
- *In case of mass abdomen—give differential diagnosis*

For example, C/O menstrual symptoms, infertility, firm mass, midline swelling, lower border not felt—*then probable diagnosis is fibroid.*

DIAGNOSIS
Mention only about clinical provisional diagnosis.

DIFFERENTIAL DIAGNOSIS
- *Full bladder* to be ruled out
- *Pregnancy*: period of amenorrhoea will be present. Uterus is enlarged, soft and pregnancy symptoms will be present. Foetal parts will be felt
- *Ovarian tumour*: usually there will not be menstrual symptoms
  Functioning tumours like sex cord stromal tumours, such as granulosa and theca cell tumours can present with menstrual symptoms (Table 5.1). Lower border usually felt—refer Case 10 on ovarian tumour
- *Adenomyosis*: size of the uterus not more than 12 weeks with uniformly enlarged uterus, which may be tender and it mostly occurs in parous women around 35–45 years. H/O heavy menstrual bleeding PV and triple dysmenorrhoea may be present
- *Endometriosis—chocolate cyst*: mass in the fornix, which may be adherent to uterus. Uterus will be normal in size. Patient may have dysmenorrhoea, menorrhagia, deep dyspareunia and infertility

Table 5.1 Differentiating Points Between Fibroid and Ovarian Tumour

	Fibroid	Ovarian Tumour
Age	Reproductive age	Extremes of age (germ cell tumour—younger age group)
Menstrual symptoms	Common	Uncommon. Except in functioning ovarian tumours (granulosa and theca cell tumour, sex cord stromal tumours)
Site	Mostly midline	Can be towards one side
Consistency	Firm	Variable (cystic to hard)
Lower border	Not felt except in pedunculated subserous fibroid	May be felt
Mobility	Side to side	May be moved in all directions
PV findings	Mass continuous with uterus; movement of cervix transmitted to the mass; groove sign absent	Uterus can be felt separately from mass; movement of cervix not transmitted; groove sign present

- *Haematometra*: there will be period of amenorrhoea. Uterus will be enlarged uniformly but soft and sometimes tender
- *Pyometra*: uniformly enlarged soft, tender uterus. Sometimes patient will be febrile
- *Endometrial carcinoma*: usually occur in older women. Uterus is usually normal in size or may be enlarged
- *Uterine sarcoma*: uterus will be enlarged but not firm and there will be rapid growth. Occurs in post-menopausal woman
- *Pelvic kidney*: lump in the abdomen will be felt during examination. An ectopic kidney may cause abdominal pain or urinary problems
- *Bicornuate uterus*: it is incidentally discovered when the pelvis is imaged. The most common symptomatic presentation is with early pregnancy loss and cervical incompetence

INVESTIGATIONS
ROUTINE AND SPECIFIC INVESTIGATIONS

- *HB, PCV*: to rule out anaemia
- *USG—abdomen and pelvis*: can actually map out all the details about fibroid and it depicts the size/site/number of fibroids/type of fibroid (submucous, intra-mural, subserous)/endometrial cavity/endometrial thickness/adnexal mass/associated adenomyosis/pressure effect on ureter—hydroureter, hydronephrosis
- *Saline infusion sonography*: can diagnose submucous fibroid (done in cases of fibroid with infertility)
- *Hysteroscopy*: both diagnostic and therapeutic (done in cases of infertility with fibroid) Submucous fibroid up to 4 cm can be resected through hysteroscopy
- *Laparoscopy*: done when fibroid is associated with infertility, to rule out tubal factor, associated endometriosis, PCOD

- *IVP*: is indicated in large fibroid, broad ligament fibroid and in cervical fibroid. There may be dilatation, kinking or alteration in the course of ureter in large, cervical and lateral fibroids
- *CT, MRI*: done when diagnosis is inconclusive with USG

CASE DISCUSSION
SYMPTOMS OF FIBROID AND THEIR CAUSES

Causes for menorrhagia in fibroid:
- Increase in endometrial surface area
- Increase in vascularity of the uterus
- Pelvic congestion
- Interference with normal uterine contractility
- Stasis and dilatation of venous plexuses
- Associated endometrial hyperplasia
- Hyperoestrogenic state
- Polymenorrhoea may be due to co-existence of cystic ovaries and PID

Intermenstrual bleeding is due to—ulceration of submucous fibroids, or fibroid polyp.

Painful menstruation is due to—congestive dysmenorrhoea—due to increase in vascularity of uterus, venous stasis, pelvic congestion.

Spasmodic dysmenorrhoea occurs in submucous myoma when uterus is trying to expel fibroid polyp.

Pelvic pain and discomfort are due to—large myoma. Woman may experience discomfort and dragging pain.

Acute pain occurs in torsion of subserous fibroid, red degeneration in fibroid with pregnancy or OC pill use, sarcomatous degeneration.

Abdominal mass—when myoma is large, it is palpable per abdomen.

Pressure symptoms:
- Urinary symptoms: anterior wall fibroid and cervical fibroid will cause urinary symptoms
- Frequency of micturition: is due to change in bladder capacity and dynamics
- Retention of urine: occurs when posterior wall fibroid is incarcerated in pouch of Douglas and due to compression of urethra
- Large fibroids on the uterine body, broad ligament, cervical fibroids can cause compression of the ureters causing hydroureteronephrosis

CAUSES FOR INFERTILITY IN FIBROID

Implantation is impaired due to the following:
- In submucous myoma, there may be thinning of the endometrium/ulceration of endometrium
- Poor vascularisation
- Distortion of cavity

Tubal factor is affected due to the following:
- Cornual fibroid can cause tubal block
- Tubal motility affected

- Impaired gamete transport
- Tube may be overstretched
- Associated PID, endometriosis

Cervical fibroid:
    Sperm transport may be impaired
    Cervix may be displaced from vaginal pool

Infertility in fibroid may be due to associated anovulation, hyperoestrogenic state, endometriosis and PID

TYPES OF SECONDARY CHANGES AND DEGENERATIONS IN FIBROID

Hyaline, cystic, atrophic, calcareous and sarcomatous changes; red degeneration occurs during pregnancy and when OCP is used.

COMPLICATIONS OF FIBROID

Torsion, infection, haemorrhage, infertility, associated endometrial carcinoma, inversion of uterus, sarcomatous degeneration.

FIBROID SHOULD BE TREATED IN THE FOLLOWING CONDITIONS

- Symptomatic fibroid
- Asymptomatic large fibroid more than 12 weeks size
- When fibroid is the cause for infertility
- Rapidly growing fibroid
- Fibroid causing pressure effects

DRUGS USED IN MEDICAL MANAGEMENT

- Drugs used for correcting anaemia—iron
- Drugs used for control of menorrhagia—NSAIDs, tranexamic acid, Ru 486: 10–25 mg daily for 3 months
- Gestrinone 2.5 mg thrice weekly
- Isoprisinol—selective progesterone receptor modulator (SPRM) 10–25 mg for 12 weeks
- GnRH analogue—inj. 3.75 mg monthly, for not more than 6 months
- Aromatase inhibitors like letrozole
- Danazol—not used nowadays due to its side-effects

USEFULNESS OF MEDICAL MANAGEMENT

    Corrects anaemia
    Cures menorrhagia
    Reduces the size and blood supply and can be used pre-operatively. Hence laparoscopic or vaginal hysterectomy is possible with less blood loss
    Decrease in size reduces the pressure symptoms

DISADVANTAGES OF MEDICAL MANAGEMENT

Side-effects of GnRH analogues do not allow treatment over indefinite period
Cost of the drugs
Tumour can re-grow after stopping the drug
Failure of treatment
Recurrence of symptoms
Surgery may be required

DISADVANTAGES OF GnRH ANALOGUES

Costly
Post-menopausal symptoms like hot flushes and osteoporosis
Re-growth after stopping the drug
Can be used only for 6 months

INDICATIONS FOR MYOMECTOMY (Fig. 5.1)

- When reproductive function is to be retained
- When fibroid is the cause for infertility and other factors are ruled out
- When fibroid is the cause for recurrent pregnancy loss
- When menstrual function is to be retained in young patient

PRE-REQUISITES FOR MYOMECTOMY

- Should be done in pre-ovulatory phase to reduce blood loss
- Other causes for infertility like tubal factors, anovulation and male infertility to be ruled out
- Adequate blood should be reserved
- Informed consent for hysterectomy should be obtained

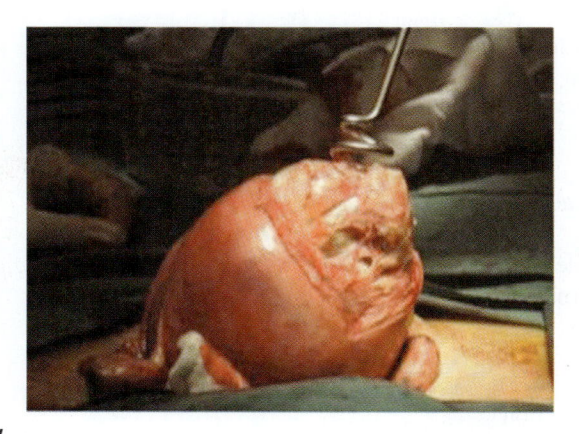

FIGURE 5.1 Myomectomy

- Need for hysterectomy in case of complication like profuse haemorrhage during myomectomy should be explained and consent to be obtained for hysterectomy
- Preliminary endometrial biopsy to be done to rule out endometrial carcinoma.

> Myomectomy can be done by hysteroscopy, laparoscopy, laparotomy.

COMPLICATIONS OF MYOMECTOMY

Haemorrhage—primary, reactionary and secondary
To reduce haemorrhage intra-operatively, the measures taken are: use of energy sources like diathermy/harmonic scalpel, inj. vasopressin in the tumour bed or application of Bonney's myomectomy clamp or tourniquet at the level of isthmus
Trauma to adjacent structures—bladder, ureter, rectum, bowel
Infection
Intestinal obstruction, paralytic ileus
Remote—adhesion
Rupture of uterus in subsequent pregnancy
Scar endometriosis

RED DEGENERATION OF FIBROID

Occurs due to thrombosis of vessels supplying fibroid and extravasation of blood pigments
Seen in fibroid complicating pregnancy or with OC pill use
Treatment: conservative—rest, analgesics and antibiotics, if necessary

> Never attempt surgery for red degeneration during pregnancy.

COMPLICATIONS IN PREGNANCY WITH FIBROID

- Recurrent pregnancy loss—submucous fibroid
- Spontaneous abortion
- Pre-term labour
- Red degeneration
- Malpresentation
- Incoordinate uterine action
- Placental abruption
- Increased operative delivery
- Post-partum haemorrhage—atonic

NEWER MODALITIES IN TREATMENT OF FIBROID

- Uterine artery embolisation
- MRI-guided high-intensity focused ultrasound (HIFU)—non-invasive

INDICATIONS FOR HYSTERECTOMY IN FIBROIDS

It depends on age, parity and symptoms.
- In women above 40 years, who have finished child-bearing function
- Fibroid associated with malignancy
- Large fibroids with pressure symptoms above 40 years
- In symptomatic fibroid, hysterectomy results in permanent cure
- In women above 50 years, prophylactic oophorectomy can be performed and in women with history of familial cancer or associated TO mass or endometriosis, it can be performed even before 50 years

MANAGEMENT (Flow chart 5.1)

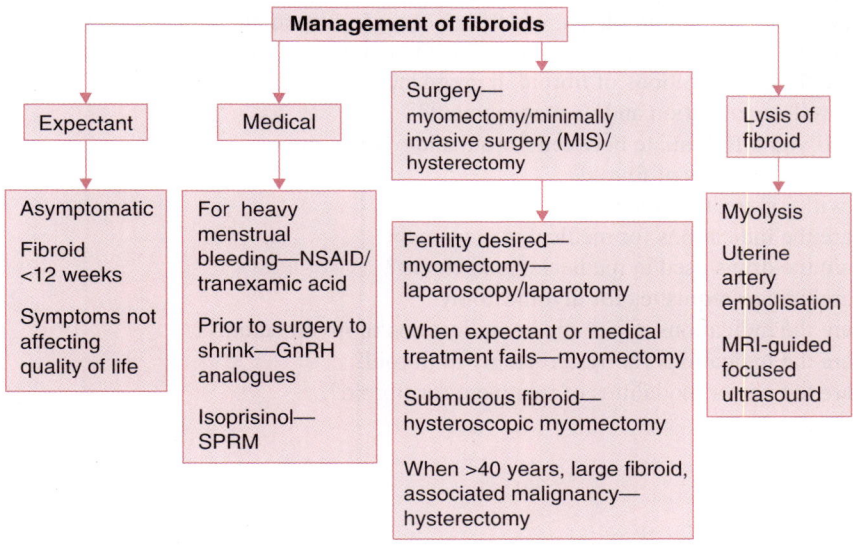

```
                        Management of fibroids
        ┌──────────┬──────────┬──────────────────────┬──────────┐
        │          │          │                      │          │
    Expectant   Medical    Surgery—              Lysis of
                           myomectomy/minimally    fibroid
                           invasive surgery (MIS)/
                           hysterectomy
```

Expectant:
- Asymptomatic
- Fibroid <12 weeks
- Symptoms not affecting quality of life

Medical:
- For heavy menstrual bleeding—NSAID/tranexamic acid
- Prior to surgery to shrink—GnRH analogues
- Isoprisinol—SPRM

Surgery:
- Fertility desired—myomectomy—laparoscopy/laparotomy
- When expectant or medical treatment fails—myomectomy
- Submucous fibroid—hysteroscopic myomectomy
- When >40 years, large fibroid, associated malignancy—hysterectomy

Lysis of fibroid:
- Myolysis
- Uterine artery embolisation
- MRI-guided focused ultrasound

FLOW CHART 5.1 Management of Fibroids

KEY POINTS

- Fibroid is a benign uterine neoplasm.
- Fibroids are seen in women with hyperoestrogenic conditions.
- Rarely new fibroids appear after menopause and it tends to shrink after menopause.
- Menstrual disturbances, infertility, pain and lump in abdomen and pressure symptoms are the clinical symptomatology associated with fibroid.
- Fibroid can undergo secondary changes like hyaline, cystic, calcareous degeneration and sarcomatous changes.
- Red degeneration, which occurs during pregnancy should be managed conservatively.

- Treatment for fibroid may be expectant, medical, MIS and surgery.
- When myomectomy is offered, woman should be counselled and informed consent to be obtained for hysterectomy because due to unforeseen circumstances, as hysterectomy may have to be performed.
- Hysterectomy is offered to women over 40 years with symptomatic fibroid, which will relieve the symptoms.
- Newer modalities in the management of fibroid are uterine artery embolisation and MRI-guided focused ultrasound.

FREQUENTLY ASKED QUESTIONS

1. What are the other names for fibroid and where does fibroid arise from?
2. What are the causes for infertility in fibroid?
3. What are the menstrual problems, which can occur in fibroid and how are they caused?
4. What are the different types of degeneration and commonest degeneration that occur in fibroid?
5. What are the complications of fibroid in pregnancy?
6. What is red degeneration and its management?
7. How will you differentiate between fibroid and ovarian tumour?
8. Differential diagnosis of fibroid?
9. When will you treat fibroid?
10. What are the indications for medical management?
11. What are the drugs used in medical management?
12. What are the pre-requisites for myomectomy?
13. What are the indications, types and complications of myomectomy?
14. What are the indications for hysterectomy in fibroid?
15. What are the newer modalities of treatment for fibroid?

CASE 6

A CASE OF CANCER CERVIX

PATIENT'S DETAILS
Name...................................... Age................. Address......................... Occupation..............
Socioeconomic Class............ Para......................

[Low socioeconomic class—more prone for cancer cervix because of early marriage, early and frequent childbirth, sexually transmitted infections (STI), poor genital hygiene]

PRESENT COMPLAINTS (MAY BE)
- Discharge PV
- Irregular bleeding PV
- Intermenstrual or continuous bleeding PV
- Post-coital bleeding

HISTORY
HISTORY OF PRESENTING ILLNESS
- Discharge PV—whether blood stained, foul smelling, amount, duration
- Post-coital bleeding PV—duration
- Intermenstrual bleeding PV—amount, duration
- Irregular bleeding PV—duration
- Pelvic pain
- Frequency of micturition, painful micturition, blood-stained urine
- Diarrhoea, rectal pain
- Low backache
- Loss of weight
- Pedal oedema
- History suggestive of STI
- History suggestive of immunosuppressive state

MENSTRUAL HISTORY
Menarche, cycles, age of menopause

To view the lecture notes log in to your account on www.MedEnact.com

MARITAL HISTORY
Age at marriage, age at first intercourse, history suggestive of multiple sexual partners

OBSTETRIC HISTORY
- Age at first pregnancy, parity, abortions
- Contraception: H/O OCP usage (increases incidence of cancer cervix)

CONTRACEPTIVE HISTORY
- Refer Case 1

PAST HISTORY
- H/O taking immunosuppressant drugs
- History suggestive of reproductive tract infections, HIV, genital warts, history suggestive of immunosuppressive state
- Pap smear if taken and it's reports

PAST SURGICAL HISTORY
Previous history of conisation for cervical intra-epithelial neoplasia (CIN)

FAMILY HISTORY
Diabetes, hypertension

PERSONAL HISTORY
Smoking, drug abuse, alcohol

EXAMINATION
GENERAL EXAMINATION
- Refer Case 1

Special attention to be paid for the following details:
- Height
- Weight
- Anaemia, cachexia
- Lymph nodes—supra-clavicular and inguinal

ABDOMINAL EXAMINATION
- Mass in lower abdomen (may be due to pyometra)
- Tenderness
- Hepatomegaly

GYNAEC EXAMINATION
External genitalia
Speculum examination
- *Cervix*—presence of growth/ulcer and the extent of growth to vagina
- Growth can be exophytic, endophytic or ulcerative
- Exophytic—cauliflower like growth, bleeds on touch, friable with indurated base
- Ulcerative—infiltrative, bleeds on touch, fixed

Bimanual pelvic examination
Uterine size, feel of cervix, growth extending onto fornices, vagina, parametrial involvement are made out.

Per rectal examination
Involvement of rectal mucosa and parametrial induration/whether induration is up to lateral pelvic wall or short of it are made out to stage disease. Parametrial induration may be due to infection and hence staging should be done after a course of antibiotics.

> Cancer cervix staging is always clinical.

SUMMARY
- Mrs.....years old....... para, with H/O irregular bleeding PV, (duration)....or discharge PV (duration)..... or post-menopausal bleeding PV
- Mention about general examination findings and speculum examination findings

DIAGNOSIS
PROVISIONAL CLINICAL DIAGNOSIS
- Cancer cervix stage—if speculum and PV examination is allowed
- If speculum examination is not done, differential diagnosis is to be given

DIFFERENTIAL DIAGNOSIS
- Cancer cervix, cervical polyp, cervical erosion, tuberculosis of cervix
- Carcinoma endometrium
- Vaginal infection, cancer vagina, vulva
- Tubal carcinoma
- Forgotten pessary with cancer vagina
- Senile vaginitis
- Atrophic endometritis in post-menopausal woman

INVESTIGATIONS

- *Urine analysis*
- *CBC*
- *Blood group and Rh typing*
- *RFT* in late stages of cancer cervix, obstructive hydroureter and hydronephrosis can result in uraemia
- *LFT*
- *X-ray of the chest*
- *Colposcopy*-directed biopsy—early stage
- *Biopsy*—if growth or ulcer is seen, biopsy from growth or at the edge of the ulcer including the normal tissue should be taken
- *USG abdomen and pelvis*, KUB—following points to be noted: uterus—(rule out pyometra) size and volume of cervical growth, ovaries, hydroureteronephrosis, pelvic and para-aortic lymph nodes
- *IVP*
- *Cystoscopy*
- *CT*—abdomen and pelvis—is included in routine investigation of caner cervix but cannot pickup lymph node less than 1 cm
- *MRI*—abdomen and pelvis—can detect lymph node enlargement, parametrial infiltration and offers better pre-treatment assessment
- *PET, FDG PET*

CASE DISCUSSION

Methods for screening cancer cervix: visual inspection with acetic acid (VIA), visual inspection with Lugol's iodine (VILI), Pap smear, liquid-based cytology (LBC), HPV testing, colposcopy.

These tests are screening test for CIN—pre-malignant lesion of cervix and malignant lesions of cervix.

- **Pap smear**: This is a screening test for pre-malignant and malignant lesions of cervix.
  The cervix is visualised after placing Cusco's bivalve speculum and the ectocervix is scraped using an Ayre's spatula and endocervix with cytobrush. The cells are smeared on a glass slide and fixed in a 1:1 mixture of 95% ethanol and ether kept in Koplik's jar. Alternatively, the smears may be fixed with fixative spray.
  They are stained using Papanicolaou's stain and examined (Fig. 6.1B).
- **LBC**: The cells are scraped using special broom and collected in a liquid medium and transported to the lab. It is processed and a smear of monolayer of cells is made and fixed. In this method, blood and other cells are removed. Hence interpretation is made easy (Figs. 6.1A and 6.2).
  Interpretation of Pap smear and Papanicolaou system—Class I–V
- **Bethesda system of reporting**:
  Abnormal results include:
  - Atypical squamous cells (ASC)
  - Atypical squamous cells of undetermined significance (ASC-US)
  - Atypical squamous cells—cannot exclude HSIL (ASC-H)

CASE DISCUSSION

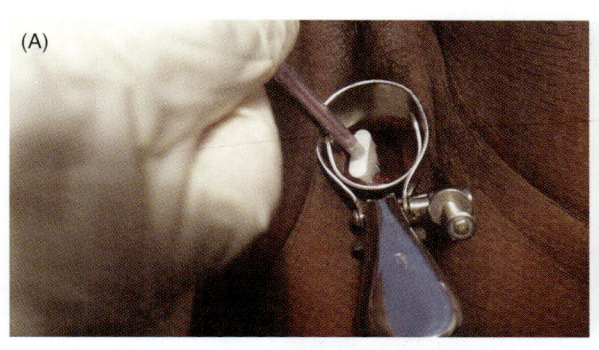

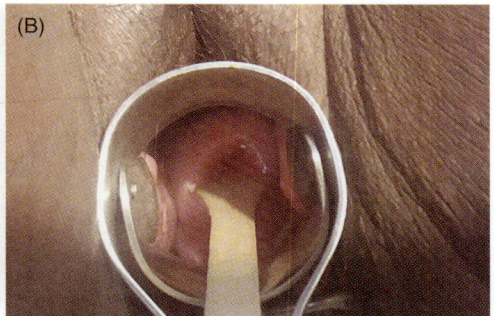

FIGURE 6.1
(A) LBC and (B) Pap smear with Ayre's spatula.
▶ Scan to play How to do Papsmear

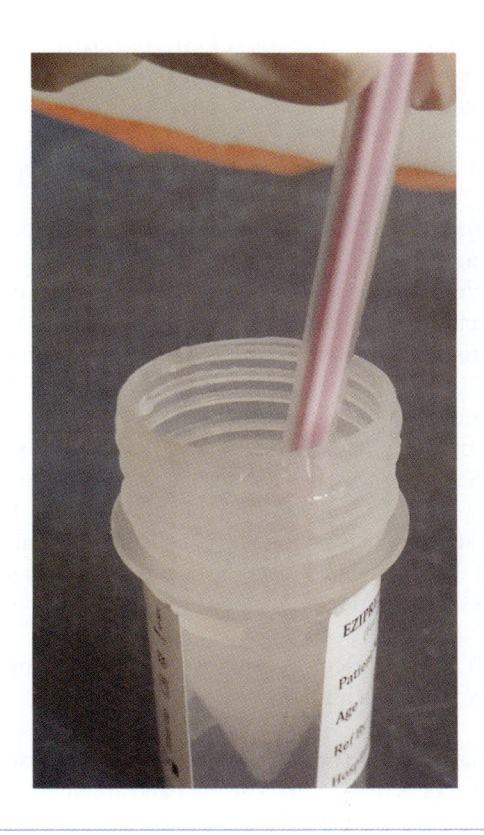

FIGURE 6.2 LBC Broom

280 CASE 6 A CASE OF CANCER CERVIX

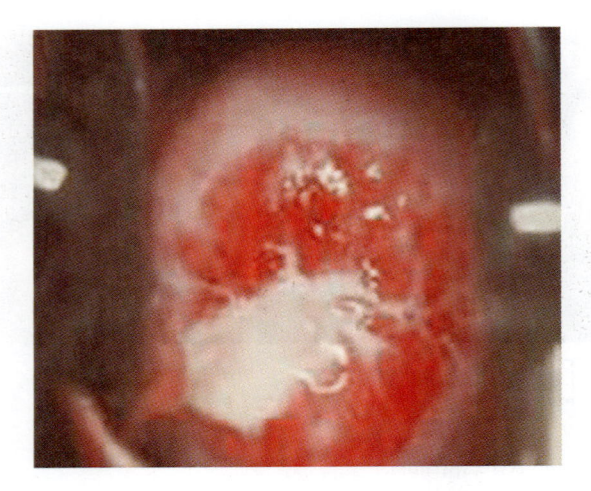

FIGURE 6.3 VIA

- Low-grade squamous intra-epithelial lesion (LGSIL or LSIL)
- High-grade squamous intra-epithelial lesion (HGSIL or HSIL)
- Squamous cell carcinoma
- Atypical glandular cells not otherwise specified (AGC-NOS)
- Atypical glandular cells, suspicious for AIS or cancer (AGC-neoplastic) adenocarcinoma in situ (AIS)
- **LSIL include CIN 1** (mild dysplasia, and changes of HPV-koilocytotic atypia)
- **HSIL include CIN 2 and CIN 3**

- *VIA*: After application of freshly prepared 3% acetic acid, cervix is visualised with hand-held magnifying lens. Acetic acid when applied to the cervix, coagulates the areas of cells with increased nuclear chromatin which will turn white. Aceto white area indicates area of dysplasia—abnormal cells (Fig. 6.3).
  If VIA is positive, it indicates CIN—abnormal cells.
- *VILI*: On application of Lugol's iodine, normal cervical epithelium which is rich in glycogen, stains mahogany brown (Schiller's test). The abnormal areas do not stain due to lack of glycogen (Fig. 6.4).
- **Transformation zone**: Is the area between the original squamocolumnar junction and new squamocolumnar junction. When atypical metaplasia with abnormal nuclear changes occurs in this area, it results in dysplasia and malignancy (Fig. 6.5).
- **Diagnosis of CIN**:
  Pap smear, LBC, VIA, VILI, speculoscopy, spectroscopy, colposcopy, cervicography, cone biopsy, Agnor, DNA study, HPV testing
- *Colposcopy*
  Cervix visualised under magnification and transformation zone is visualised.
  Presence of acetowhite area, punctuation, mosaic area and atypical vascular pattern denotes abnormal epithelium and CIN and directed biopsy can be taken.

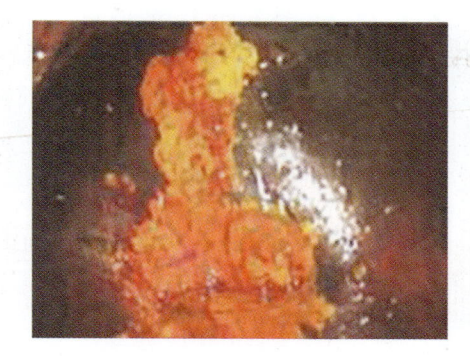

FIGURE 6.4 VILI

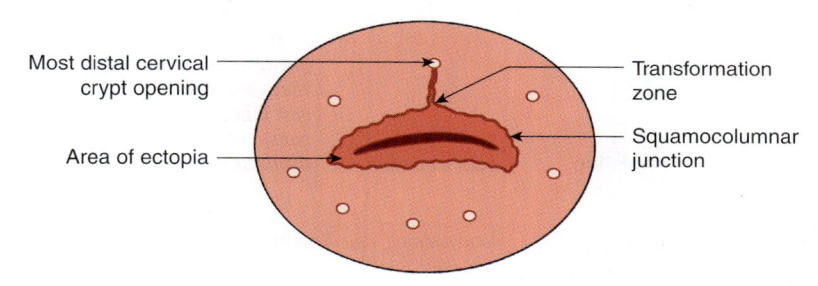

FIGURE 6.5 Transformation Zone

MANAGEMENT
PRE-INVASIVE LESIONS OF CERVIX (Flow chart 6.1)
Treatment of LSIL/CIN 1:
  Spontaneous regression possible, advised follow up Pap tests every 6 months; if persistent, needs treatment
  Treatment of HSIL/CIN 2 and CIN 3—ablation or excision methods
  Ablative treatment can be undertaken when the transformation zone can be visualised completely (cryocautery, electrocautery, laser ablation).
  Excision methods range from local treatment (LLETZ, LEEP NETZ) to hysterectomy.
  Conisation is diagnostic and therapeutic and undertaken in young women desirous of children.

Hysterectomy is advocated:
- In old women
- Where margins are not free
- Recurrent disease
- With other associated symptoms

CASE 6 A CASE OF CANCER CERVIX

```
A. Pap smear
    ↓
LSIL (treat infection and test for HPV)
    ↓
Follow up yearly
    ↓
If persists → Treat as HSIL

B. If Pap smear—HSIL
    ↓
Colposcopy and directed biopsy
    ↓
┌───────────┬───────────────┬─────────────────────┐
Ablation    Local excision   Radical (when margins
                             are not free, in
                             recurrent disease)

Electrocautery  Conisation    Trachelectomy
Cryocautery     LLETZ         Simple hysterectomy
Laser ablation  LEEP          Follow up
Follow up       NETZ
                Follow up
```

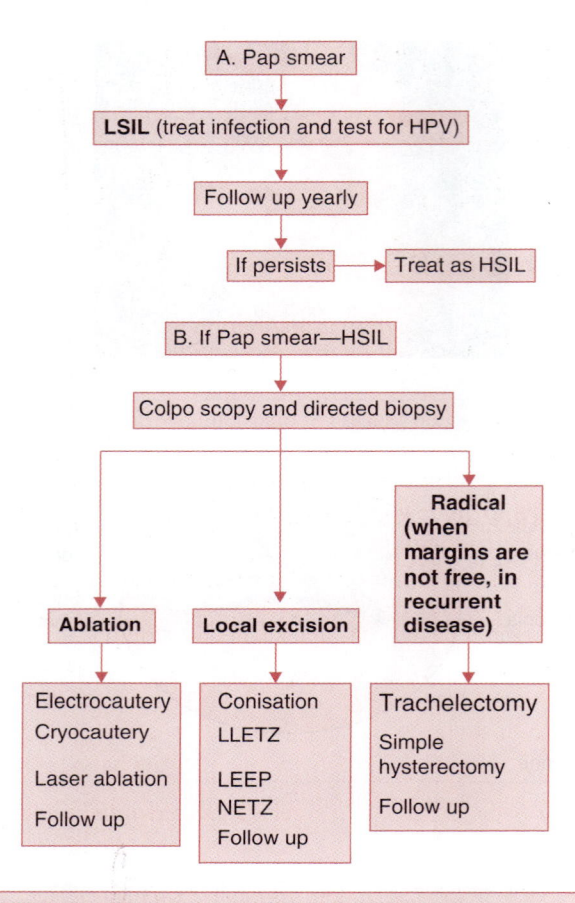

LLETZ: Large loop excision of transformation zone
LEEP: Loop electrosurgical excision procedure
NETZ: Needle excision of transformation zone and conisation

FLOW CHART 6.1 Management of Pre-Invasive Lesions of Cervix

MALIGNANT LESIONS OF CERVIX—CANCER CERVIX

- **Pathology of cancer cervix:**
  The more common variety is squamous cell carcinoma originating from the squamocolumnar junction. Endocervical cancers arise from endocervical mucus membrane; 95% of cervical cancers are squamous cell carcinoma and 5% adenocarcinoma.
- **Lymphatic drainage of cervix:**
  - *Primary group*: para-cervical, parametrial, internal iliac, external iliac, common iliac, obturator
  - *Secondary group*: pre-sacral, para-aortic

- **Spread of cancer cervix**:
  Direct contiguous spread, lymphatic (permeation and embolism) and blood spread, intra-peritoneal implantation
- **Risk factors for cancer cervix**:
  - HPV infection
  - STI, HSV, HIV infection
  - Coitus before the age of 18
  - Multiple sexual partners
  - Multi-parity
  - Low SE class, poor hygiene
  - COC use, alcohol, drug abuse
  - Immunosuppression
- **HPV virus and cancer cervix risk factors**:
  - High oncogenic risk—HPV 16, 18, 31, 33
  - Low oncogenic risk—HPV 6, 11, 35, 45, 56, 58
  - Persistent infection is the cause of cancer cervix in 70%–90% of cases
- **Down-staging of cancer cervix**:
  In this process, paramedical persons are trained to detect the disease early by simple speculum examination and visualisation of cervix and refer the cases to higher centres, if any abnormality is found

STAGING OF CANCER CERVIX

By clinical staging, when in doubt, the earlier stage should be selected:
- *Stage 1*: carcinoma strictly confined to cervix can be diagnosed only by microscopy
  - *1A1*—confined to cervix, <3 mm stromal invasion, lateral extension <7 mm, no LVSI
  - *1A2*—confined to cervix, >3–5 mm stromal invasion, lateral extension not more than 7 mm, with LVSI
- *Stage 1B*: visible lesion confined to cervix and microscopic lesion >1A2
  - *1B1*—visible <4 cm in size
  - *1B2*—visible >4 cm in size
- *Stage 2*: extension into parametrium not up to pelvic side wall, and vagina up to the upper two-third of vagina
  - *2A*—involvement of upper vagina
  - *2B*—involvement of medial parametrium not up to pelvic side wall
- *Stage 3*: extension into parametrium up to pelvic side wall, involving the lower one-third of vagina
  - *3A*—involving the lower one-third of vagina
  - *3B*—extension into parametrium up to pelvic side wall
- *Stage 4*:
  - *4A*—involving the bladder, rectum, spreads beyond the pelvis
  - *4B*—widespread with distant metastasis
  - Micro-invasive stages: 1A1 and 1A2
- *Early stage cancer cervix*: 1A1, 1A2, 1B, 2A
- *Late-stage cancer cervix*:
  - Stages 2B, 3, 4

EARLY DISEASE OF CANCER CERVIX

It can be treated by radical hysterectomy and also by radiotherapy with similar outcome. Both surgery and radiotherapy yield identical cure rate 70%–90%.

SURGICAL MANAGEMENT FOR CANCER CERVIX (Table 6.1)

- *Stage 1A1*: Lymph node involvement, 0.5%
  - Young women—diagnostic and therapeutic conisation with clear margins (before conservative treatment, MRI mapping for local extension and lymph node involvement)
  - Older women—simple hysterectomy—Type 1. Lifelong follow up is advised but lymphadenectomy is not required
- *Stage 1A2*:
  - Stromal invasion (3–5 mm)—only 5% lymph node involvement
  - Young women—vaginal radical trachelectomy + pelvic lymphadenectomy laparoscopically
  - Older women—extended hysterectomy (Type 2 modified radical hysterectomy) with pelvic lymphadenectomy
  - *Fertility conservation treatment* includes trachelectomy 80%; removal of cervix 80%; upper vagina and Mackenrodt's will be cut on either side. Before surgery, blue dye should be injected into cervical tissue and if obturator gland (sentinel node) is not involved, no further lymphadenectomy is needed
- *Stage 1B1 and 2A (treatment options are similar)*:
  - Stromal invasion (>5 mm), <4 cm size
  - Stage 1B, 2A—Type 3 radical Wertheim's hysterectomy/Shauta Mitra vaginal hysterectomy
  - Primary radiotherapy
  - Combined surgery and radiotherapy
- *Stage 1B2*:
  - In bulky tumour >4 cm with large volume, higher incidence of lymph node metastasis, 44%, hence recurrence rate is *high*
  - *Different options for Stage 1B2*—they require pre-operative chemoradiation or neoadjuvant chemotherapy followed by radical hysterectomy or radical hysterectomy with lymphadenectomy followed by radiation are considered
  - Neoadjuvant chemotherapy is used with the rationale of reducing tumour volume prior to surgery or radiotherapy

Table 6.1 Different Types of Hysterectomy

Type 1: Simple Hysterectomy (Extra Fascial)	Type 2: Modified Radical Hysterectomy (Extended Hysterectomy)	Type 3: Radical Hysterectomy
Uterus, cervix are removed but parametrium and para-cervical tissues not removed	Uterus, cervix and cuff of vagina with parametrial, para-cervical tissues are removed, medial to ureters with pelvic lymphadenectomy	Uterus, cervix, cuff of vagina, parametrium up to the pelvic side wall and para-cervical tissues are removed with pelvic lymphadenectomy

- *Stage 2B, 3 and 4A (advanced disease)*
  - Chemoradiation, chemotherapy at the time of radiotherapy makes cancer cells more sensitive to radiation. Cisplatin is used along with radiotherapy
  - Palliative radiotherapy and exenteration surgery in advanced cases
- *Stage 4B*
  - Palliative radiation or palliative chemotherapy

ADVANTAGES OF SURGERY OVER RADIOTHERAPY

- Surgery is done in young women with no co-morbid conditions
- Accurate staging is possible/ovaries can be preserved
- Surgery is done if fibroids/adnexal masses co-exist
- Preservation of ovaries and retention of pliable vagina

WERTHEIM'S HYSTERECTOMY ALSO KNOWN AS MEIG OBAYASHI TYPE 3 OR RADICAL HYSTERECTOMY

- Abdominal procedure
- Removal of entire uterus with cervical growth along with cuff of vagina and both adnexa
- Pelvic lymph nodes (external, internal and common iliac nodes, obturator nodes removed)
- Parametrium up to the pelvic side wall and para-cervical tissues are removed
- Ureters are dissected and mobilised to remove the parametrium

SCHAUTA MITRA'S HYSTERECTOMY—VAGINAL APPROACH

- Removal of entire uterus with growth and adnexa
- Most of the vagina
- Medial portion of parametrium
- Extra-peritoneal pelvic lymphadenectomy done either before or after by laparoscopy

COMPLICATIONS OF SURGERY

- Anaesthetic complications
- Surgical mortality—1%
- Haemorrhage
- Injury to ureter and adjacent organs
- Bladder atony
- Sepsis, lymph cyst formation, lymphoedema, paralytic ileus, thromboembolism

RADIOTHERAPY

It is a modified Manchester technique by brachytherapy and teletherapy.
- *Brachytherapy*—In this form of radiotherapy, the source is placed close to the tumour, a central uterine and two vaginal ovoids in the vaginal vault are kept and radioactive caesium 137 pellets are used by remote control after loading technique. This irradiates the primary growth and the parametrium and the obturator nodes for 48 h

- *Teletherapy*—In this form of radiotherapy, the source is placed at a distance to the tumour (external therapy), irradiates mainly the parametrium and the pelvic lymph nodes over a period of 4–6 weeks
- **Point A**—2 cm above and 2 cm lateral to cervical canal—gets 7000–8000 cGy, theoretically corresponds to the point where the uterine artery and ureter cross
- **Point B**—2 cm cephalic and 5 cm from uterine axis laterally and at the same level as point A—gets 6000 cGy by teletherapy, over 4–6 weeks, 20 sittings
  This point corresponds to obturator gland
- *Contraindications for radiotherapy are*: PID, ovarian tumours, myoma, prolapse uterus
- *Complications of radiotherapy*: anaemia, diarrhoea, proctitis, rectal stricture, ovarian failure, pyometra, vaginal fibrosis, bladder and bowel fistula, skin burns, avascular necrosis of femoral head
- **Prevention of cancer cervix**:
    - *Primary prevention*:
      HPV vaccines bivalent and quadrivalent
      Age of administration: 9–13 years; it can be given up to 25 years (before first sexual activity)
      Dose: three doses at 0, 2, 6 months; protection—up to 10 years
      Continue screening even after vaccination. Women are advised to continue screening by Pap smear, which is a secondary prevention of cancer cervix
    - *Secondary prevention*:
      Periodic screening tests for pre-invasive lesions of cervix and appropriate treatment

KEY POINTS

- The most common gynaec cancer is cancer cervix in India.
- Pre-cancerous lesion in cervix occurs 10–15 years earlier hence screening can reduce the incidence.
- Persistent HPV infection can cause cancer cervix in 70%–90% but when immune system is intact 90% women can get rid of it.
- CIN is diagnosed by cytological screening.
- Treatments for CIN are local destructive methods like cryosurgery, electrocoagulation, laser ablation or excision of abnormal tissue by conisation, LLETZ, LEEP, NETZ or hysterectomy.
- Cancer cervix is mostly related to HPV infection and prophylactic HPV vaccines are available now.
- Classic signs of cancer cervix are growth, bleeds on touch, induration, friability and fixity.
- Staging is clinical staging, CT scan for lymph node metastasis and MRI for parametrial involvement and tumour volume are undertaken.
- Management of cancer cervix is based on age, stage of disease, size of tumour and associated co-morbid condition.
- Stage 1A1 is treated by therapeutic conisation or Type 1 hysterectomy; Stage 1A2 is treated by Type 2 radical hysterectomy; 1B1 and 2A treated with Type 3 radical hysterectomy and pelvic lymphadenectomy or chemoradiation; Stage 1B2 by pre-operative chemoradiation or neoadjuvant chemotherapy followed by radical hysterectomy or radical hysterectomy with lymphadenectomy followed by radiation; Stage 2B, 3 and 4 is treated with chemoradiation.

FREQUENTLY ASKED QUESTIONS

1. What is CIN, pathogenesis of cancer cervix?
2. What is down-staging of cancer cervix?
3. What are the methods for screening of cancer cervix?
4. What is colposcopy? What are the different patterns you can get?
5. How do you treat CIN?
6. What are the risk factors for cancer cervix?
7. What is the lymphatic drainage of cervix?
8. What is staging of cancer cervix and modes of spread of cancer cervix?
9. What is the definition of micro-invasive cancer cervix?
10. What are early and late disease of cancer cervix?
11. Up to what stage surgery can be done for cancer cervix? What are the types of hysterectomy?
12. What are the treatment modalities available for cancer cervix?
13. What is chemoradiation?
14. What are the contraindications for radiotherapy?
15. What are the advantages of surgery over RT for cancer cervix?
16. What are the complications of Wertheim's hysterectomy and radiotherapy?
17. What are brachytherapy and teletherapy?
18. What are point A and point B and what is their significance?
19. How to prevent cancer cervix?
20. What is the role of HPV vaccination?

CASE 7

A CASE OF INFERTILITY

PATIENT'S DETAILS

Name.. Age.................. Address........................... Occupation..............
Socioeconomic Class.......................... Para

HISTORY
HISTORY OF PRESENTING ILLNESS

C/O inability to conceive/anxious to conceive—duration

The following history is to be elicited:
- Intake of hormones to regularise cycles, drugs for ovulation induction.
- White discharge PV, fever and pain in abdomen are symptoms of PID, which may cause tubal block.
- Pruritus vulva, genital ulcers may indicate STI leading to tubal block.
- Chronic cough, fever, loss of weight, treatment for cervical lymphadenopathy suggestive of tuberculosis, which may cause tubal block.
- Intolerance to cold, constipation, hoarseness of voice, lethargy, history of weight gain are symptoms of hypothyroidism causing anovulation.
- Weight loss, tremors, palpitation—hyperthyroidism.
- Weight gain, acne, hirsutism, irregular menstrual cycle—diagnostic of PCOD.
- Amenorrhoea, abnormal milk secretion—anovulation due to hyperprolactinaemia.
- Previous contraception—OCP, IUCD.
- Previous abdominal and pelvic surgery, appendicitis/surgery or medical treatment for ectopic gestation; all these can cause adhesions, tubal block.
- Previous history of procedures like hysterosalpingogram (HSG), laparoscopy, follicle study and induction of ovulation.
- Prolonged illness/drug intake for psychiatric disorders.
- *In case of secondary infertility, following additional history has to be elicited*—whether conceived spontaneously or after induction of ovulation in previous pregnancy.
- H/O previous pregnancy, abortions, H/O post-abortal/puerperal curettage—may cause Asherman's syndrome—may lead to secondary infertility.

To view the lecture notes log in to your account on www.MedEnact.com

MENSTRUAL HISTORY

- *Cycles*: regular cycles with pain and mid-cycle pain/profuse mucoid discharge PV—probably ovulatory cycles
- *Pain*: H/O painful menstruation—congestive or spasmodic type of dysmenorrhoea can occur in fibroid
- History suggestive of triple dysmenorrhoea occurs in endometriosis, which may be the cause for infertility
- History suggestive of congestive dysmenorrhoea—PID endometriosis
- *Flow*: infrequent cycles, scanty menstruation, period of amenorrhoea followed by profuse periods—anovulation probably due to PCOD
- H/O profuse periods may be due to fibroid, endometriosis, PID
- Oligomenorrhoea—thyroid dysfunction
- H/O pre-menstrual syndrome (usually present in ovulatory cycle)

MARITAL HISTORY

- Duration of marriage.
- How long she is living with her husband?

COITAL HISTORY

The following history is to be elicited:
- Frequency of intercourse—normal 3–4 days/week
- Painful coitus—superficial—vulvovaginitis
- Deep—endometriosis, PID
- Vaginismus
- Knowledge of fertile period and ovulation

ANDROLOGICAL HISTORY—MALE PARTNER

- Age
- Occupational history
- Working in places exposed to high temperature/radiation
- Work with frequent travel, shift duties
- H/O heavy smoking, alcohol, drug abuse
- Genital ulcers, dysuria
- Mumps in adolescence—mumps orchitis
- Chronic chest infection suggestive of bronchiectasis, tuberculosis—tuberculous epididymo-orchitis
- Trauma to genitals
- Diabetes
- Chronic intake of anti-hypertensives, antacids, anti-psychiatric drugs can cause hyperprolactinaemia
- Surgery in inguinal region, urethra and surgery for hydrocoele can cause injury to vas deferens
- Sexual dysfunction—erectile dysfunction, premature ejaculation
- Absence of ejaculate, cloudy urine after ejaculation—suggestive of retrograde ejaculation

OBSTETRIC HISTORY

In case of secondary infertility, following history has to be elicited:
- Previous pregnancy whether conceived after treatment for infertility
- If H/O previous abortion, post-abortal H/O curettage
- Previous surgery for ectopic pregnancy/previous delivery by LSCS may lead to adhesions leading to tubal block
- If previous delivery is present—H/O puerperal sepsis may cause tubal block resulting in secondary infertility

CONTRACEPTIVE HISTORY
- Refer Case 1

PERSONAL HISTORY
- Refer Case 1

FAMILY HISTORY
- Diabetes
- Hypertension

EXAMINATION
GENERAL EXAMINATION
- Refer Case 1

Special attention to be paid for the following details:
- *Build*: obese (PCOD)/hypothyroidism
- Hirsutism, acanthosis nigricans, acne, pallor
- *Breast*: milk secretion (hyperprolactinaemia)
- *Thyroid*: swelling, goitre

ABDOMINAL EXAMINATION
- *Scar*: may be due to previous investigations for infertility, like laparoscopy either diagnostic or operative/appendicectomy/ectopic gestation
- *Mass*: may be due to fibroid (may be the cause for infertility)
- *Tenderness*: may be due to PID (salpingitis can cause tubal block, adhesions, kinking of tubes, altered tubal motility, the peri-ovarian, peritubal adhesions and peritoneal factor—which may result in infertility)

GYNAEC EXAMINATION
External genitalia
- Whether hymen is intact

Speculum examination
- *Speculum examination is done to inspect the following findings if present:*
    - Vaginal septum, discharge
    - Cervix—discharge

Bimanual pelvic examination
- Uterus—size, mobility, tenderness noted
- Enlarged uterus may be due to fibroid, adenomyosis
- Mobility—fixed retroversion in PID and endometriosis
- Fornices—tenderness may be due to PID or endometriosis
- Adnexal mass may be due to endometrioma, TO mass, ovarian tumour

SUMMARY
- Name....Age....married for....years....anxious to conceive.........how many years
- Mention about relevant history, general examination, systemic examination findings

PROVISIONAL DIAGNOSIS
Mrs.................. married for.................. years.................. anxious to conceive. A case of primary/secondary infertility for evaluation

INVESTIGATIONS
MALE PARTNER
- *Seminal analysis*
  Collect semen in wide-mouthed container after 3–5 days of abstinence. If abnormal, repeat after 2–3 months.
  Spermatogenesis takes 74 days, and transit of spermatozoa through the epididymis and vas deferens takes 12–15 days. Sperms are stored in the ampulla of vas and then ejaculated. Sperm count reflects the health of man 74 days earlier.
- *Thyroid function test*
- *Serum prolactin*—increased prolactin can cause sexual dysfunction
- *Serum testosterone*
- *Anti-sperm antibody*
- *Blood sugar*
- *In retrograde ejaculation*: post-coital voiding urine to be tested for sperms
- *Scrotal USG*: evaluation of testes and epididymis
- *Doppler* study of scrotum for varicocele
- *Testicular biopsy* is done to differentiate between primary testicular failure and obstruction of vas deferens in case of azoospermia
- *Transrectal ultrasound*: visualisation of prostate

- *Karyotyping*: chromosomal study is done in azoospermia, 47XXY Klinefelter's syndrome is associated with azoospermia

FEMALE PARTNER

Tests for ovulation
- *BBT*: There will be dip followed by raise in basal body temperature by 0.5–1°F due to thermogenic effect of progesterone after ovulation and indicates ovulation has occurred
  Pitfalls—It is retrospective and does not indicate impending ovulation
- *Ultrasound for follicular study*: To monitor follicle growth from day 10 to 16. Follicle reaches 18–20 mm just prior to ovulation
- *LH surge*—occurs 24–36 h prior to ovulation, mid-menstrual serial urinary LH assay done to know LH surge
- *Mid-luteal serum progesterone*: >5 ng/mL confirms ovulation; peak 15 ng/mL
- *Cervical mucus—Fern test*—Ferning is present prior to ovulation due to crystallisation of NaCl under the effect of oestrogen. Ferning disappears after ovulation under the effect of progesterone
- *Spinnbarkeit*—Stretchability of cervical mucus up to 10 cm due to the effect of oestrogen just prior to ovulation and this quality is lost after ovulation.
- *Pre-menstrual endometrial biopsy*:
  - To find out secretory changes which indicates ovulation
  - To find out luteal phase defect (there will be lag of 2 days between the endometrial histopathology and the date of menstrual cycle)
  - To rule out tuberculous endometritis
- *Hormonal assay in anovulation*:
  - FSH, LH: Day 2/3
  - T4, T3, TSH
  - Serum prolactin

Tests for tubal patency
- *HSG*:
  Done on day 8–10 of menstrual cycle; advantage—outpatient procedure. Viscous water-soluble dye/50% iodine with 6% polyvinyl alcohol is used. It is a permanent record.
  HSG gives information about uterine contour, uterine malformation, septa, polyp, submucous fibroid and tubal patency, site of tubal block/hydrosalpinx.
  Bilateral tubal block with beaded tubes and extravasation of dye could be due to tuberculosis.
- *Saline infusion sonography—SION test*: can diagnose polyps, septa, tubal patency or block.
- Diagnostic laparoscopy with chromotubation:
  - Methylene blue dye is injected into cervical canal and flow of the dye through the tubes and collection of dye in pouch of Douglas is visualised.
  - Laparoscopy is useful also to diagnosis myoma, uterine anomalies, peritubal adhesions, tubal block, fimbrial condition, hydrosalpinx, PCOD, TO mass, adhesions, abdominal tuberculosis, endometriosis.
  - Laparoscopy can be combined with operative procedures like adhesiolysis and ovarian drilling.
  - Laparoscopy can be both diagnostic and therapeutic.
- *Hysteroscopy*:
  - Cornual ostia can be visualised.

- Other benefits: both diagnostic and therapeutic.
  Septum can be resected, submucous fibroid and endometrial polyp can be removed.

> 'Gold standard' investigation in infertility—hysterolaparoscopy.

- *Salpingoscopy via laparoscope.*
- *Falloposcopy*: via hysteroscopic transcervical can visualise tubal lumen. Under guidance, tubal cannulation can be done.

Other tests
- *Post-coital test (Sim's or Huhner's test)*—done 1–2 days before ovulation.
  After 2–12 h of coitus, cervical mucus is aspirated and examined under microscope. Presence of 10–50 motile sperms/HPF, indicates normal sperm motility and mucus penetrating capacity. Presence of immobile sperms may be due to immunological factors (anti-sperm antibodies).
  It can assess cervical mucus qualities, spinnbarkeit, ferning.
  It can be done when husband is not willing for seminal analysis.
- *Semen cervical mucous contact test*
- *Sperm penetration test, Miller–Kurzrok test*

CASE DISCUSSION
DEFINITION OF INFERTILITY
Apparent failure of a couple to conceive after 1 year of unprotected regular coitus. Nowadays the word subfertility is used for infertility.

STERILITY
- Absolute inability to conceive.
- **Primary infertility**: conception has never occurred.
- **Secondary infertility**: patient fails to conceive after prior conception.

CAUSES OF INFERTILITY
- Male factor: 30%–40%
- Female factor: 40%–45%
- Both: 10%
- Unexplained: 10%

CAUSES FOR FEMALE INFERTILITY
- *Vaginal causes*: 5%
- *Cervical causes*: 5% (amputation of cervix, conisation, Fothergill's surgery, LEEP procedure)
- *Uterine causes*: 10% (fibroid, intra-uterine adhesions, TB endometritis, congenital abnormalities, Asherman's syndrome, endometrial polyps)
- *Ovarian causes*: 30% [anovulation, luteal phase defect (LPD), PCOD]
- *Tubal causes*: 30% (infections like chlamydial, gonococcal, tuberculous infection, post-abortal and puerperal infection, endometriosis, abdominal or pelvic surgery, previous ectopic gestation)

- *Peritoneal causes*: 5% (endometriosis, adhesion, TO mass)
- *Unexplained*: 15%

MALE FACTOR EVALUATION
WHO criteria 2010—semen analysis
- Volume: 2 mL, Ph: 7.2–7.8
- Viscosity <3 (scale 0–4)
- Sperm concentration: 20 million/mL
- Total sperm count >40 million per ejaculate or more
- Motility >50% or more with progressive motility
- Morphology >14%; strict criteria 4%
- Viability >75% or more (50%)
- White blood cells <1 million/mL
- Round cells <5 million/mL
- Sperm agglutination <2 (scale of 0–3)

Terminology
- <20 millions/mL—oligozoospermia
- No sperms in semen—azoospermia
- Decreased motility—asthenospermia
- Abnormal morphology—teratospermia
- Dead sperms—necrospermia
- Absence of semen—aspermia

Latest WHO recommendations for normal semen analysis reference values
- Volume: 1.5–5 mL
- Ph > 7.2
- Viscosity <3 (scale 0–4); sperm concentration >20 million/mL
- Total sperm number >40 million per ejaculate; percent motility >50%
- Forward progression >2 (scale 0–4); normal morphology >50%; normal round cells <5 million/mL
- Sperm agglutination <2 (scale 0–3)

Causes for low volume
- Incomplete abstinence or collection
- Abnormalities in the seminal vesicles
- Partial vas obstruction
- Retrograde ejaculation
- Hypogonadism

Aetiology of male infertility

Pre-Testicular	Testicular Causes	Post-Testicular Causes
Hypothalamic, pituitary disorders, thyroid dysfunction adrenal disorders, liver failure	Chromosomal abnormalities, local conditions like varicocele, trauma, orchitis, exposure to heat and toxins in work place, substance abuse, smoking	Block in vas deferens, congenital vas aplasia, erectile dysfunction, anti-sperm antibodies

CASE 7 A CASE OF INFERTILITY

MANAGEMENT
- Counselling the couple about the basics of reproduction, fertile period, frequency of coitus
- Identify and treat the cause

MALE PARTNER
General
- Avoidance of smoking, alcohol, drug abuse
- Improvement of general health
- Cold scrotal bath
- Treatment of genital tract infections and endocrinopathies
- In hypogonadotropic hypogonadism:
    Clomiphene citrate 25 mg/day for 3 months
    Inj. HCG 5000IU IM once weekly

Management of Male Infertility (Flow chart 7.1)

```
                        Male infertility
                       /              \
          Abnormal semen          Normal semen
            parameters              parameters
                |                       |
        Pre-testicular, testicular   Post-testicular
        and post-testicular
```

Abnormal semen parameters	Normal semen parameters
Hypogonadal hypopituitarism: Clomiphene—25 mg daily for 25 days for 3–6 cycles	Erectile dysfunction: Sildenafil—25–100 mg—1 h before coitus
Pituitary inadequacy: HMG 150-IU thrice/week for 6 months	Premature ejaculation: selective serotonin reuptake inhibitors—30–60 mg—1 h before coitus
Hypothalamic failure—GnRH	IUI, if fails IVF ICSI
Grade 2 and 3 varicocele need surgical intervention	
Block in vas deferens, congenital vas aplasia—micro-surgical vas anastomosis/IVF	
Azoospermia—IVF, ICSI with sperms retrieved by PESA, MESA	

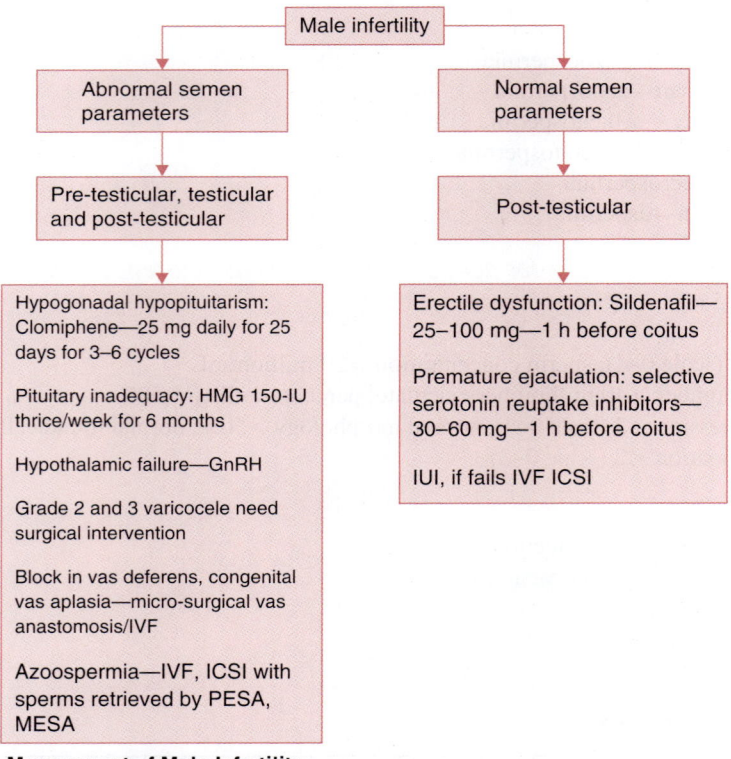

FLOW CHART 7.1 Management of Male Infertility

Intra-uterine insemination—husband's semen—AIH
Indications:
- Oligozoospermia

- Asthenospermia
- Presence of anti-sperm antibodies
- Agglutination of sperms
- Sexual dysfunction
- Hypospadias
- In retrograde ejaculation, sperm retrieved from post-coital voiding urine is used

Intra-uterine insemination—donor semen—AID
Azoospermis: IUI with donor's semen can be undertaken with consent from the couple; in vitro fertilisation (IVF), intra-cytoplasmic sperm injection (ICSI) can be offered with successful sperm retrieval by microsurgical epididymal sperm aspiration (MESA), or percutaneous epididymal sperm aspiration (PESA).

FEMALE PARTNER
Management of female infertility

Ovulation Cause	Tubal Cause
Ovulation-inducing drugs: *Clomiphene citrate*: CC 50–150 mg/day from 2nd day for 5 days *Gonadotrophins*: *Human menopausal gonadotrophin*—HMG has FSH and LH activity; can be used alone or with CC, monitor serum oestradiol, start with 75 IU/day from 5th day continued depending on response *Human chorionic gonadotrophin*—HCG has LH activity to trigger ovulation when follicular diameter 18–20 mm *Recombinant FSH*: Drugs which enhances ovulation: Insulin sensitisers: Metformin 500 mg t.i.d. Aromatase inhibitors—Letrozole When not responding, IVF with donor ovum or adoption *Hyperprolactinemia*: • Bromocryptine—start with 1.25 mg at bedtime and gradually increase to 2.5 mg twice daily • Cabergoline—0.5 mg once/twice weekly PCOS—metformin 500 mg twice or thrice a day and ovulation induction drugs	*Proximal tubal occlusion*: Hysteroscopic cannulation Radiologically guided tubal cannulation Tubo-cornual anastomosis *Distal tubal occlusion*: Salpingostomy Fimbrioplasty Laparoscopic adhesiolysis IVF: best option in many cases Secondary infertility in women undergone sterilisation—block at isthmus or ampulla—resection and anastomosis

Assisted reproductive technology (ART) includes IVF with embryo transfer (ET), in selective cases, ICSI.

ART though costly, brings a ray of hope for the infertile couples and has helped women to have children. Ovum donation and surrogacy are also advocated in selective cases of IVF.

IVF and ET
- Bilateral tubal block or absent tubes
- Endometriosis
- Immunological factor for infertility
- Unexplained male and female infertility
- Severe male factor infertility

ICSI and IVF
- Azoospermia
- Severe oligoasthenoteratozoospermia
- Unexplained infertility
- Previous failed IVF

KEY POINTS

- Infertility is prevalent among 10%–15% of reproductive couples.
- Infertility may be caused by male or female or combined factor.
- Male infertility factors may be due to pre-testicular, testicular and post-testicular factors.
- Female infertility factors may be due to anovulation, uterine factors, tubal factors, cervical factors and peritoneal factors.
- Basic investigations include seminal fluid analysis, test for ovulation, test for tubal patency.
- Unexplained infertility is seen in 10% of the couple.
- Hysterolaparoscopy can be used to evaluate uterus, tubes, ovaries and peritoneal factors.
- Ovulation induction drugs are used along with follicular study for anovulation.
- Tubal block requires IVF since following tuboplasty, chances for ectopic gestation is high.
- Treatment of choice is IUI for cervical factor and ejaculatory dysfunction.
- ICSI is another option for male infertility.
- Prognosis of infertility has improved after assisted reproductive techniques.

FREQUENTLY ASKED QUESTIONS

1. What are primary and secondary infertility?
2. What are the causes for male infertility?
3. What are the causes for female infertility?
4. When will you investigate a case of infertility?
5. How will you investigate male partner?
6. What are the investigations for female infertility?
7. What is the tubal factor for infertility and its investigations?
8. What are the tests for ovulation?
9. What are the uterine and cervical factors for infertility?
10. What are the drugs used for induction of ovulation and dose?
11. What is ART?
12. What are the indications for ART?

CASE 8

A CASE OF PRIMARY AMENORRHOEA

PATIENT'S DETAILS
Name.. Age................. Address........................... Occupation.............
Socioeconomic Class......................... Para

HISTORY
HISTORY OF PRESENTING ILLNESS
C/O not yet attained menarche and non-development of secondary sexual characters or C/O Not attained menarche but secondary sexual characters have developed

The following history is to be elicited:
- Cyclical pain abdomen/retention of urine may be due to cryptomenorrhoea as a result of imperforate hymen and vaginal agenesis
- Weight loss, chronic cough—tuberculosis/juvenile diabetes/chronic illness/mumps
- Swelling in inguinal region (testis may be present in inguinal region in testicular feminization syndrome)
- Lymphedema at birth (Turner's syndrome)
- Deficit in smelling, hearing, defective field of vision, mental retardation (MR)—hypothalamo pituitary cause
- Hoarseness or deepening of voice/abdominal mass/head injury/encephalitis in the past/delayed milestones

FAMILY HISTORY
- Age of menarche in siblings, mother
- H/O primary amenorrhea in maternal aunt (X-linked recessive trait—in testicular feminization syndrome)

EXAMINATION

GENERAL EXAMINATION

- Refer Case 1

Special attention to be paid for the following details:
- Height, weight, BMI
- Build, stature and nourishment
- Arm span, height ratio
- Hirsutism
- Galactorrhoea
- Short stature, webbed neck, cubitus valgus, shield chest, high palate, low set ears—Turner's syndrome

EXAMINATION FOR BREAST DEVELOPMENT

Tanner's staging

EXAMINATION OF AXILLARY AND PUBIC HAIR

Sparse pubic hair and well-developed breast occur in testicular feminization syndrome

EXAMINATION OF THYROID

CVS, RS, CNS examination
Abdominal examination
- Abdominal striae in cases of obesity and Cushing's syndrome
- Mass—haematometra
- Swelling in inguinal region may be due to presence of testis in androgen insensitivity syndrome

GYNAEC EXAMINATION

External genitalia:
- Pubic hair—present/absent or sparse
- Development of labia majora/minora/clitoromegaly
- Hymen—bluish bulge (cryptomenorrhoea)/presence or absence of vagina

PER-RECTAL EXAMINATION

- *To find out*:
  - Presence or absence of uterus
  - Size of uterus
  - Uterine mass (haematometra)

SUMMARY

- Name....Age.....C/O not yet attained menarche with or without secondary sexual characters
- Mention about special features in general and local examination

DIAGNOSIS
- Primary amenorrhoea—for evaluation

INVESTIGATIONS
ROUTINE
Complete blood count

SPECIFIC INVESTIGATIONS
- *USG: abdomen, pelvis and KUB area*
  To find out anomalies of genitourinary system
  Uterus—to find out presence or absence of uterus, haematocolpos haematometra, haematosalpinx
  Ovaries—streak ovaries, primary ovarian failure
- *Serum FSH, LH, prolactin (PRL)*
- *Thyroid profile*
- *Testosterone, DHEAS*
- *17OH progesterone*
- *Karyotyping*
- *X-ray skull—lateral view for sella turcica*
- *CT/MRI brain*

CASE DISCUSSION
DEFINITION OF PRIMARY AMENORRHOEA
Absence of menstruation by the age of 16 years regardless of development of secondary sexual characters.

In recent years, the age limit is decreased by one year to 15 years, as the age of menarche is advancing

PRIMARY AMENORRHOEA
It is now defined as absence of menses by 13 years of age when there is no development of secondary sexual characters or absence of menses by 15 years of age when there is development of secondary sexual characters.
- ***Thelarche***: *8 years/**pubarche**: 10 years/**menarche**: 12–13 years*
- During puberty there is growth spurt, then breast budding and almost simultaneously pubic hair appears
- Menarche occurs within 1 year of peak growth velocity, within 2 years of earliest pubic hair growth and breast changes and bone age of about 13 years

TANNER'S STAGING OF BREAST DEVELOPMENT
Stage 1—infantile, elevation of papilla only
Stage 2—the bud stage, enlargement of areola

CASE 8 A CASE OF PRIMARY AMENORRHOEA

Table 8.1 Various Causes for Primary Amenorrhoea

Hypergonadotropic hypogonadism (48.5% of cases)	Hypogonadotropic hypogonadism (27.8%)	Eugonadotropic (with normal gonadotropins; 23.7%)
The hypergonadotropic hypogonadism category includes patients with abnormal sex chromosomes (i.e., Turner syndrome)	Hypogonadotropic hypogonadism includes isolated GnRH deficiency, hypopituitarism, hyperprolactinaemia	Eugonadism may result from anatomic abnormalities or intersex disorders. Anatomic abnormalities include congenital absence of the uterus and vagina and cervical atresia—Mullerian agenesis, cryptomenorrhoea. Intersex disorders include androgen insensitivity syndrome (testicular feminisation syndrome), 17-ketoreductase deficiency (adrenogenital syndrome).

Stage 3—similar to that of a small adult breast
Stage 4—areola and papillae enlarge to form a secondary mound
Stage 5—secondary mound disappears, typical adult breast with rounded contour
Pubic hair development has 1–5 stages.

PRIMARY AMENORRHOEA—CAUSES (TABLE 8.1)
- *Cryptomenorrhoea*

EUGONADOTROPHIC PRIMARY AMENORRHOEA
- It occurs due to imperforate hymen or vaginal agenesis
- Not attained menarche, cyclical pain abdomen, abdominal mass, retention of urine and tense bulging bluish hymen—in case of imperforate hymen

Treatment:
- Cruciate incision and drainage of haematocolpos in case of imperforate hymen (Fig. 8.1A and B)

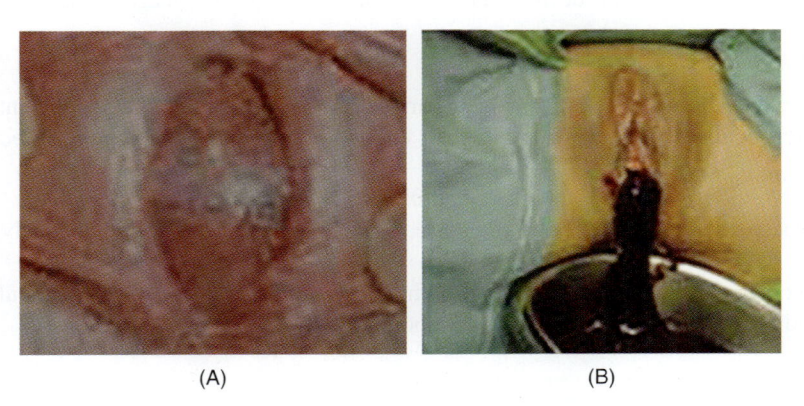

(A)   (B)

FIGURE 8.1 Drainage of Haematocolpos

(A) Tense bluish hymen. (B) drainage of haematocolpos.

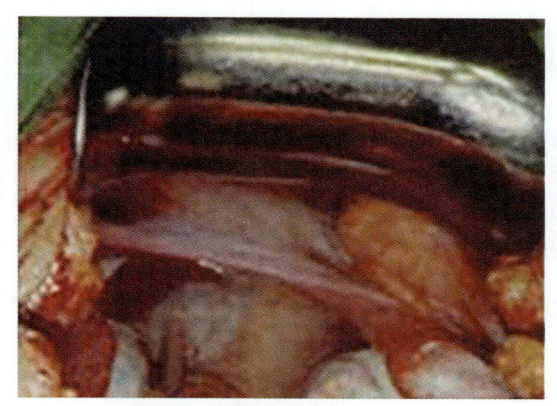

FIGURE 8.2 Uterus Absent and Ovaries Present—Mullerian Agenesis

- *Mullerian agenesis (Mayer-Rokitansky-Kuster-Hauser syndrome) eugonadotropic primary amenorrhoea (Fig. 8.2)*
    - Normal height
    - Presence of secondary sexual characters
    - Ovaries present
    - Normal values of gonadotropins—FSH, LH and oestradiol
    - Uterus and vagina absent
    - Karyotype 46XX
    - In 15%, congenital renal anomalies and 5% skeletal anomalies may be present
  Treatment:
    - Counselling
    - Vaginoplasty before sexual activity
    - Reproduction—biological child by surrogacy

TESTICULAR FEMINIZATION SYNDROME

- Phenotype—female. Genotype 46 XY
- Well developed breasts, small areola. No axillary and pubic hair
- Absent uterus short blind vagina
- Gonads in inguinal region/abdomen

Treatment:
- Counselling—assigning the sex of rearing
- Gonadectomy after full sexual development by age 18–20 years because of malignant potential of gonads

ADRENOGENITAL SYNDROME

- 46XX
- Hirsutism, clitoromegaly
- Increased 17OH Progesterone/increased urinary pregnanediol

CASE 8 A CASE OF PRIMARY AMENORRHOEA

Treatment:
- Synthetic corticosteroids, prednisolone 2.5 mg b.i.d.

TURNER'S SYNDROME (Fig. 8.3)—HYPERGONADOTROPIC HYPOGONADISM
- Short stature
- Absent secondary sexual characters
- Shield chest, webbed neck, cubitus valgus
- Streak ovaries
- Primary ovarian failure—high gonadotropins—FSH and LH
- Low oestradiol
- Uterus, vagina normal
- Karyotype—45XO

Treatment:
- Oestrogen is started for the development of secondary sexual character at the age of 10 at very low dose as bone growth is better at lower oestrogen level to avoid premature epiphyseal closure.
- Cyclical oestrogen and progesterone started at the age of 13 for secondary sexual character and withdrawal bleeding.

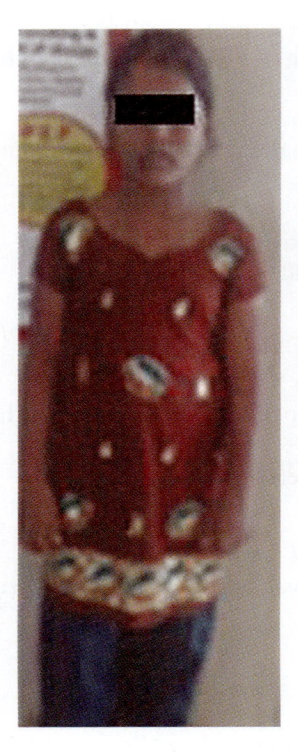

FIGURE 8.3 Turner's Syndrome

- Growth hormone for growth and height.
- Patient can have normal sexual activity.
- Patient can conceive by IVF with donor ovum.

HYPOGONADOTROPIC HYPOGONADISM
- Decreased FSH, LH short stature, obesity
- Loss of olfactory function—Kallman's syndrome, MR, retinitis pigmentosa

Treatment:
- Cyclical oestrogen and progesterone
- Gonadotrophins for ovulation induction

HYPERPROLACTINAEMIA—INCREASED PROLACTIN (PRL)
(See Flow chart 8.1)
Treatment:
- Bromocriptine, cabergoline

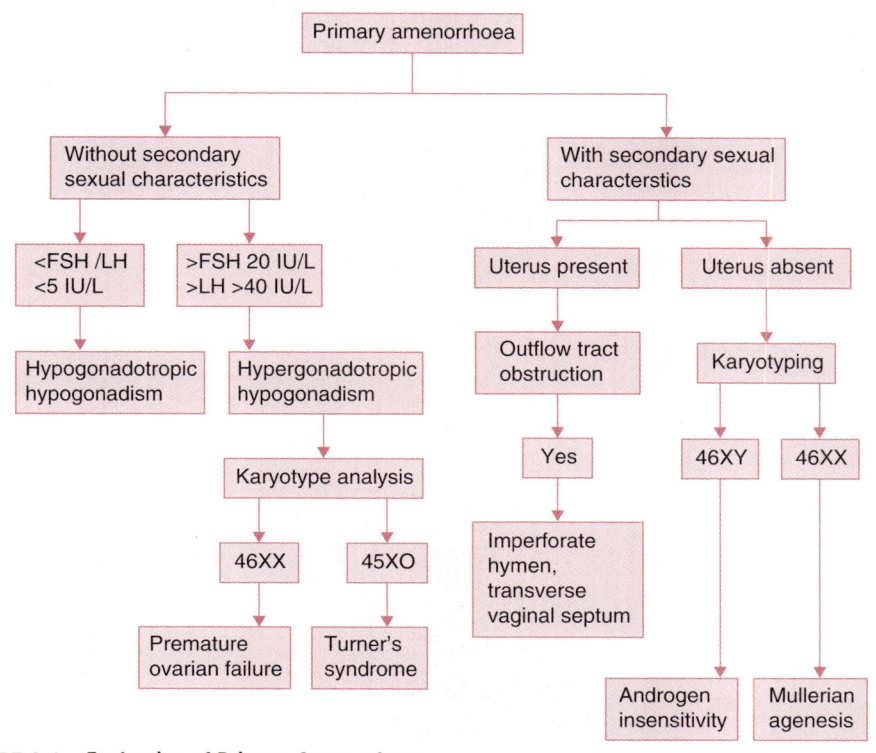

FLOW CHART 8.1 Evaluation of Primary Amenorrhoea

CASE 8 A CASE OF PRIMARY AMENORRHOEA

KEY POINTS
- Pregnancy, lactation and menopause are the physiological causes for amenorrhoea.
- Normal hypothalamic—pituitary ovarian function will results in secondary sexual characteristics.
- Hypothalamo pituitary ovarian axis dysfunction, developmental defect of genital tract, chromosomal pattern abnormality are the common causes for Primary amenorrhoea.
- In Turner's syndrome ovaries are absent or streaks hence oestrogen is started for the development of secondary sexual characters at the age of 10.
- For outflow obstruction surgery is needed.

FREQUENTLY ASKED QUESTIONS
1. Define primary amenorrhoea?
2. When do you investigate a case of primary amenorrhoea?
3. What is Tanner's staging for breast development?
4. Counselling in testicular feminisation syndrome?
5. Features of Turner's syndrome and management?
6. Common causes for primary amenorrhoea?
7. What is cryptomenorrhoea and how do you treat it?

A CASE OF SECONDARY AMENORRHOEA

CASE 9

PATIENT'S DETAILS
Name... Age.................. Address............................ Occupation..............
Socioeconomic Class.......................... Para..........................

HISTORY
Complaints of absence of menstruation for............... months

HISTORY OF PRESENTING ILLNESS
The following history is to be elicited:
- Period of amenorrhoea
- Loss or gain in weight
- Intolerance to cold, constipation, hoarseness of voice, lethargy, hypothyroidism
- Drug intake for withdrawal bleeding
- Inappropriate milk secretion (may be due to hyperprolactinaemia—galactorrhoea amenorrhoea syndrome)
- Acne, hirsutism, weight gain, infertility [may be present in polycystic ovarian syndrome (PCOS)] acne, hirsutism and change in voice (occurs in adrenal disorders or virilising tumours of ovary)
- Loss of appetite, vomiting—anorexia nervosa
- Stress, strenuous exercise
- Headache, visual disturbances (may be due to pituitary adenoma)
- Intake of anti-psychiatric drugs, anti-hypertensives, OC pills
- Dryness of vagina, hot flushes (occurs in premature ovarian failure)

MENSTRUAL HISTORY
- Onset of menarche, cyclicity, duration of flow, association with pain, clots

PAST OBSTETRIC HISTORY
- Parity, abortions

- H/O PPH, shock (Sheehan's syndrome)
- Puerperal sepsis, post-abortal or puerperal curettage (Asherman's syndrome)

PAST MEDICAL HISTORY
- Tuberculosis, diabetes, chronic renal disease, treatment with chemotherapy or radiotherapy

PAST SURGICAL HISTORY
Refer Case 1

FAMILY HISTORY
- Diabetes, hypertension, thyroid dysfunction
- H/O menstrual irregularities or premature menopause in siblings, mother, aunts

PERSONAL HISTORY
Refer Case 1

EXAMINATION
GENERAL EXAMINATION
- Refer Case 1

Special attention to be paid for the following details:
- Height, weight, BMI
- Acne, hirsutism
- Galactorrhoea
- Thyroid—goitre
- Cervical lymph nodes, scar from previous tuberculous sinus

CVS, RS, CNS EXAMINATION
ABDOMINAL EXAMINATION
- Abdominal striae (may be due to Cushing's)
- Mass (may be due to virilising tumours of ovary)

GYNAEC EXAMINATION
- *External genitalia*: look for clitoromegaly
- *Speculum examination*: may reveal normal findings
- *Bimanual pelvic examination*:
  - Cervix

- Uterus, size, mobility, tenderness
- Adnexal mass (may be due to ovarian mass or TO mass due to tuberculosis)
- POD nodules (in cases of ovarian mass)

SUMMARY
- Name...Age...C/O amenorrhoea....months....relevant past and present history
- Mention about general examination, abdominal examination and gynaec examination positive findings

PROVISIONAL DIAGNOSIS
- Name...years...old, para, live, with....period of amenorrhoea, with previous regular/irregular cycles for evaluation of secondary amenorrhoea

INVESTIGATIONS
ROUTINE INVESTIGATIONS
Specific investigations
- Complete blood count
- *USG*—abdomen and pelvis for uterus, endometrial thickness, ovaries—presence of follicles, PCOD
- *Free T3, T4, TSH*
- *Prolactin*
- *Day 2/3—FSH, LH*
- *DHEAS, free testosterone*
- *Fasting blood sugar/fasting insulin*—2 h oral GTT in cases of PCOS
- *CT/MRI brain/X-ray sella turcica*—when indicated
- *Endometrial biopsy*—if TB endometrium is suspected
- *HSG or hysteroscopy*—to rule out Asherman's syndrome

CASE DISCUSSION
DEFINITION OF SECONDARY AMENORRHOEA
Absence of menstruation for 6 months or for a period 3 times the length of the previous menstrual cycles in women who have previously menstruated

MANAGEMENT

Evaluate and find the cause for secondary amenorrhoea and appropriate treatment is to be given.

CASE 9 A CASE OF SECONDARY AMENORRHOEA

CAUSES OF SECONDARY AMENORRHOEA
- *Ovarian*: PCOD, resistant ovarian syndrome, radiotherapy, chemotherapy virilising tumours of ovary
- *Nutritional*: anorexia nervosa, bulimia
- *Uterine*: Asherman's syndrome, tuberculous endometritis
- *Pituitary*: Sheehan's syndrome
- *Hyperprolactinaemia*
- *Hypothalamic*: vigorous exercise, stress
- *Other endocrine causes*: thyroid dysfunction, Cushing's disease, Addison's disease

PROGESTERONE CHALLENGE TEST (HELPS TO FIND OUT LEVEL OF FAULT)
- Withdrawal bleeding PV following progesterone administration indicates presence of endogenous oestrogen (denotes uterus primed with oestrogen).
- If there is no withdrawal bleeding PV combination of oestrogen and progesterone is given.
- If still there is no withdrawal bleeding PV—it denotes end organ failure—tuberculous endometritis, Asherman's syndrome.

PCOS/PCOD
Diagnostic criteria:
- *Rotterdam's criteria*—any two of the following three:
  - Oligo and/or anovulation
  - Hyperandrogenism
  - Polycystic ovaries
- *Clinical features*
  - Obesity, oligomenorrhoea, infertility, acne, hirsutism
  - Acanthosis nigricans—thick pigmented skin over nape of neck, inner thigh (Fig. 9.1)
- *Investigations*
  - USG—presence of peripherally arranged multiple small follicles
  - Each follicle 2–9 mm, 12 or more in number—necklace pattern or string of pearl appearance

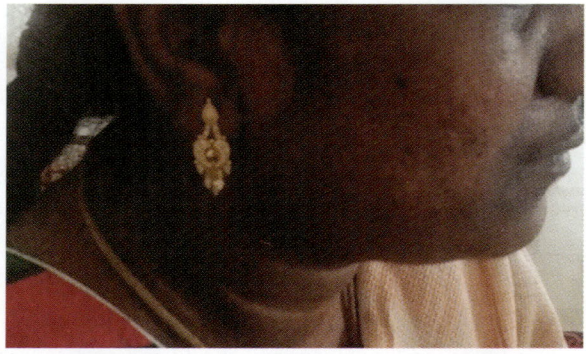

FIGURE 9.1 Acanthosis Nigricans

- Ovarian volume >10 cm^3
 - Altered LH/FSH ratio >3:1
 - Serum hormone binding globulin (SHBG) level is reduced
 - Testosterone >150 ng/dL
 - Fasting insulin level >25 m IU/mL
 - Laparoscopy—bilateral polycystic ovaries
- *Long-term sequelae of PCOS*
 - Metabolic syndrome—diabetes mellitus, dyslipidemia, hypertension, coronary heart disease
 - Endometrial cancer, breast cancer
- *Treatment*
 - Weight reduction/life style modification
 - OCP and Metformin—adolescent and in unwed women and in those who do not wish to conceive
 - Metformin and ovulation induction—when PCOD is associated with infertility
 - Clomiphene citrate—50 mg/day for 5 days from day 2 to 6
 - If ovulation does not occur, dose can be increased up to 150 mg day
 - Clomiphene with HCG—(HCG 5,000 or 10,000 units is given when follicle is around 18–20 mm)
 - Clomiphene + HMG 75 IU units with HCG
 - When medical treatment fails, laparoscopic ovarian drilling can be done

HYPERPROLACTINAEMIA

- Prolactin level 25 ng/mL
- Up to 200 ng/mL—may be due to microadenoma, in the absence of thyroid dysfunction
- More than 200 ng/mL—indicates macroadenoma
- *Causes*
 - Increased PRL due to prolactionoma/hypothyroidism/drugs like methyl dopa/phenothiazines, metoclopramide, cimetidine
- *Treatment*
 - Microadenoma—medical–bromocriptine 1.25 mg/day gradually increased or cabergoline 0.25 mg once or twice weekly
 - Macro adenoma—treatment is surgery

TREATMENT OF SECONDARY AMENORRHOEA DUE TO OTHER CONDITIONS

- *Hypothyroidism*: thyroid hormone replacement
- *Eating disorders, stress*: counselling, psychotherapy
- *Exercise-induced amenorrhoea*: moderation of activity
- *Virilising tumours of ovary*: surgery

TREATMENT OF HIRSUTISM

- OCP containing cyproterone acetate
- Anti-androgens—spironolactone, flutamide

CASE 9 A CASE OF SECONDARY AMENORRHOEA

PREMATURE OVARIAN FAILURE

- *Causes*
  - Genetic, autoimmune, smoking, radiotherapy, chemotherapy
  - Symptoms: Women present with menopausal symptoms—vasomotor, urogenital symptoms
- Diagnosis
  - FSH >40 IU/mL, E2 < 20 pg/mL
- Treatment
  - Oestrogen and progesterone replacement and prevention of osteoporosis

See (Flow chart 9.1)

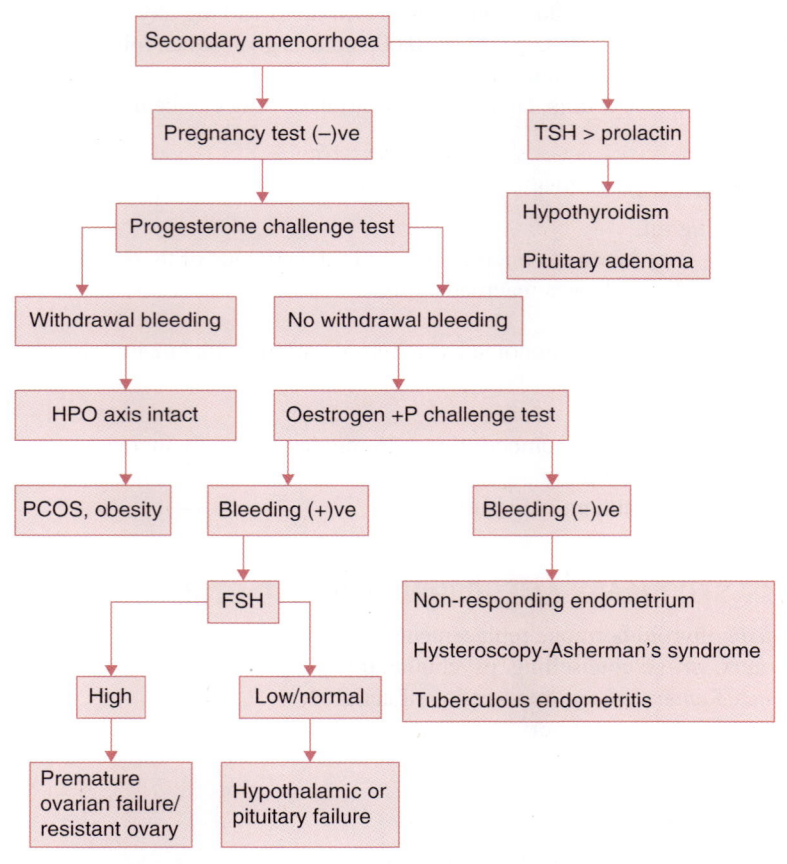

```
Secondary amenorrhoea
    │
    ├──────────────────────────────┐
    ▼                              ▼
Pregnancy test (−)ve          TSH > prolactin
    │                              │
    ▼                              ▼
Progesterone challenge test   Hypothyroidism
    │                         Pituitary adenoma
    ├──────────────┐
    ▼              ▼
Withdrawal    No withdrawal
bleeding      bleeding
    │              │
    ▼              ▼
HPO axis      Oestrogen +P challenge test
intact             │
    │         ┌────┴────┐
    ▼         ▼         ▼
PCOS,     Bleeding   Bleeding
obesity    (+)ve      (−)ve
              │         │
              ▼         ▼
             FSH     Non-responding endometrium
           ┌──┴──┐   Hysteroscopy-Asherman's syndrome
           ▼     ▼   Tuberculous endometritis
         High  Low/normal
           │     │
           ▼     ▼
      Premature  Hypothalamic or
      ovarian    pituitary failure
      failure/
      resistant ovary
```

FLOW CHART 9.1 Evaluation of Secondary Amenorrhoea

KEY POINTS
- Absence of menstruation for 6 months in a regularly menstruating woman is secondary amenorrhoea.
- Abnormalities in hypothalamic pituitary ovarian axis ,non responding endometrium, thyroid dysfunction, psychological factors can cause secondary amenorrhoea.
- PCOS is the most common cause of secondary amenorrhoea.
- In PCOS when progesterone is given, withdrawal bleeding occurs since endometrium is oestrogenised.
- When there is no withdrawal bleeding after oestrogen and progesterone it indicates endometrium is not responding (end organ failure) and the commonest cause is Asherman's syndrome and tuberculous endometritis.

FREQUENTLY ASKED QUESTIONS
1. Definition of secondary amenorrhoea.
2. Diagnostic criteria for PCOD.
3. Investigations and management of PCOD.
4. Long-term sequelae of PCOD.
5. Common causes of secondary amenorrhoea.
6. Investigations and management of secondary amenorrhoea.
7. Diagnosis and treatment of premature ovarian failure.

CASE 10

A CASE OF OVARIAN TUMOUR

PATIENT'S DETAILS

Name.. Age.................. Address.......................... Occupation..............
Socioeconomic Class......................... Para

(Age: Germ cell tumours—occur in younger age group/epithelial tumours—occurs in elderly age group.............. Para—Nulliparous are more prone for ovarian tumour)

PRESENT COMPLAINTS

Patient may come with following complaints:
- Loss of appetite, vomiting, dyspepsia
- Weight loss and cachexia
- Abdominal discomfort
- Abdominal distension/abdominal mass—with sudden increase in size may be due to malignancy
- Pressure symptoms (pedal oedema, varicosity of lower limbs, urinary symptoms like retention, frequency, constipation)
- Breathlessness or respiratory symptoms when there is pleural effusion, abdominal distension or lung metastasis
- Occasionally women may present with irregular bleeding PV or post-menopausal bleeding PV, which may be due to feminising tumour of ovary
- Usually menstrual symptoms will be absent in other types of ovarian tumours
- Defeminising symptoms like oligomenorrhoea, amenorrhoea, breast changes followed by virilising symptoms like acne, hirsutism, temporal baldness, voice changes, clitoromegaly may be present—due to virilising tumours of ovary—arrhenoblastoma

Acute pain occurs in the following situations and patient may present as an emergency:
1. Torsion ovarian cyst
2. Rupture of the cyst
3. Haemorrhage into the cyst
4. Infection
5. Malignant changes

To view the lecture notes log in to your account on www.MedEnact.com

CASE 10 A CASE OF OVARIAN TUMOUR

> Ovarian tumours are mostly asymptomatic and hence detected at late stage.

HISTORY
MENSTRUAL HISTORY
- Usually there will be no menstrual abnormality
- Menorrhagia can occur in feminising sex cord stromal tumours like granulosa and theca cell tumours, which may result in precocious puberty, post-menopausal bleeding PV
- Amenorrhoea and virilising symptoms may be the features of—virilising sex cord stromal tumours, Sertoli–Leydig cell tumour—arrhenoblastoma

PAST OBSTETRIC HISTORY
- Parity—in Nulliparous woman, according to theory of incessant ovulation, there may be increased risk of ovarian malignancy
- Contraceptive history—use of OCP protects against ovarian malignancy

FAMILY HISTORY
- H/O ovarian malignancy, breast carcinoma, colon cancer, uterine cancer in the family to be elicited
- BRCA1 and BRCA2—mutations in this gene is responsible for hereditary ovarian cancer
- Familial Lynch 11 syndrome [hereditary non-polyposis colorectal cancer (HNPCC)]—high risk for endometrial and ovarian carcinoma

PAST MEDICAL HISTORY
- History of repeated treatment taken for induction of ovulation
- Tuberculosis (to differentiate encysted tuberculosis of abdomen from ovarian mass)

PAST SURGICAL HISTORY
- Surgical treatment for previous ovarian tumour

PERSONAL HISTORY
- Use of talc, H/O working in asbestos factory (risk factor for ovarian tumour)

EXAMINATION
GENERAL EXAMINATION
- Refer Case 1

Special attention to be paid for the following details:
- Anaemia, cachexia, pedal oedema
- BMI and weight—weight loss

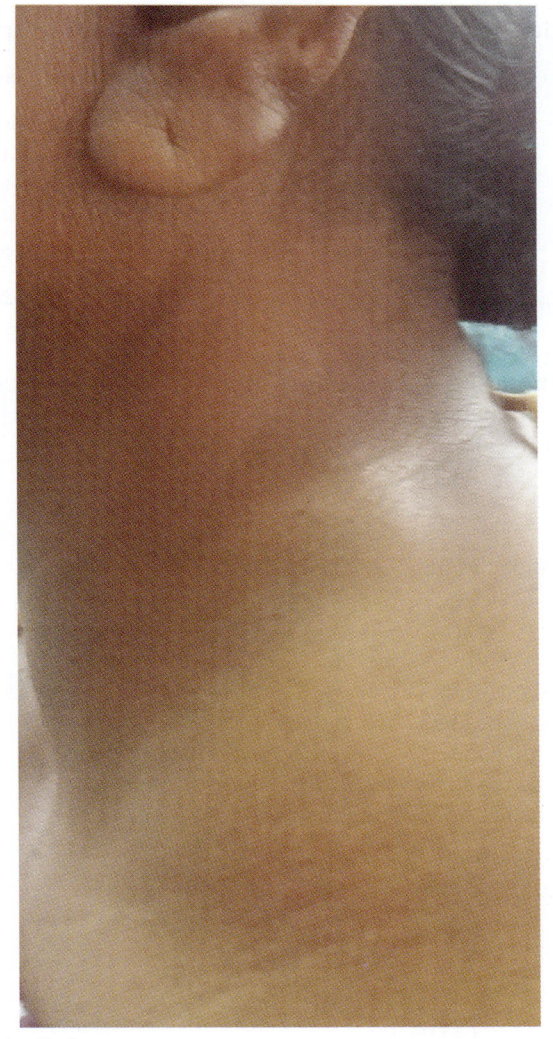

FIGURE 10.1 Supraclavicular Node

- In addition to general lymphadenopathy, supraclavicular lymph node enlargement to be looked for (Fig. 10.1)
- *Breast and thyroid examination*: breast cancer and ovarian tumour can co-exist

ABDOMINAL EXAMINATION

It includes inspection, palpation, percussion, auscultation.
- *Inspection*: describe the site, size of the mass, presence of engorged veins, position of umbilicus, skin over swelling (may be stretched and shiny)

Table 10.1 Clinical Differentiation Between Benign and Malignant Ovarian Tumours

	Benign	Malignant
Growth	Slow growing	Fast growing
Consistency	Cystic/tense	Firm and hard, varying
Site	Mostly unilateral	May be bilateral
Mobility	Mobile	Fixed
Contour	Well defined	Ill defined
Presence of ascites	Absent	Present

- *Palpation*: size of the mass/site of the mass/unilateral or bilateral/shape/consistency/margins/whether lower border felt/mobility/fixity
- *Benign tumours* (Table 10.1):
  - Mostly unilateral
  - Mobile
  - Cystic
  - Smooth surface without ascites
- *Malignant tumours*:
  - Mostly bilateral
  - Irregular surface
  - Hard or variable in consistency
  - May be fixed and may be associated with ascites
  - Presence of hepatosplenomegaly, any other mass in the abdomen
- *Percussion*: dull over the mass, may be resonant at the flanks
  - In ascites—dull in flanks, shifting dullness will be present

SPECULUM EXAMINATION
- To visualise cervix, vagina

BIMANUAL PELVIC EXAMINATION
This is done to find out the following:
- Position of cervix
- Uterine size, mobility
- Whether mass felt per abdomen is felt through fornix
- Size of the mass, consistency, tenderness, whether other fornix is free
- Whether uterus is made out separately from the mass
- Whether movement of cervix is transmitted to the mass and vice versa
- Groove sign is positive in ovarian tumour—definite groove will be felt between the uterus and the mass
- Nodules felt through posterior fornix (secondary deposits)

PER RECTAL EXAMINATION
- To find out nodules in pouch of Douglas (deposits in case of malignant ovarian tumour), extra luminal mass

SUMMARY
- Name……...……... Age………Para……C/O……….mass abdomen/dyspepsia......for.......months
- Mention about relevant past history, general examination findings, local examination findings and then differential diagnosis of mass abdomen is given

DIAGNOSIS
- Mention only about clinical provisional diagnosis and how the diagnosis was arrived at. *For example*: woman may not have menstrual problems, can come with mass or distension of abdomen.
- P/A mass may not be in midline, lower border may be felt, may be tense, cystic/variable/hard in consistency, with or without ascites. The previously mentioned findings are indicative of ovarian tumour.

INVESTIGATIONS
ROUTINE INVESTIGATIONS
Specific
Imaging
- ***Ultrasonography of abdomen and pelvis***
  - Ovarian cyst which is unilocular, unilateral, cystic, clear or multiloculated with thin septa—may be benign
  - Features of malignancy in ovarian tumour—multilocular/bilateral/thick septa/internal echoes/papillary excrescences/increased vascularity/presence of ascites
- ***Doppler***—to assess blood flow and vascularity (Table 10.2)
- ***CT*** detects tumour of size 1.5–2 cm
- ***MRI*** detects tumour size of <1 cm and also done to assess lymph node involvement and extent of the tumour
- ***Paracentesis***: tapping of ascitic fluid for cytological examination for malignant cells
- ***IVP***: due to pressure effect—hydronephrosis, hydroureter may be present
- ***Endoscopy: upper GI endoscopy/colonoscopy***—to rule out GI pathology in case of malignant ovarian tumours
- ***Tumour markers***
  - CA 125 > 35 U/mL in post-menopausal women—suspect malignancy—epithelial tumours
  - CA 125 > 200 U/mL in pre-menopausal—suspect malignancy (other causes—endometriosis, TB, colon cancer)

Table 10.2 Doppler Findings in Benign and Malignant Ovarian Mass

Benign	Malignant
• Less or absent diastolic flow • Higher PI • Higher RI • Peripheral flow	• More diastolic flow • More vascular • Low PI • Low RI • Elevated peak systolic velocity • Increased impedance • Central flow

PI, Pulsatility index; RI, resistance index.

- CA 19.9
- CA 15.3
- CEA—mucinous, Brenner and endometroid tumours
- AFP, HCG—embryonal carcinoma
- HCG, LDH—germ cell tumour
- Mixed dysgerminoma
- AFP—endodermal sinus tumour
- HCG—choriocarcinoma
- *X-ray of chest*: to identify right side hydrothorax (Meig's syndrome), lung secondaries

CASE DISCUSSION
FUNCTIONAL CYSTS OF OVARY

Ovarian enlargement may be non-neoplastic and are due to functional cysts namely follicular cyst, corpus luteum cysts and theca lutein cysts

The functional cysts are <5–7 cm in size. Spontaneous regression happens.

When not regressed—3–6 cycles of OCP can be given.

BENIGN TUMOURS OF OVARY

Benign neoplasms may be epithelial, sex cord stromal and germ cell tumours and need surgery as they are prone for complications.

In younger age, ovarian cystectomy or oophorectomy is done, preserving the uterus and other ovary (biopsy of the ovary, when needed).

DIFFERENTIAL DIAGNOSIS OF MASS ABDOMEN

- *Ascites*: In ascites on percussion, flanks are dull and resonant at midline, shifting dullness may be present. When patient lies on one side, flanks will become resonant.
- *Encysted tuberculosis*: History of oligomenorrhoea/amenorrhoea may be present. Evening rise of temperature/history of tuberculosis in the past and history of tuberculosis in other family members may be present. Cyst will be fixed. Tympanic note over mass will be present.

- *Fibroid*: Menstrual problems are common and mostly, occur in reproductive age group. Fibroids are firm in consistency and are mostly midline swelling. Lower border is not made out. Side-to-side mobility will be present (Refer Case 5). On bimanual pelvic examination, mass will be continuous with uterus, and movement of cervix will be transmitted to mass and vice versa. Groove sign is absent.
- *Pregnancy*: H/O amenorrhoea and signs of pregnancy will be present; uterus will be enlarged and soft; foetal parts will be felt.
- *Full bladder*
- *Functional ovarian cyst*: Simple unilocular cyst <5 cm made out in USG and it will usually resolve by itself. If it does not resolve, OCP can be given for 3–6 cycles.

RISK FACTORS FOR OVARIAN MALIGNANCY

- Early menarche, late menopause
- Nulliparity, infertility
- Prolonged use of ovulation induction drugs
- Use of talc in perineum
- Previous PCOS
- Family H/O cancer of ovary, breast, endometrium, colon, HNPCC syndrome, BRCA1, BRCA2 gene mutation carriers
- High-fat diet
- Tamoxifen therapy

CAUSES FOR OVARIAN CYST TORSION (Flow Chart 10.1)

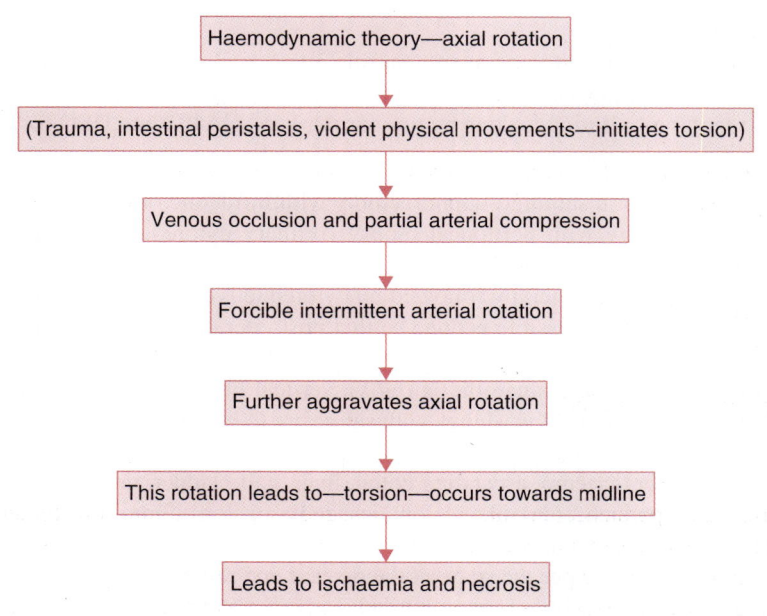

```
Haemodynamic theory—axial rotation
        ↓
(Trauma, intestinal peristalsis, violent physical movements—initiates torsion)
        ↓
Venous occlusion and partial arterial compression
        ↓
Forcible intermittent arterial rotation
        ↓
Further aggravates axial rotation
        ↓
This rotation leads to—torsion—occurs towards midline
        ↓
Leads to ischaemia and necrosis
```

FLOW CHART 10.1 Cause for Ovarian Cyst Torsion

COMPLICATIONS OF OVARIAN TUMOUR
- Torsion—long pedicle (in post-natal period, dermoid can undergo torsion)
- Rupture—rapid growth or during labour
- Pseudomyxoma peritonei (due to rupture of benign or malignant mucinous tumour of ovary)
- Haemorrhage
- Infection—may occur in post-natal period
- Malignancy

MANAGEMENT
MANAGEMENT OF MALIGNANT OVARIAN TUMOURS

> Staging laparotomy and surgery is the primary or gold standard for treating malignant ovarian tumours.

- *Pre- or post-operative chemotherapy*: has shown to improve the survival rate
- *Radiotherapy* is not used nowadays due to side-effects of radiation to adjacent organs, as total abdominopelvic radiation is needed. In advanced cases, neoadjuvant chemotherapy is given and, surgery is to be performed after 3–6 cycles of chemotherapy
- *Second look surgery or interval cytoreductive surgery*: performed after 3–6 cycles of chemotherapy, in patients when primary attempt at cytoreduction was suboptimal to find out the response to chemotherapy and proceed with removal of residual tumour burden

Conservative surgery
- *In Stage 1a1*: tumour confined to one ovary, capsule intact, unilateral salpingo-oophorectomy is done in young women who wish to preserve child-bearing function.
  In follow up, regular monitoring is done by tumour markers, CA125 and USG for ovaries.

Early stages (Stage 1 and 11): *staging laparotomy and primary cytoreductive surgery*—total abdominal hysterectomy with bilateral salpingo-oophorectomy with infracolic omentectomy with pelvic and para-aortic lymphadenectomy with peritoneal biopsy (primary cytoreductive surgery) followed by chemotherapy or radiotherapy when necessary.
Late stages: pre-operative chemotherapy followed by cytoreductive surgery or debulking surgery; removal of as much of tumour as possible is done so that post-operative chemotherapy or radiotherapy will have better effect.
Staging laparotomy: under general anaesthesia (G/A), vertical liberal incision is made and abdomen is opened. Ascitic fluid or peritoneal washings with saline are to be sent for cytological examination.
- Systematic exploration in clockwise direction of the following structures are done: uterus, both ovaries, paracolic gutter, caecum, ascending colon, liver, gall bladder, under surface of Rt. and Lt. hemidiaphragm, stomach, transverse colon, descending colon, sigmoid colon, rectum, small bowel, omentum, para-aortic nodes.
- Then surgery is proceeded as per the stage of the disease and removal of as much of tumour as possible is done to leave very little tumour burden.

FERTILITY SPARING TREATMENT (CONSERVATIVE TREATMENT)
- Done in early stage with Stage 1A Grade 1—in young women, who desire fertility
- Unilateral oophorectomy is done and patient has to be followed up

CHEMOTHERAPEUTIC AGENTS IN OVARIAN MALIGNANCY
- Cisplatin, carboplatin, paclitaxel and cyclophosphamide are used as single agent or in various combinations in epithelial cancer.

KEY POINTS
- Ovarian enlargement can be due to functional cysts, inflammation, metaplastic and neoplastic tumours (benign or malignant).
- Ovarian enlargement can occur in all age groups. In pre-menarchal group, 10% are malignant; in reproductive group, 15% are malignant; in post-menopausal, 50% are malignant.
- Functional cysts are <5–7 cm and it will regress after some time. When not regressed, 6 cycles of OCP can be given.
- Epithelial tumours account for 80%.
- Benign tumours are 80% and 20% are malignant, 20% are secondary deposits from primary growths elsewhere.
- Ovarian tumours are symptomless for long time.
- Ovarian tumours seldom cause menstrual disturbances.
- Complications of ovarian tumour are torsion, rupture, malignancy, infection, pseudomyxoma peritonei, haemorrhage.
- Risk factors for ovarian malignancy are older age group, nulliparity, early menarche, late menopause, family history of ovarian, breast, colon malignancy.
- Women with malignant disease will be cachectic, supraclavicular node may be palpable, abdominal mass, ascites, nodules in pouch of Douglas may be present.
- Women with malignant ovarian disease will be evaluated with USG, Doppler, CA125 and CT and MRI will be required for nodal and distant metastasis.
- Staging of the disease is done by staging laparotomy.
- Early stages (Stage 1 and 11): staging laparotomy and primary cytoreductive surgery is advocated.
- Late stages: pre-operative chemotherapy followed by cytoreductive surgery or debulking surgery and post-operative chemo or radiotherapy are offered.

FREQUENTLY ASKED QUESTIONS
1. What is functional cyst? Up to what size it is called functional cyst?
2. How do you differentiate between fibroid and ovarian tumour clinically?
3. What are the risk factors for developing ovarian tumour?
4. What are the symptoms in torsion of the ovarian cyst?
5. What is the cause for torsion?

CASE 10 A CASE OF OVARIAN TUMOUR

6. What are the causes for pain in ovarian tumour?
7. How do you differentiate benign and malignant ovarian tumour?
8. What is FIGO classification?
9. What is staging laparotomy?
10. What is the role of chemotherapy and agents commonly used?
11. What is neoadjuvant chemotherapy?
12. What is the role of conservative treatment for Stage 1a1?
13. What is cytoreductive (debulking) surgery?
14. What is the management for benign ovarian cyst?
15. What are the management options for malignant ovarian tumour?
16. What is second look laparotomy or laparoscopy?

A CASE OF POST-MENOPAUSAL BLEEDING PV

CASE 11

PATIENT'S DETAILS

Name..................................... Age................. Address.......................... Occupation..............
Socioeconomic Class....................... Para.........................

Nulliparous—more prone for ovarian and endometrial carcinoma *Multiparous*—carcinoma cervix

Bleeding PV any time after 1 year of amenorrhoea, in the menopausal age is considered as post-menopausal bleeding PV

PRESENT COMPLAINTS

Following history pertaining to present illness to be elicited:
- C/O bleeding PV
- Onset
- How many years after menopause, bleeding started?
- Duration—continuous or intermittent
- Frequency, amount (mild, moderate or profuse), number of pads soaked, associated clots, associated with pain
- H/O similar episodes in the past
- Offensive discharge PV (may be due to cancer cervix, pyometra)
- Blood-stained discharge PV or not (blood stained may be due to cancer cervix and vagina, cervical polyp)
- Post-menopausal bleeding PV may be associated with menopausal symptoms like frequency of micturition, urgency and stress incontinence, palpitation and hot flushes.
- History of taking menopausal hormone therapy (MHT)—oestrogen/progesterone taken or local oestrogen applications
- Tamoxifen therapy taken for breast carcinoma to be elicited which can increase risk of endometrial and ovarian cancer
- History of oral contraceptive pill use in the past will protect—against cancer endometrium and ovary, but increases the risk of cancer cervix
- Previous investigations and treatment for post-menopausal bleeding (USG, Pap smear, fractional curettage, hysteroscopy)
- Post-coital bleeding PV—may be due to cancer cervix/cervical polyp
- Post-menopausal bleeding PV with mass abdomen (fibroid, endometrial carcinoma, pyometra with cancer cervix, feminising ovarian tumour)

CASE 11 A CASE OF POST-MENOPAUSAL BLEEDING PV

- Post-menopausal bleeding PV with mass descending per vaginum (carcinoma of cervix, decubitus ulcer, cervical polyp, cervical polyp turning malignant)
- Post-menopausal bleeding PV with loss of appetite, loss of weight (ovarian malignancy, cancer cervix, endometrial carcinoma)

HISTORY
PAST MENSTRUAL HISTORY
- Elicited as usual (early menarche and late menopause predisposes to ovarian and endometrial malignancy)
- History suggestive of PCOD—irregular, infrequent cycles—anovulation and unopposed oestrogen exposure—risk factor for endometrial carcinoma

MENOPAUSAL HISTORY
- Details to be obtained—age of menopause, sudden or gradual, menopausal symptoms, H/O MHT

PAST OBSTETRIC HISTORY
- Refer Case 1

CONTRACEPTIC HISTORY
- Refer Case 1

PAST MEDICAL & SURGICAL HISTORY
- Refer Case 1

MARITAL HISTORY
- Duration of marriage/onset of sexual activity (early marriage, multiple sexual partners can lead to cancer cervix)
- H/O infertility, H/O induction of ovulation (frequent/repeated)—*high risk for ovarian malignancy*

FAMILY HISTORY
- Breast, ovarian, colon, endometrial carcinoma runs in the family
- BRCA1 and BRCA2—mutations in this gene is responsible for hereditary ovarian cancer
- Familial lynch 11 syndrome [hereditary non-polyposis colorectal cancer (HNPCC)]—high risk for endometrial and ovarian carcinoma

PERSONAL HISTORY
- Smoking, drug abuse, alcohol

EXAMINATION

GENERAL EXAMINATION

- Refer Case 1
  Special points to be noted:
  - Pallor/pedal oedema/supraclavicular node
  - *Build*: obesity—risk factor for endometrial carcinoma (corpus cancer syndrome—obesity, diabetes, hypertension, endometrial carcinoma)
  - *Cachexia*—indicates malignancy
  - *Vitals*—hypertensive—prone for endometrial carcinoma
  - *CVS/RS/CNS*—examination

ABDOMINAL EXAMINATION

- To be done in the usual manner
- Palpate for abdominal mass/hepatosplenomegaly/ascites
- Percussion—if ascites is present

INSPECTION OF EXTERNAL GENITALIA

Vulval lesion—ulcer, growth, lump, discharge

SPECULUM EXAMINATION

- Inspection of vagina and cervix should be done for—senile vaginitis (vaginal wall reddish with discharge)/vaginal ulcer, growth
- Inspection of cervix—look for ulcer/growth/polyp/discharge/bleeding through os. If growth or ulcer is present—size, site to be noted

BIMANUAL PELVIC EXAMINATION

- Ulcer or growth in cervix—find out if it is friable/bleeds on touch and induration is present or not
- Size of uterus (enlarged in endometrial carcinoma/cancer cervix with pyometra)
- Fixity (in cancer cervix)
- Fornices—adnexal mass felt through fornices (may be ovarian mass) and to assess parametrical involvement in cancer cervix

PER RECTAL EXAMINATION

- Involvement of rectal mucosa—in cancer cervix
- Induration of parametrium and uterosacral ligament—in cancer cervix, nodules in pouch of Douglas, in ovarian malignancy

SUMMARY

- Name....Age...Para.. C/O ....post-menopausal bleeding PV... for.....days/months
- Mention about relevant general examination, abdominal examination findings and then differential diagnosis is given

DIAGNOSIS
Post-menopausal bleeding PV for evaluation
Mrs.. Age.................. Nulliparous/Multiparous...............................
A case of Post menopausal bleeding for evaluation

INVESTIGATIONS
ROUTINE INVESTIGATIONS

> Based on the clinical diagnosis: appropriate investigations are to be done.

For example, if endometrial carcinoma is suspected:
- **Transvaginal USG**—for endometrial thickness >4 mm (normal is less than 4 mm in post-menopausal women) to be evaluated
  - Size of uterus/pyometra/to rule out endometrial polyp/to rule out ovarian mass
- **Doppler study** of the endometrial growth
- **Pap smear**
- **OP endometrial aspiration biopsy** with 90%–98% diagnostic accuracy, adequate samples in 95%
- **Fractional curettage with ectocervix biopsy or hysteroscopy and directed biopsy**—more accurate in identifying endometrial lesions (polyps, myoma, growth)
- **CT and MRI** to assess myometrial invasion and lymph node involvement
- **X-ray of chest**—lung metastasis

Relevant investigations are done based on clinical diagnosis, investigations for cancer cervix, ovarian tumour, AUB—(refer cancer cervix Case 6, ovarian tumour Case 10, AUB Case 3.)

CASE DISCUSSION
MENOPAUSE
- It is cessation of ovarian activity and is clinically defined as cessation of menstruation for a period of 12 months
- Age of menopause: 45–50 years; average: 47 years

MENOPAUSAL SYMPTOMS
- Vasomotor—hot flushes, sweating, insomnia, irritability, depression, 'empty nest syndrome'; urogenital symptoms—dysuria, urge and stress incontinence, called as 'urethral syndrome', vaginal dryness
- Osteoporosis, skin changes, coronary vascular disease

MANAGEMENT OF MENOPAUSAL SYMPTOMS
- Counselling, diet, weight-bearing exercises
- *MHT:* Oestrogen with progesterone when uterus is present
  - Oestrogen alone in hysterectomised woman
  - Tibolone

MENOPAUSAL HORMONE THERAPY BENEFITS
- Improvement of menopausal symptoms, bone mineral density, and cardioprotective effect
- Risks: slightly increased risk in long term use of MHT—breast cancer, stroke, thromboembolism

Timing of investigation
After the age of 40 years, if vaginal bleeding occurs after 6 months of amenorrhea/bleeding PV in post-menopausal woman/continuation of menstruation even after age of 52 years should be investigated.

CAUSES FOR POST-MENOPAUSAL BLEEDING PV

Causes	Condition
Vulval causes	Vulval carcinoma
Vaginal causes	Senile vaginitis/forgotten pessary/foreign body/carcinoma of vagina
Cervical causes	Cervical polyp/decubitus ulcer/carcinoma of cervix, tuberculous ulcer
Uterine causes	Atrophic endometrium/senile endometritis/endometrial hyperplasia/endometrial polyp/endometrial carcinoma, sarcoma of uterus
Ovarian causes	Feminising ovarian tumour—sex cord stromal tumours (granulosa and theca cell tumour)/Brenner tumour
Tubal cause	Tubal carcinoma
Other causes	Exogenous hormones—MHT

RISK FACTORS FOR ENDOMETRIAL CARCINOMA
- Anovulation, unopposed oestrogen exposure
- Early menarche, late menopause, nulliparity, infertility, PCOD
- MHT with oestrogen therapy, tamoxifen therapy, feminising ovarian tumours
- Family H/O cancer endometrium, HNPCC syndrome
- Corpus cancer syndrome—obesity, diabetes, hypertension, endometrial cancer

TREATMENT OF ENDOMETRIAL CARCINOMA
- FIGO staging of endometrial carcinoma is surgical

> Primary surgery—TAH with BSO with omentectomy and pelvic and para-aortic lymph node sampling is the corner stone treatment in the early stage endometrial carcinoma.

- *Early stage-endometrial carcinoma*: staging laparotomy followed by total abdominal hysterectomy with bilateral salpingo-oopherectomy (TAH with BSO) with omentectomy with pelvic and para-aortic lymphadenectomy followed by adjuvant radiotherapy or chemotherapy when necessary and rarely hormone therapy (depends on surgicopathological findings and staging)
- *Route of hysterectomy*: nowadays vaginal route is preferred and laparoscopic vaginal hysterectomy is preferred with laparoscopic lymphadenectomy is preferred. (Portal site metastasis can occur in laparoscopic surgeries) or post-operative radiotherapy in diabetic, obese and in case of prolapse uterus
- *The prognostic factors for endometrial carcinoma*: are tumour grade, size, histologic type, depth of myometrial invasion, patient's age, surgicopathologic evidence of extra-uterine disease spread
- *In patients with Grade 1 and 2*, with no myometrial invasion or any other risk factors, no additional treatment is needed
- *In high-risk woman*: post-operative vaginal brachytherapy and external radiation are advocated
- *In cases of advanced disease*: adjuvant chemotherapy is the treatment advocated

EVALUATION OF POST-MENOPAUSAL BLEEDING PV (Flow Chart 11.1)

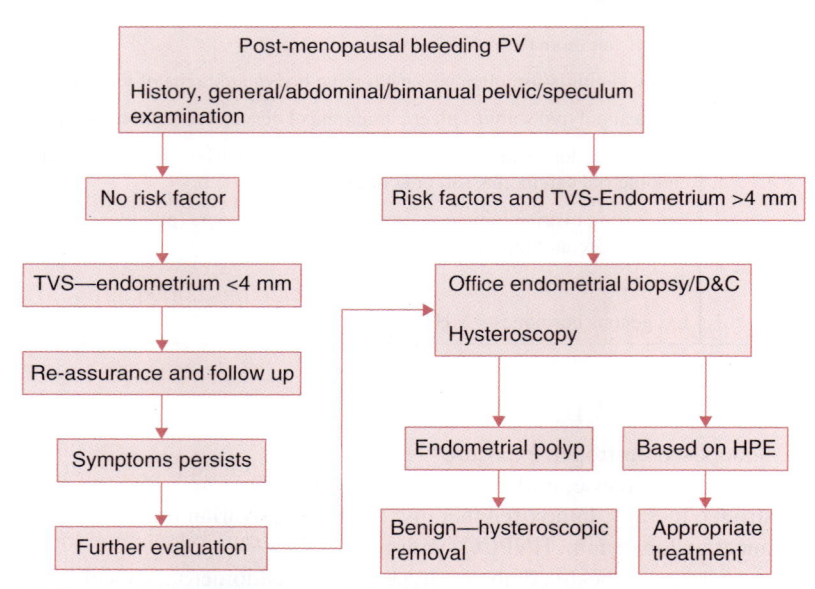

FLOW CHART 11.1 Evaluation of Post-Menopausal Bleeding PV

KEY POINTS

- Menopause is defined as cessation of menstruation for 12 months or more.
- Bleeding occurring after menopause should be evaluated carefully.
- In post-menopausal bleeding PV, 30% is due to cancer.

- Various causes for post-menopausal bleeding PV are senile vaginitis/vulvitis/vaginal tumour/cervical cancer/polyp/senile endometritis/endometrial cancer/functioning ovarian tumour/urethral caruncle/carcinoma bladder/endometrial polyp and exogenous oestrogen therapy.
- All causes for post-menopausal bleeding PV are not due to malignancy, but excluding malignancy must be the main aim of investigations.
- Management of post-menopausal bleeding PV is directed towards the cause.

FREQUENTLY ASKED QUESTIONS

1. Define menopause.
2. What is the mean age of menopause?
3. What are the menopausal symptoms?
4. What are the drugs used in HRT, their advantages and risks?
5. What are the causes for post-menopausal bleeding PV?
6. What is corpus cancer syndrome?
7. How will you investigate a case of post-menopausal bleeding PV?
8. How will you do fractional curettage?
9. What are the risk factors for endometrial carcinoma?
10. Management of endometrial carcinoma?
11. Questions from cancer cervix and ovarian carcinoma may be asked.

A CASE OF URINARY INCONTINENCE

CASE 12

PATIENT'S DETAILS
Name……………….....……… Age……..... Address…………….……… Occupation………………
Socioeconomic Class………......…. Para……......

C/O involuntary loss of urine/dribbling of urine

PRESENT COMPLAINTS
Following history is to be elicited:
- Duration/continuous or intermittent/amount of leakage/associated with cough, sneezing, intense desire to pass urine/frequency of urination/burning micturition/difficulty in urination
- Mass abdomen and involuntary loss of urine
- Surgery in the perineum/vagina/pelvis/abdomen
- Excoriation in vulval region
- Trauma to pelvis

HISTORY
MENSTRUAL HISTORY
- Elicited as usual; cyclical haematuria or 'menuria' can occur in cases of uterovesical fistula following a caesarean section

MARITAL HISTORY
- Refer Case 1

PAST OBSTETRIC HISTORY
- Duration of labour/type of delivery/conducted by qualified person/condition of baby at birth—alive, deeply asphyxiated, dead
- **Obstetric vesicovaginal fistulas** can occur after prolonged obstructed labour, after caesarean in deeply engaged head and difficult forceps delivery and in destructive operational deliveries
- Due to pressure to the bladder base by the engaged head and the pubic bone
- Vesicovaginal fistula develops after a period of 7–10 days due to devascularisation

PAST SURGICAL HISTORY
- Dribbling of urine following abdominal, vaginal, laparoscopic hysterectomy, surgery for ovarian cysts, radical surgery for gynaec malignancy like Wertheims hysterectomy
- Surgery done for endometriosis, large fibroids, broad ligament and cervical fibroids
- Whether dribbling of urine started immediately after surgery or 7–10 days later (in transection or cut injuries dribbling occurs immediately or after a period of 7–10 days in cases of devascularisation)

PAST MEDICAL HISTORY
- Radiotherapy for pelvic malignancy

PAST SURGICAL HISTORY
- Refer Case 1

FAMILY HISTORY
- Refer Case 1

EXAMINATION
GENERAL EXAMINATION
- Refer Case 1

Special attention to be paid for the following:
Short stature, obese women (prone for obstructed labour)
CVS and RS examination: bronchiectasis, cor pulmonale can cause chronic cough, which will lead to stress urinary incontinence
CNS examination: spinal cord lesions, multiple sclerosis—may present with retention with overflow urinary incontinence

ABDOMINAL EXAMINATION
- Done as usual
- Abdominal mass to be ruled out

EXTERNAL GENITALIA EXAMINATION (Fig. 12.1)
- Excoriation of vulva, groin due to continuous dribbling of urine and irritation and watery discharge with urinary smell.
- Urine is normally odourless when in bladder; when it is dribbling and in contact with bacteria, the smell of ammonia is present.

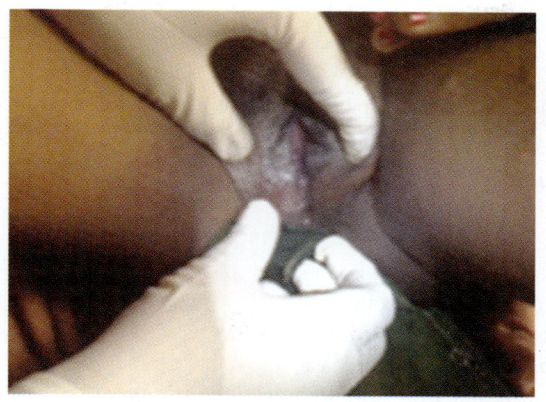

FIGURE 12.1 Excoriation of Vulva—VVF

- Obstetric fistula may be associated with complete perineal tear.
- In cases of stress urinary incontinence, examination is done with full bladder. Patient is asked to cough and leakage of urine is noted.
- If test is positive, Marshall and Bonney's test is done.
- *Marshall and Bonney's test*: two fingers are placed in the vagina at the urethrovaginal junction on either side of urethra and bladder neck region is elevated. Patient is asked to cough or strain and absence of leakage is indicative of good outcome after surgery.

SPECULUM EXAMINATION
- The fistulous opening can be seen, after retracting the posterior vaginal wall.
- A knee chest position or Sim's lateral position is helpful to visualise the fistulous opening.

BIMANUAL PELVIC EXAMINATION
The size and site of fistula is noted. Palpation is done for pliability of the vagina, scaring around fistula, fixity of the fistula to the pubic bone to assess the prognosis for surgical repair.

SUMMARY
Name……………………..……… Age……. Para…………….. C/O involuntary loss of urine/dribbling of urine……………….for……………days/months

Mention about relevant history, general examination, abdominal examination findings and then differential diagnosis is given

DIAGNOSIS
A case of urinary incontinence for evaluation

INVESTIGATIONS

Appropriate investigations are done as per the type of urinary incontinence.

- *Urine analysis and culture*
- *USG of abdomen, KUB area and pelvis*
- *IVP*
- *Cystoscopy and*
  - Intra-venous indigo carmine excretion test
  - ureteric catheterisation—in *ureterovaginal fistula*
- **Methylene** Blue swab test to diagnose VVF
- *In stress urinary incontinence and urge urinary incontinence*:
  - Urodynamic study
  - Uroflowmetry
  - Urethrocystometry
- *Urethroscopy*
- *Micturition cystourethrography*
- *MRI and neurophysiological studies*

CASE DISCUSSION

- **Urinary continence** is maintained by the intra-urethral pressure that is higher than the intra-vesical pressure at rest and with stress. The urethral closure pressure is the difference between the urethral and vesical pressure, which is more than 20 cm of water.
  - **Stress urinary incontinence** is involuntary loss of urine associated with straining activities that increase the intra-abdominal pressure, such as coughing, sneezing and the amount of loss is minimal. There is no prior urge to void, she is aware of the leak.
  - **Urge urinary incontinence** is involuntary loss of urine associated with intense desire to pass urine. The amount of loss is always considerable. It can occur in acute cystitis, and in cases of detrusor instability.
  - **True urinary incontinence** is due to urinary fistulae—Vesico Vaginal Fistula and Uretero Vaginal Fistula, and there is continuous involuntary loss of urine.
  - **Retention with overflow urinary incontinence** is common after surgery on perineum and vagina and in post-partum period. It can occur in cases of space occupying lesions of pelvis, retroverted gravid uterus, cervical fibroid, posterior wall fibroid and ovarian tumours impacted in pouch of Douglas, and in urethral obstructive conditions.
    Autonomous bladder due to neurological causes can present with retention with overflow urinary incontinence.
  - **Genuine stress urinary incontinence is** defined as involuntary loss of urine when the intra vesical pressure exceeds the intra-urethral pressure in the absence of the detrusor activity.

- **Causes of stress urinary incontinence (GSI) or urethral sphincter Detrusor:**
  - Descent of the bladder neck and the proximal urethra due to distortion of the urethro vesical anatomy and there is no increase in intra-urethral pressure during increased intra-abdominal pressure during straining and
  - There is lowered intra urethral pressure at rest.
- **Causes of urge urinary incontinence:**
  - Detrusor instability or detrusor overactivity: causes motor urge incontinence.
  - Sensory urge incontinence due to cystitis, trigonitis, and foreign body, stone or neoplasm in bladder.
- **Urodynamic study:**
  Uroflometry: normal flow rate is 15–25 mL/s
  Cystometry: Normal findings are intra vesical pressure is 0–15 cm H_2O, first sensation of urination at 150–200 mL, capacity of bladder 400–600 mL, residual urine less than 50 mL, absence of systolic detrusor contraction, no leakage on coughing.
  In GSI: Cystometry evaluation is normal and abnormal in detrusor instability and sensory urge incontinence. Cystometry confirms the diagnosis of detrusor instability, but genuine stress urinary incontinence is a diagnosis of exclusion.
- **Management genuine stress urinary incontinence:**
  Conservative treatment; pelvic floor exercise, vaginal cone therapy
  Surgical treatment; the principle of surgery is to elevate and restore the bladder neck and the proximal urethra as intra-abdominal structures and strengthening the support of the bladder neck and the proximal urethra.
  Kelly's cystourethroplasty.
  Retro pubic colpo suspension, Marshall Marchetti Krantz operation, Burch colpo suspension. Presently, sling operations are done by placing a sling around urethra to lift it back into a normal position and to exert pressure on the urethra.
- **Urge urinary incontinence**
  Detrusor instability—medical therapy—anticholinergic drugs, musculotropic relaxants, tricyclic antidepressants.
- **True urinary incontinence:** anatomical repair to be done in fistula.

FREQUENTLY ASKED QUESTIONS
1. Define genuine stress urinary incontinence.
2. Types of urinary incontinence and causes.
3. Investigations and management of stress urinary incontinence.
4. Causes for urinary fistulae and symptoms.

VIVA VOCE EXAMINATION IN GYNAECOLOGY

CASE 13

1. **Artery forceps**
   This is curved artery forceps, an instrument used for catching/clamping the bleeding vessels. It is also used for grasping tissues at the time of operation (opening and closing the peritoneum). The tip is curved and inner surface has serrations. In straight artery forceps, the tip is straight (Fig. 13.1).

2. **Allis forceps**
   This instrument is used for grasping structures like rectus sheath or fascia while opening and closing abdominal wall in operations like tubectomy, LSCS, laparotomy, abdominal hysterectomy. It is also used for holding vaginal wall during vaginal hysterectomy and to hold the margins of vagina in vault closure in abdominal hysterectomy.
   Long Allis can sometimes be used to hold the tissue when taking wedge biopsy of vulva. Sometimes this is used to hold the lip of cervix (Fig. 13.2).

3. **Babcock's forceps**
   This instrument is used for grasping tubular structures like fallopian tube in tubectomy as in modified Pomeroy's operation. It can also be used to hold ureter, appendix etc. The tip is blunt and atraumatic as there is no sharp tooth (Fig. 13.3).

4. **Ayre's spatula**
   It is used for taking Pap smear for screening of carcinoma cervix. It is made of wood so that cells can adhere to the porous surface of carcinoma cervix. The long end is inserted into cervical canal and rotated 360 degree. The exfoliated cells obtained are smeared on glass slide and fixed in fluid in Koplick's jar, which contains ether and alcohol in equal amount. The other broad end is used for obtaining cells from lateral vaginal wall for knowing the hormonal status (Fig. 13.4).

5. **Cusco's speculum**
   It is a self-retaining double-bladed vaginal speculum, used for routine examination of cervix to visualise lesions like polyp, erosion, cancer cervix, for VIA, VILI, colposcopy, biopsy cervix. Only few procedures like taking of Pap smear, insertion and removal of copper T can be done because of limited opening of the blades (Fig. 13.5).
   Advantage: self-retaining, so no need for assistant to hold the speculum
   Disadvantage: vaginal walls cannot be visualised

6. **Doyen's retractor**
   This instrument is used for retracting bladder during abdominal operations like LSCS, abdominal hysterectomy, laparotomy (Fig. 13.6A).
   Deaver's retractor is used for retraction of deep visceral structures. Right angle retractor is used for tubectomy (Fig. 13.6B).

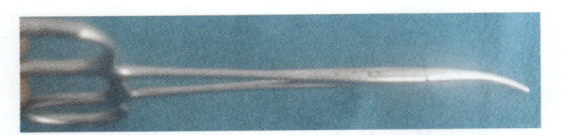

340 CASE 13 VIVA VOCE EXAMINATION IN GYNAECOLOGY

FIGURE 13.1 Artery Forceps

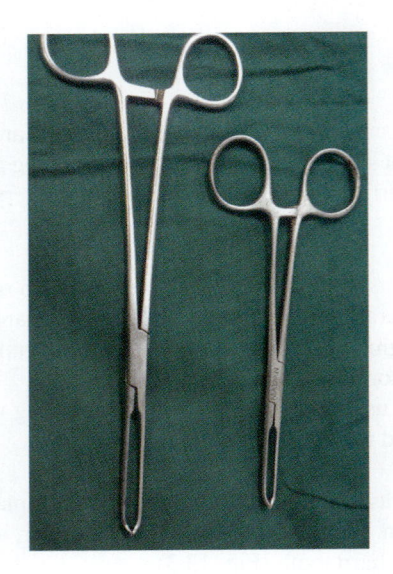

FIGURE 13.2 Allis Forceps

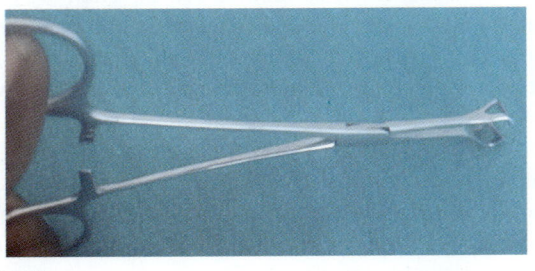

FIGURE 13.3 Babcock's Forceps

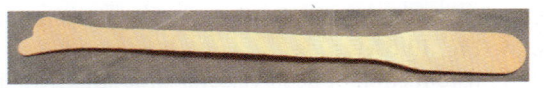

FIGURE 13.4 Ayre's Spatula

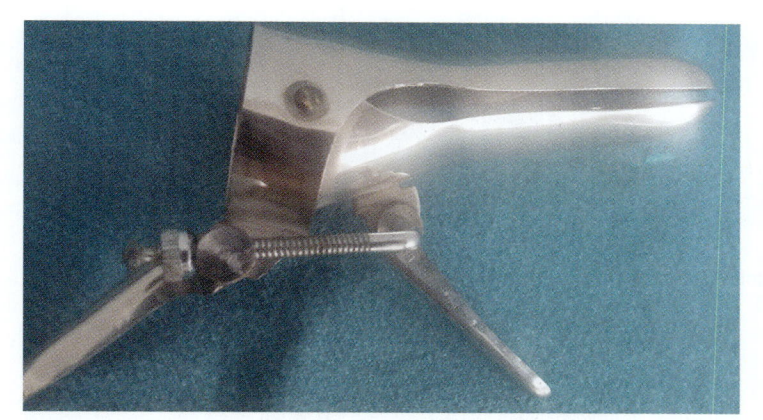

FIGURE 13.5 Cusco's Speculum

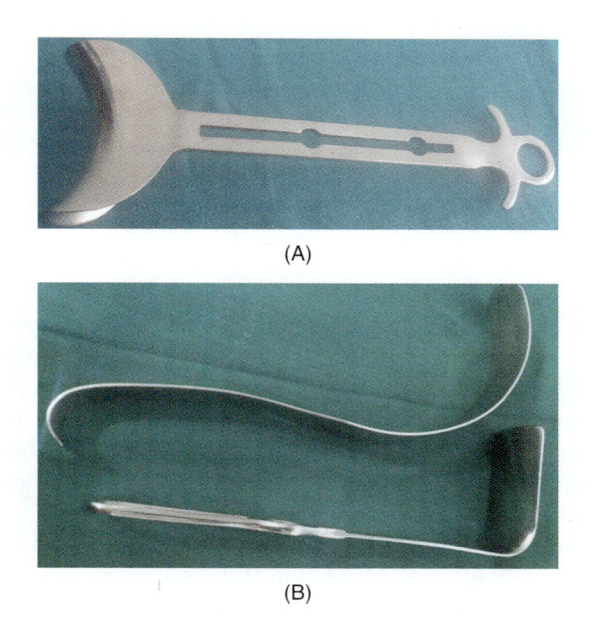

(A)

(B)

FIGURE 13.6
(A) Doyen's retractor and (B) Deaver's right angle retractor.

7. **Kocher's forceps**
   This instrument is used for holding the pedicles during hysterectomy. The tips of the blades have teeth so that the tissues do not slip. The blades can either be straight or curved. This instrument is used in hysterectomy to clamp pedicles, which are then transfixed. This can also be used for artificial rupture of membranes (ARM) (Fig. 13.7).

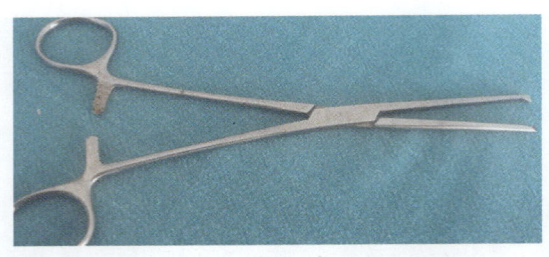

FIGURE 13.7 Kocher's Forceps

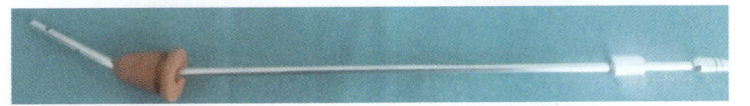

FIGURE 13.8 Rubin's Cannula

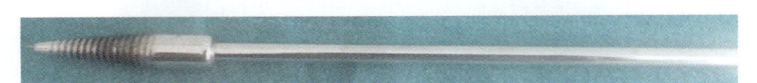

FIGURE 13.9 Leech Wilkinson's Cannula

8. **Rubin's cannula**
   This cannula is used for tubal patency test for infertility like hysterosalpingography (HSG) or chromopertubation in laparoscopy. In HSG, radio-opaque iodine (urographin) is used (it is colourless to naked eye but on X-ray, it is opaque). During laparoscopy methylene blue dye is injected through the cannula. This cannula has a rubber guard, which is adjusted according to the length of the cervical canal. It prevents backward leak of the dye. These tests are performed during HSG, laparoscopic chromopertubation and also after tuboplasty to find out the patency of the tubes (Fig. 13.8).
9. **Leech Wilkinson's cannula**
   This cannula also is used for tubal patency test in HSG and laparoscopic chromopertubation. It is straight instrument with conical tip with serrations. This cone is screwed into the cervix to prevent the backflow of dye (Fig. 13.9).
10. **Sim's speculum**
    Sim's speculum is used in the OPD for inspection of vagina and cervix. It retracts anterior and posterior vaginal walls. The blades have different breadth. It is used in gynaec OPD for following procedures: taking Pap smear, insertion and removal of copper T, taking swabs, HSG (Fig. 13.10). Its use in gynaec operations: D&C, cervix biopsy, vaginal hysterectomy, Fothergill's operation, repair of vesicovaginal fistula, hysteroscopy.
    Advantage: wide area for inspection; instrumentation is easy
    Disadvantage: needs assistant (not self-retaining); patient must be brought to the edge of the table

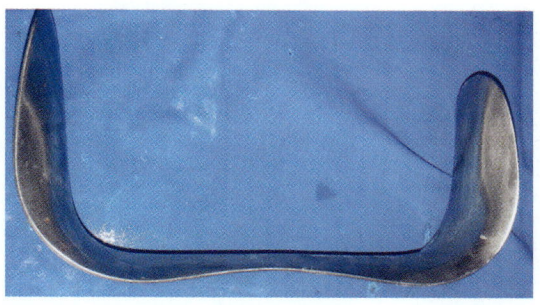

FIGURE 13.10 Sim's Speculum

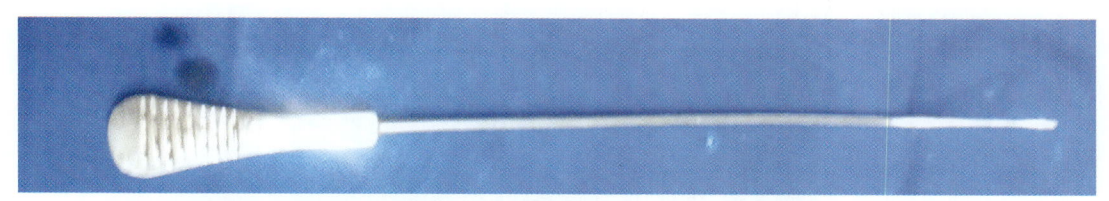

FIGURE 13.11 Uterine Sound

11. **Uterine sound**
    With this instrument, uterine length and direction can be made out. It's a long instrument with blunt tip (to avoid perforation). About 5 cm from the tip is a bend to make an angle of 30 degree. It has markings on it for measurements. The angle helps to negotiate curvature of the uterus (anteflexion or retroflexion). It helps to find out if uterus is anteverted or retroverted so that perforation can be avoided while dilating the cervix with dilators. It is used for measuring uterocervical length, length of the cervix for diagnosing infravaginal elongation of the cervix by measuring depth of fornix, to feel for any pathology inside the uterine cavity like fibroid (submucous), polyp, congenital anomalies like septa or bicornuate uterus, adhesions or synechiae/to feel for the misplaced IUCD. During Fothergill's operation, length of the cervix is measured before surgery to assess how much of cervix has to be amputated. Before advent of USG, it was used to diagnose misplaced IUCD by taking X-ray lateral view of pelvis with sound in situ (Fig. 13.11).
12. **Needle holder**
    This instrument is used for grasping needle at the time of suturing. The inner surface of tip has serrations and a small grove for firm grasp of the curved needle. The box joint is placed very close to tip to give adequate pressure because of the lever effect (Fig. 13.12).
13. **Vulsellum**
    This instrument is used for grasping the cervix (usually anterior lip of the cervix is grasped). It is a long instrument with gentle curve so that the line of vision is not obstructed. The tip of the blades have 3–4 serrations to hold and steady the cervix in procedures like insertion of IUCD, cervical biopsy, D&C, first trimester MTP with suction evacuation, Fothergill's

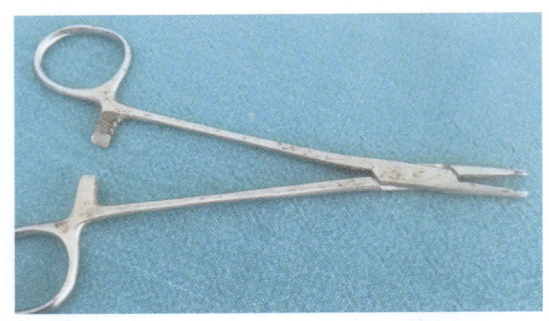

FIGURE 13.12 Needle Holder

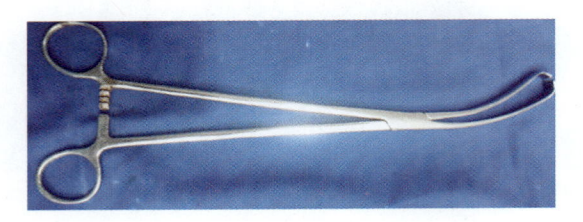

FIGURE 13.13 Vulsellum

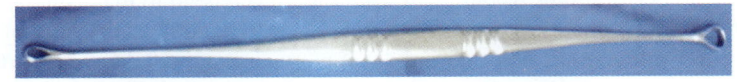

FIGURE 13.14 Uterine Curette

operation, vaginal hysterectomy. Posterior lip of the cervix is grasped for performing colpotomy, culdocentesis and to demonstrate enterocoele. Since the serrations are sharp, it is not used in pregnancy as it may cause cervical tears and lacerations and bleeding, instead, sponge holding forceps is used to grasp the cervix in pregnancy (Fig. 13.13).

14. **Uterine curette**
    It is sharp at one end, blunt at another end or it may be sharp at both ends. Sharp end is used for taking endometrial biopsy in gynaec conditions like infertility, TB endometritis, AUB. Blunt end is used in obstetric conditions to find out whether uterine cavity is empty following surgical evacuation in MTP and in spontaneous abortion (Fig. 13.14).

15. **Mathew Duncan's dilator**
    Mathew Duncan dilator is used to dilate the cervix in non-pregnant state, during procedures like dilatation and curettage, hysteroscopy, Fothergill's surgery, intra-cavitary radiotherapy in cancer cervix, to dilate cervix to drain pyometra (Fig. 13.15).

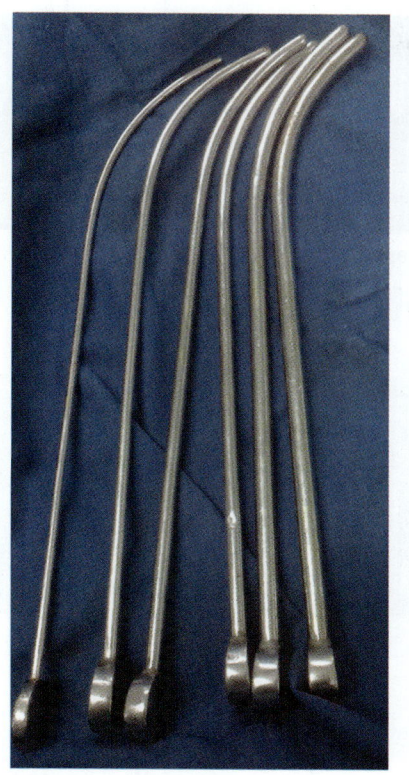

FIGURE 13.15 Mathew Duncan's Dilator

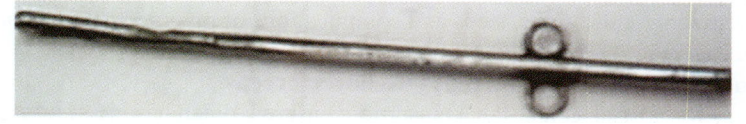

FIGURE 13.16 Female Metal Catheter

16. **Female metal catheter**
    It is used prior to surgical procedures like D&C, fractional curettage and during major vaginal operations to empty the bladder. It is also useful during vaginal hysterectomy to check the extent of cystocoele (Fig. 13.16).
17. **Punch biopsy forceps: Biopsy is taken as outpatient procedure without anaesthesia**
    Site of biopsy is either from growth/ulcer or suspected area by using Schiller's test (iodine negative area) or by using VIA (acetowhite positive area in the cervix). Colposcopy-directed biopsy is taken as outpatient procedure without anaesthesia from growth or ulcer in the cervix, and biopsy of vulval growth or biopsy of ulcer vulva (Fig. 13.17).

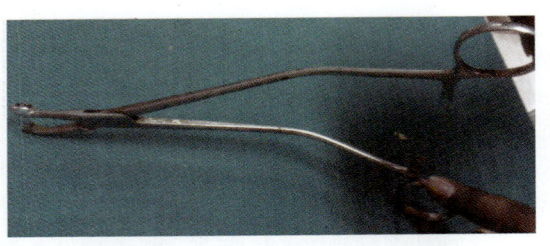

346 CASE 13 VIVA VOCE EXAMINATION IN GYNAECOLOGY

FIGURE 13.17 Punch Biopsy Forceps

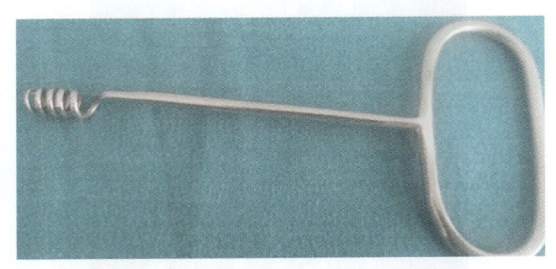

FIGURE 13.18 Myoma Screw

18. **Myoma screw**
    It has a screw with sharp edge on one end and handle at the other end. It is used in fixing the myoma after the capsule is cut open and traction is given while myoma is enucleated out from its bed during myomectomy. It can also be used to fix uterus during hysterectomy.
    Questions: regarding indications, steps and complications of myomectomy can be asked. Refer Case 5 on fibroid (Fig. 13.18).
19. **Post-placental IUCD insertion forceps—Kelley's forceps**
    Insertion steps for post-placental IUCD insertion: ensure woman has given informed consent. Ensure sterile equipments are ready.
    Complete active management of third stage of labour: confirm the woman's willingness for IUCD insertion. Examine to rule out post-partum haemorrhage and extensive lacerations. Visualise cervix using speculum. Clean cervix and vagina TWICE with povidone iodine solution. Grasp anterior lip of cervix with ring forceps. Hold IUCD with placental forceps inside its packing. Insert forceps with IUCD through cervix up to lower uterine cavity. Avoid touching the vagina. Place hand on suprapubic area, fingers towards fundus. Gently push uterus upwards to straighten uterine cavity. Move placental forceps with IUCD upward following the contour of the uterine cavity till the fundus is reached. Open and slightly tilt forceps inwards to release the IUCD at fundus. Keeping uterus stabilised, slowly sweep the forceps along the side wall of the uterus. Keeping uterus stabilised, withdraw forceps slowly keeping it slightly open. Ensure IUCD threads are not visible at the cervical os (Fig. 13.19).

GYNAEC SURGERIES 347

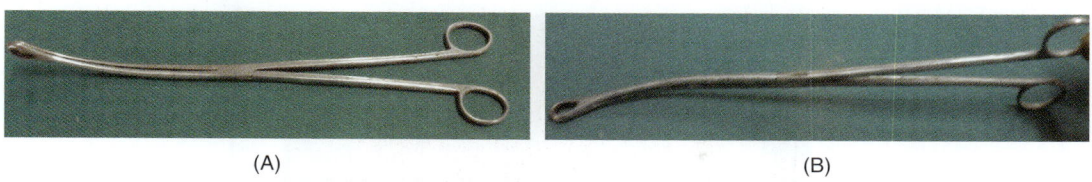

FIGURE 13.19 Post-Placental IUCD Insertion Forceps—Kelley's Forceps

GYNAEC SURGERIES

Steps of vaginal hysterectomy with PFR—anaesthesia—spinal/epidural/GA:

Inverted T-shaped incision is made on the anterior vaginal wall. Anterior vaginal wall is reflected (Fig. 13.20). Bladder is pushed up (Fig. 13.21). Incision is continued posteriorly, posterior vaginal wall reflected and pouch of Douglas is opened (Fig. 13.22). Uterus is delivered anteriorly (Fig. 13.23) after opening uterovesical fold of peritoneum.

Uterus is removed by clamping, cutting and ligating from below upwards the following structures:

1st clamp: Mackenrodt's ligaments, uterosacral ligaments (Fig. 13.24A)
2nd clamp: Uterine vessels
3rd clamp: Tubes, ovarian and round ligaments, on both sides (Fig. 13.24B)

Peritoneum is closed by extraperitonising the stumps. The 1st and 3rd stumps are approximated. Sutures are brought out through vaginal wall, which are tied after closing the anterior vaginal wall. Anterior colporrhaphy is done by plicating pubovesicocervical fascia (Fig. 13.25) from both sides and support to the bladder is strengthened in the midline. Anterior vaginal wall is closed after excising redundant vaginal wall. Posterior colpoperineorrhaphy is done by making incision in mucocutaneous

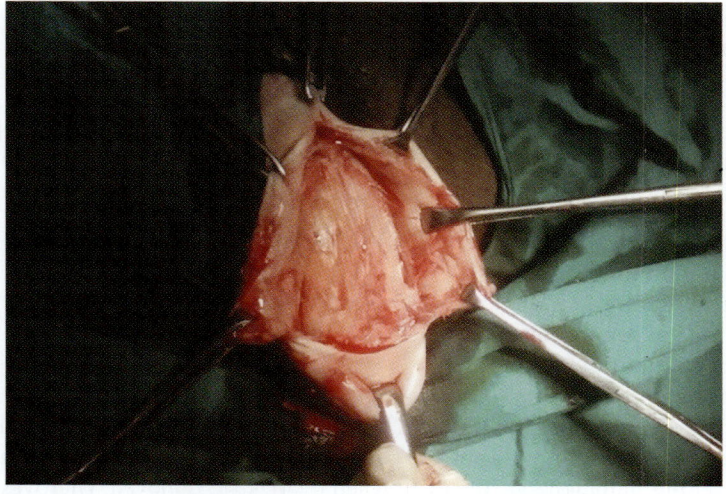

FIGURE 13.20 Anterior Vaginal Wall Is Reflected

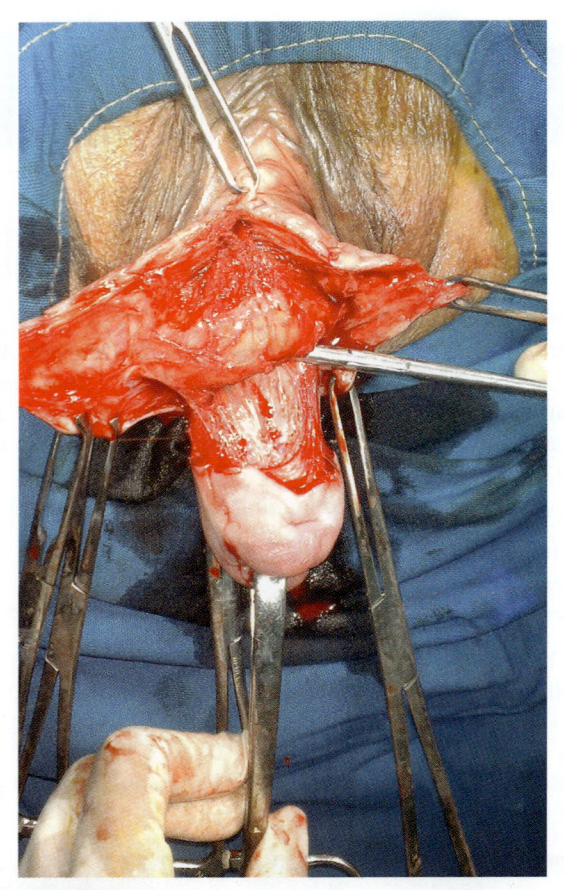

FIGURE 13.21 Bladder Is Pushed Up

junction and reflexion of posterior vaginal wall is done. Levator ani muscles are approximated from both sides and redundant vaginal wall excised and posterior vaginal wall is closed (Fig. 13.26). Superficial muscles and fascia are sutured with interrupted sutures and perineal skin is sutured (Fig. 13.27).

Steps of Total abdominal hysterectomy (TAH) with bilateral salpingo-oophorectomy—anaesthesia—spinal/epidural/GA
- Incision—Pfannenstiel—suprapubic transverse incision
- Vertical—midline or paramedian
- Rectus incised, rectus muscle retracted
- Parietal peritoneum is opened

    1st clamp: should be applied on (Fig. 13.28) round ligament—clamped, cut and ligated.
    2nd clamp: applied medially (Fig. 13.29) on ovarian ligaments and tubes when ovaries are retained/over infundibulopelvic ligament when ovaries are removed. Uterovesical fold of peritoneum is opened and bladder is pushed down (Figs 13.30 and 13.31).

GYNAEC SURGERIES 349

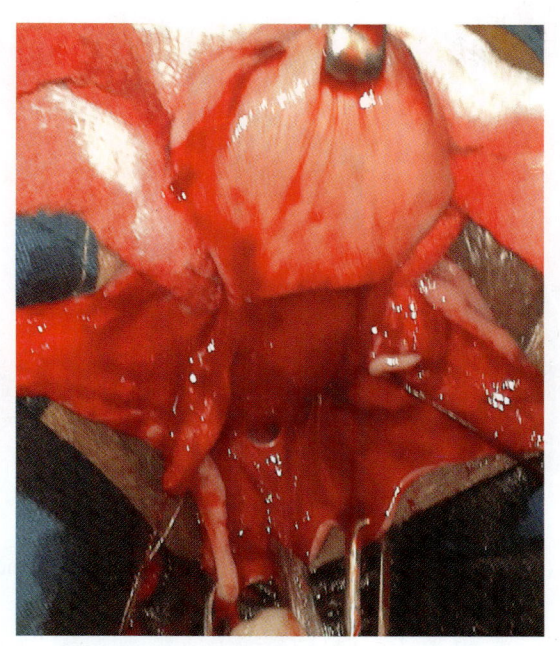

FIGURE 13.22 Pouch of Douglas

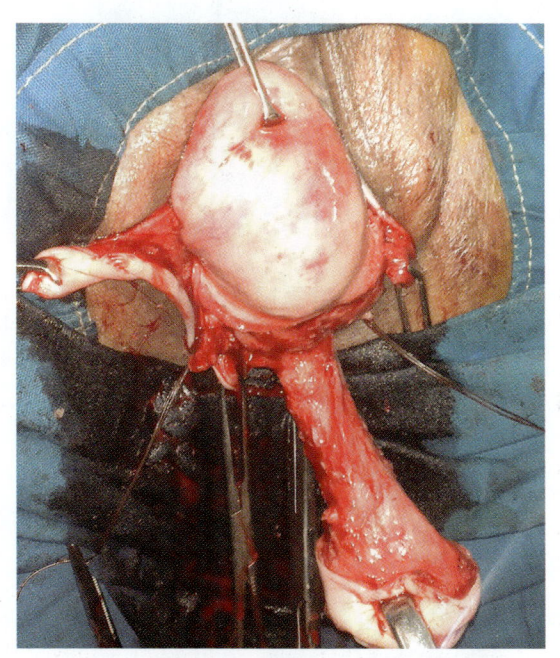

FIGURE 13.23 Uterus Delivered Anteriorly Meckenrod's clamp and ligated

FIGURE 13.24

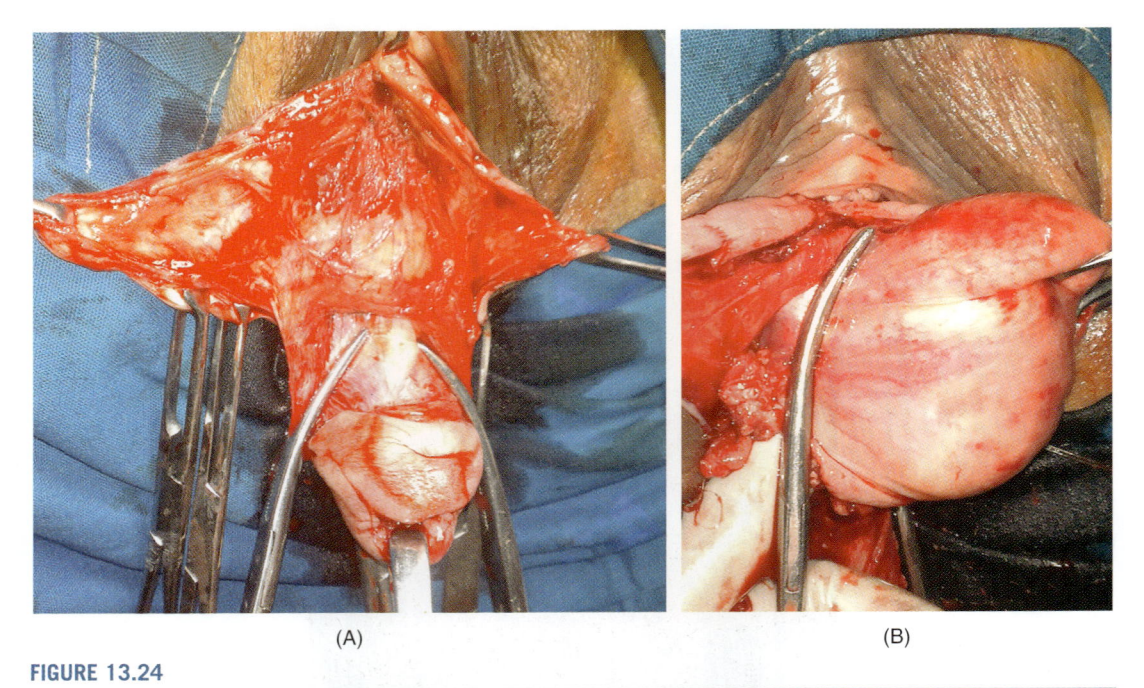

(A) Clamp on Meckenrod's, (B) clamp—tubes, ovarian and round ligaments, on both sides.

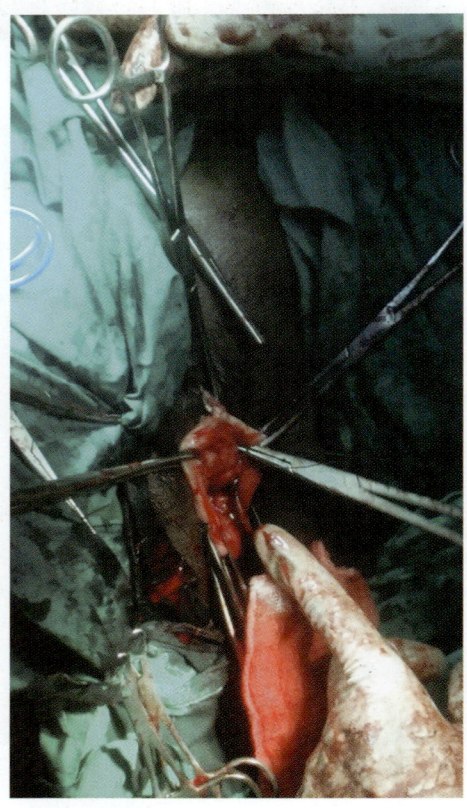

FIGURE 13.25 · **Plicating Pubovesicocervical Fascia**

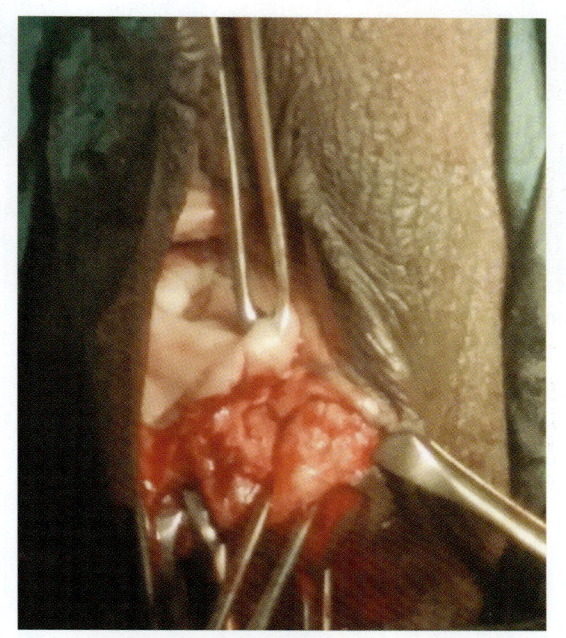

FIGURE 13.26 In Posterior Colpoperineoraphy-Leavator Ani-Approximated

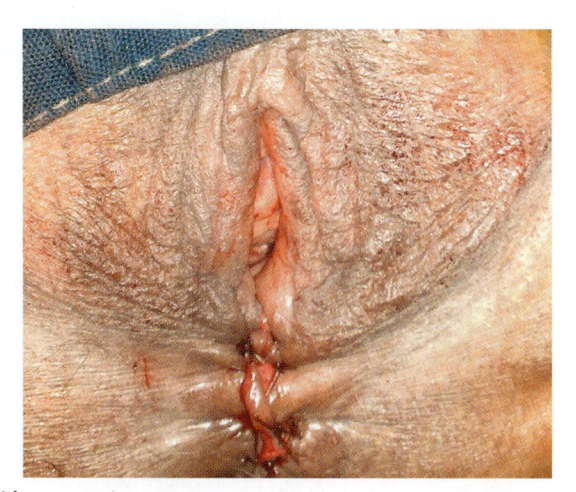

FIGURE 13.27 Perineal Skin

3rd clamp: applied on uterine vessels and stumps are cut and ligated (Fig. 13.32).
4th clamp: applied on Mackenrodt's and uterosacral ligaments (Fig. 13.33).

Uterus with tubes and ovaries will be removed in TAH with BSO or uterus will be removed in TAH. Vault is closed (Fig. 13.34) and abdomen is closed in layers.

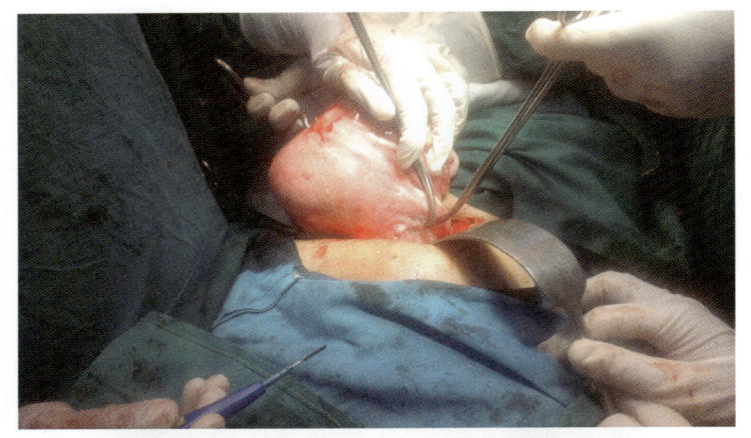

FIGURE 13.28   Round Ligament

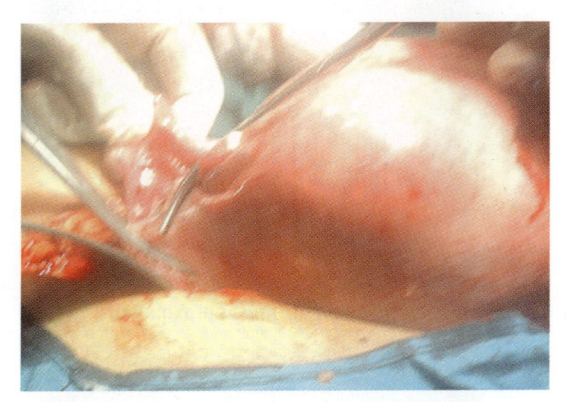

FIGURE 13.29   Ovarian Ligament

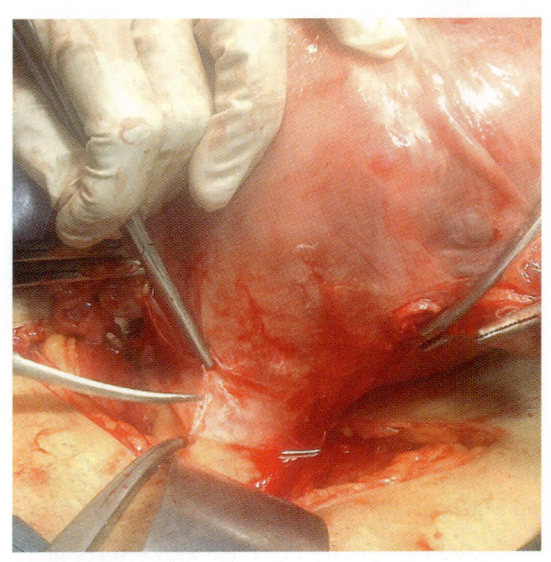

FIGURE 13.30   Uterovesical Fold

GYNAEC SURGERIES 353

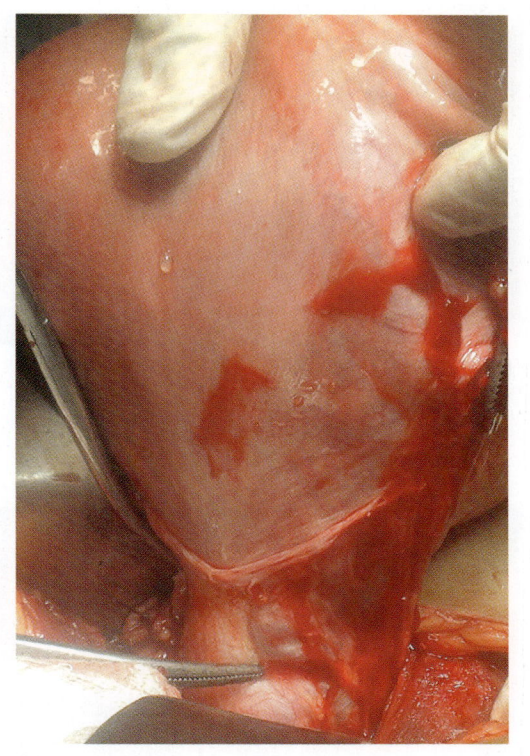

FIGURE 13.31 Bladder Pushed Down

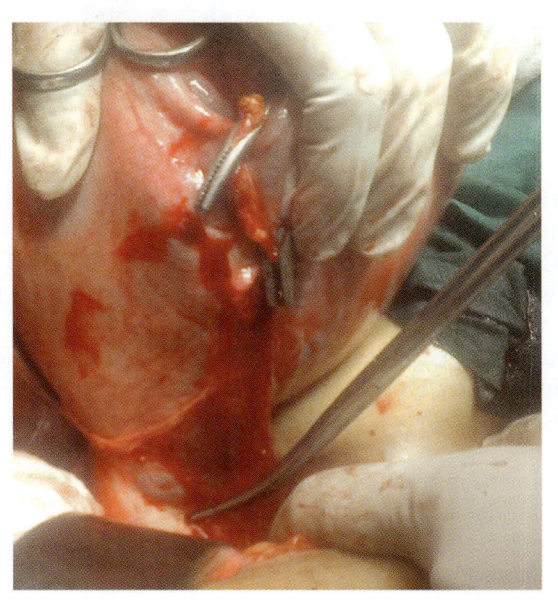

FIGURE 13.32 Uterine Artery

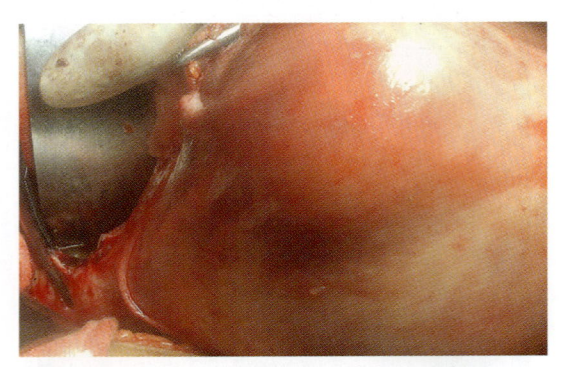

FIGURE 13.33 Mackenrodt's Ligament

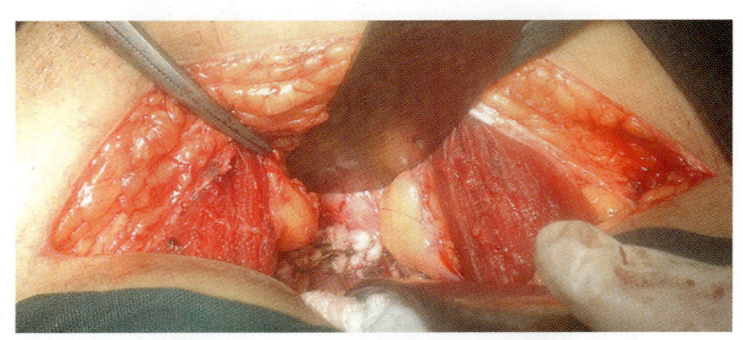

FIGURE 13.34 Vault Closed

Steps of Fothergill's with PFR: Anaesthesia—spinal/epidural/GA

First step: D&C—dilatation helps in easy cervical lip formation and allows drainage of blood and prevents haematometra. Curettage helps to rule out endometrial pathology (Fig. 13.35).

Second step: vaginal wall reflected as in vaginal hysterectomy. Mackenrodt's ligaments (Fig. 13.36) clamped, cut and ligated.

Third step: amputation of cervix (Fig. 13.37) after taking the haemostatic stitch.

Fothergill's stitch: suture taken through vaginal wall, Mackenrodt's ligament on one side, through anterior surface of cervix and through opposite Mackenrodt's ligament and vaginal wall and tied at the end (Fig. 13.38).

Fourth step: lip formation (Fig. 13.39A–B)—Strumdorf suture

Fifth step: anterior colporrhaphy.

Sixth step: posterior colpoperineorrhaphy.

Finally patency of the cervix is checked (Fig. 13.40).

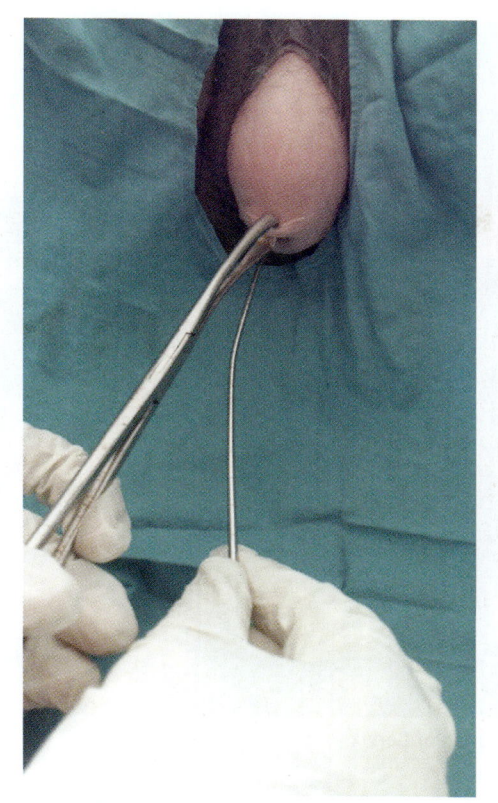

FIGURE 13.35 First Step—D&C—Dilatation

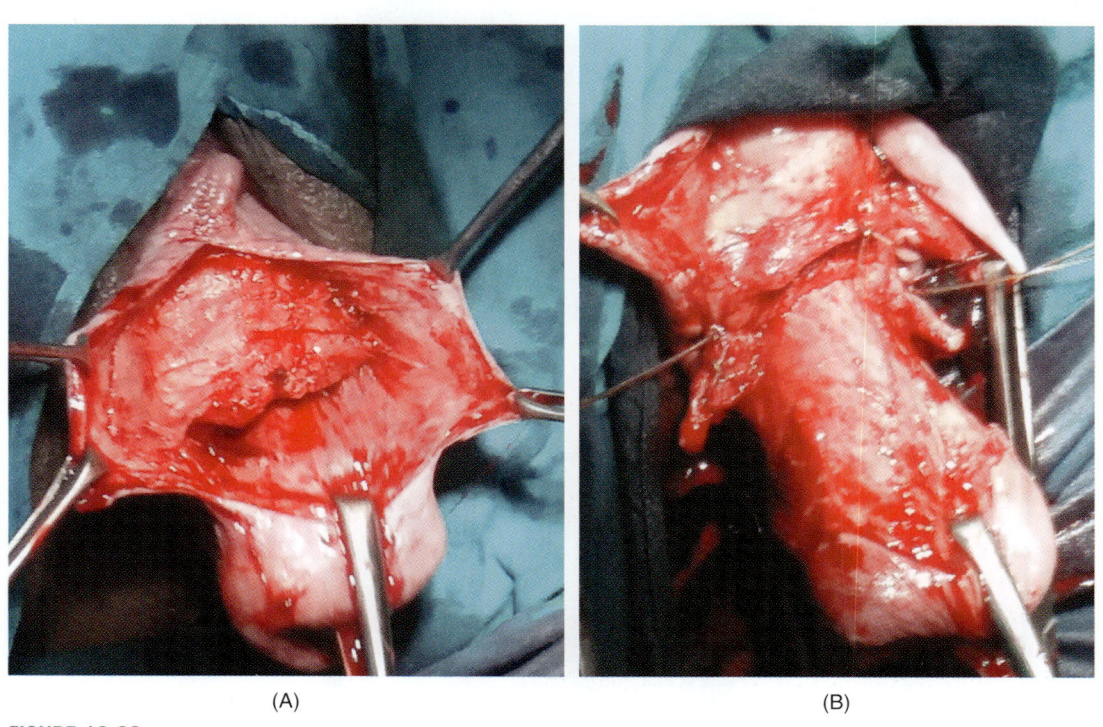

(A) (B)

FIGURE 13.36

(A) Step 2—vaginal wall reflected and (B) step 2—a Mackenrodt's cut and clamped.

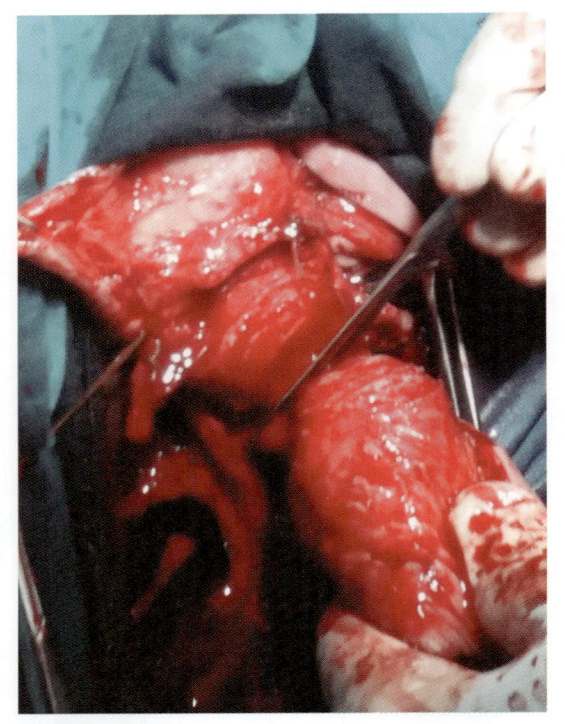

FIGURE 13.37   Step 3—Amputation of Cervix

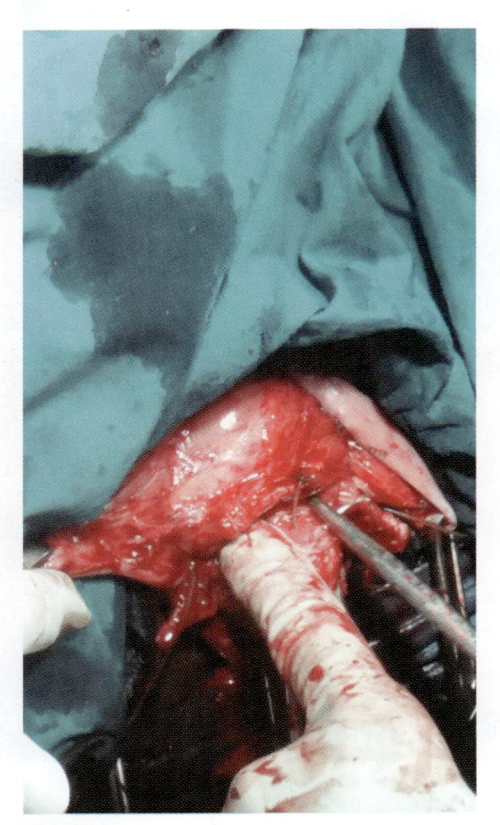

FIGURE 13.38   Step 4—Fothergill's Stitch

GYNAEC SURGERIES 357

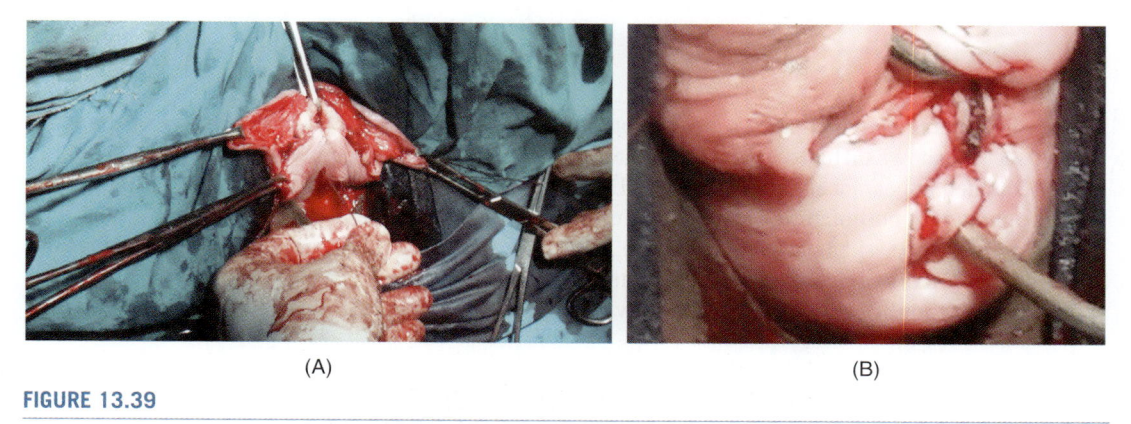

FIGURE 13.39
(A) Step 5—lip formation and (B) both lips of cervix are formed.

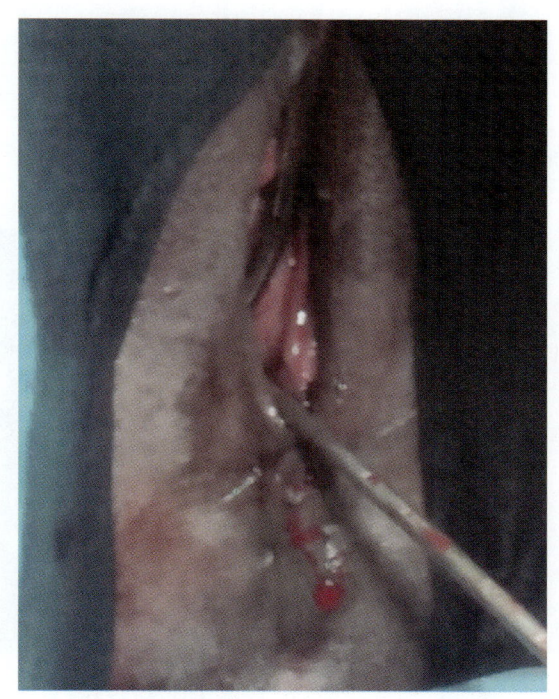

FIGURE 13.40 Finally Patency of Cervix Checked

358 CASE 13 VIVA VOCE EXAMINATION IN GYNAECOLOGY

SPECIMENS

1. **Adenomyosis**
   This is a specimen which shows cut section of uterus with cervix—total hysterectomy specimen. Cut section shows diffused symmetric increase in the thickness of the myometrium with trabeculated appearance without capsule. Dark haemorrhagic areas are seen scattered discretely throughout the musculature. Hence this is an adenomyosis specimen (Fig. 13.41).
   Questions will be asked on symptoms, signs, differential diagnosis and management of adenomyosis.

2. **Multiloculated ovarian cyst with thick septa**
   Specimen of multiloculated ovarian cyst with thick septa and unilateral (Fig. 13.42A–B).

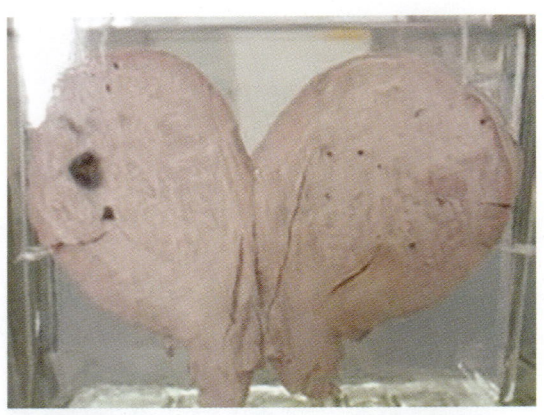

FIGURE 13.41 Adenomyosis

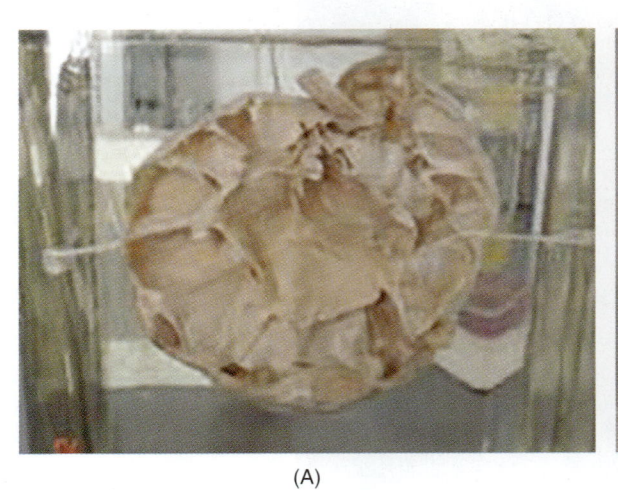

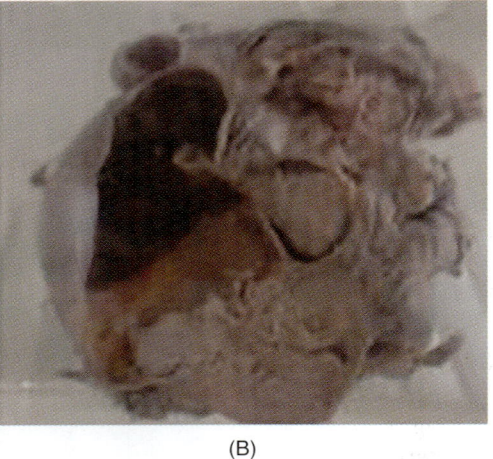

(A)   (B)

FIGURE 13.42
(A–B) Multiloculated cyst thick septa.

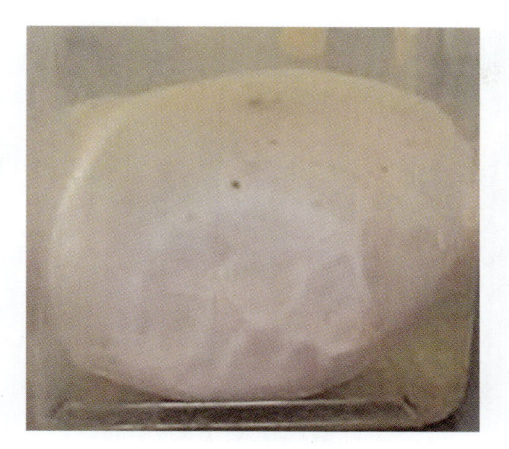

FIGURE 13.43 Ovarian Cyst

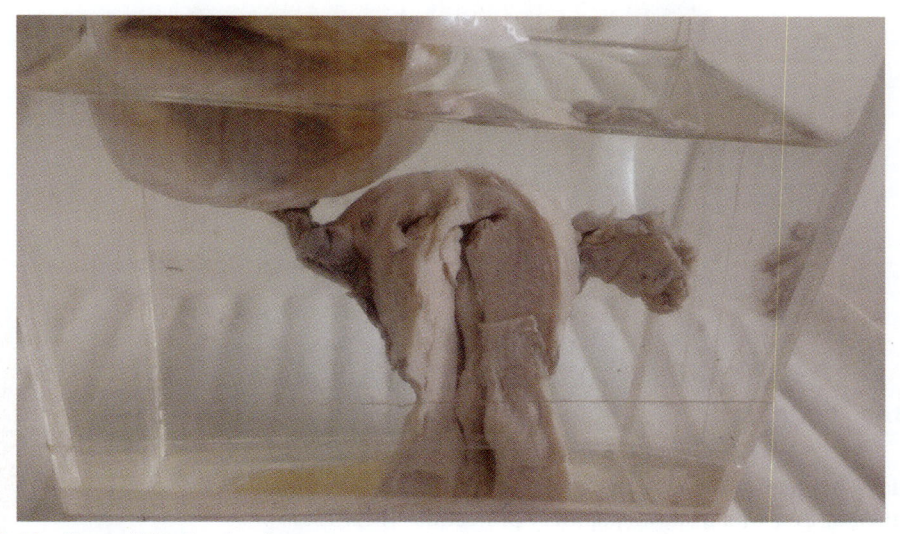

FIGURE 13.44 Uterus With Ovarian Cyst

3. **Ovarian cyst**
   Specimen of ovarian cyst—probably benign cyst of the ovary—unilateral ovariotomy specimen (Fig. 13.43).
4. **Uterus with ovarian cyst**
   Specimen of uterus with cervix with gangrenous ovarian cyst most probably due to torsion (Fig. 13.44).

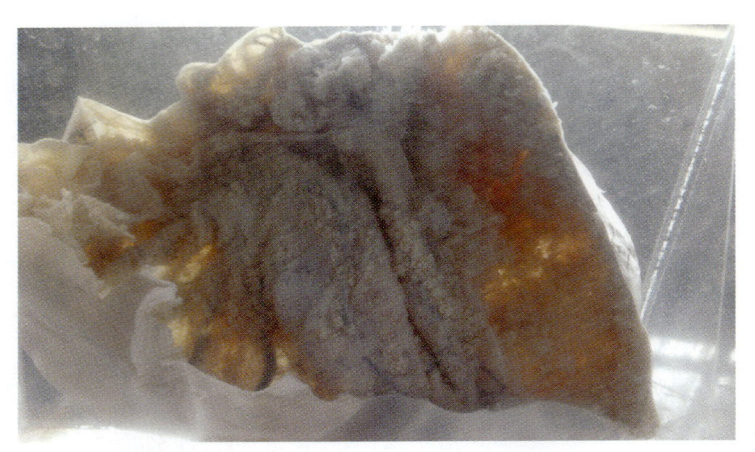

FIGURE 13.45 Papillary Projections

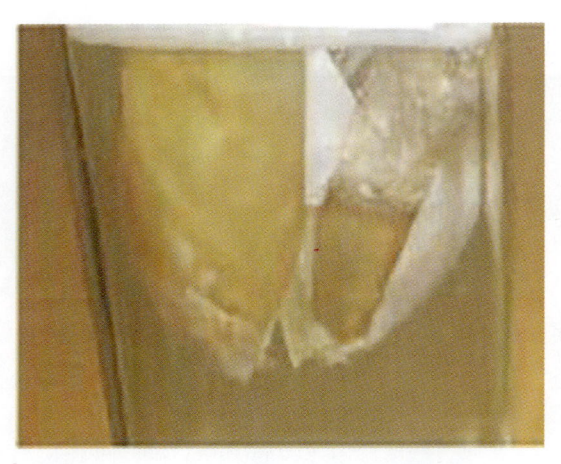

FIGURE 13.46 Dermoid Cyst

5. **Papillary projections**
   Specimen of cyst which shows papillary projections (Fig. 13.45).
6. **Dermoid cyst or dermoid**
   Specimen of cut section of uniloculated ovarian cyst with rolled up sebaceous material—probably dermoid cyst (Figs 13.46 and 13.47).
   Questions will be asked on classification, causes, signs and symptoms, causes for torsion, complications, investigations and management of ovarian tumour.
7. **Fibroid**
   Specimen of cut section of enlarged uterus and cervix with intramural three masses, which shows whorled appearance with thick pseudocapsule whitish, with distortion of uterine cavity and hence it is intramural fibroid (Fig. 13.48).
   Questions will be asked on signs, symptoms, complications and management of fibroid.

SPECIMENS **361**

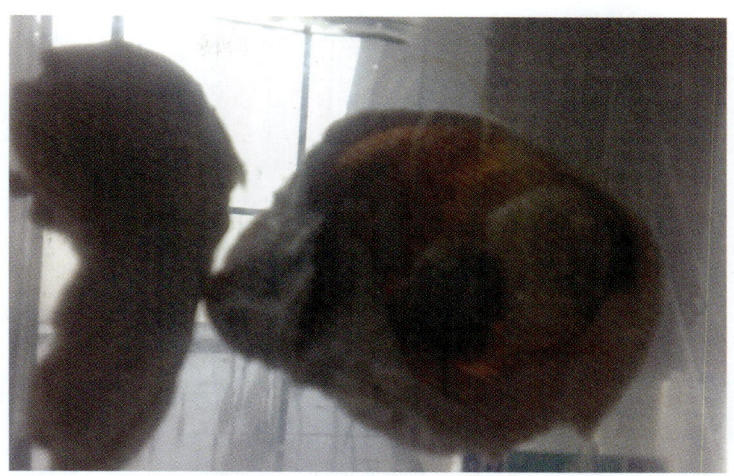

FIGURE 13.47   Dermoid

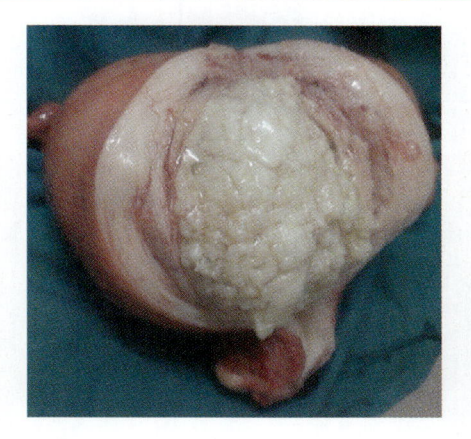

FIGURE 13.48   Fibroid

8. **Cervical polyp**
   This specimen shows enlarged uterus with a polyp in the cervical region with thick stalk (Fig. 13.49).
9. **Endometrial polyp**
   Specimen of cut section of enlarged uterus with endometrial polyp arising from fundus of uterus. This polyp has thin stalk (Fig. 13.50).
   Questions will be asked on common symptoms of cervical and endometrial polyp and their management.
10. **Ectopic gestation**
    Specimen of partial salpingectomy, which shows tube which is enlarged, congested with ruptured site with irregular edges—may be due to ruptured ectopic gestation (Fig. 13.51).
    Questions will be on asked on aetiology, signs and symptoms, investigations, diagnosis and management.

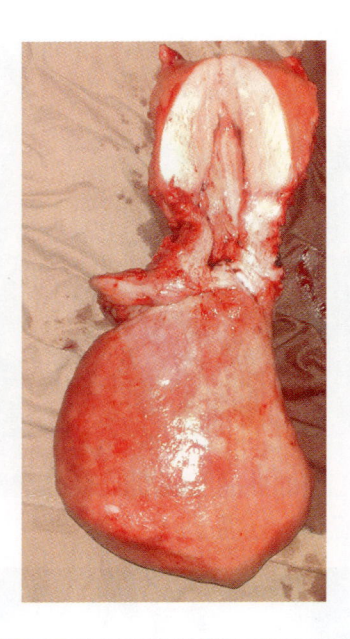

FIGURE 13.49 Cervical Polyp

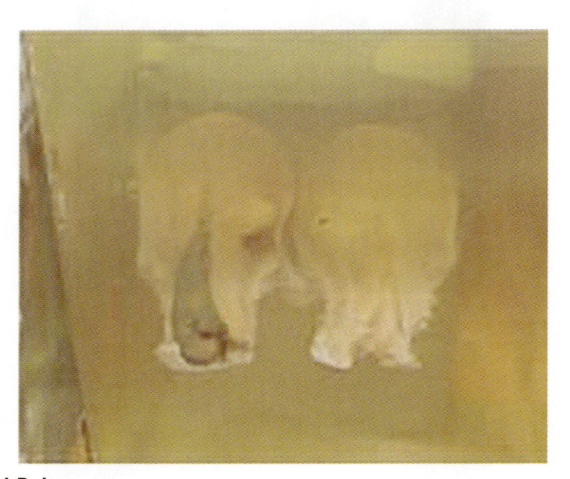

FIGURE 13.50 Endometrial Polyp

11. IUCD—copper T

Cu-T is an intrauterine contraceptive device which belongs to medicated bioactive device. It is CuT 380A. It is T-shaped made of polyethylene, with barium sulphate added for radio-opacity. CuT 380A carries 380 mm^2 surface area of copper (Fig. 13.52). Stem has 314 mm^2 and each horizontal arm has 33 mm^2 of copper. It has inserter and plunger—4.4 mm to insert the Cu-T. Effective life: 10 years; release per day: 50 µg of copper.

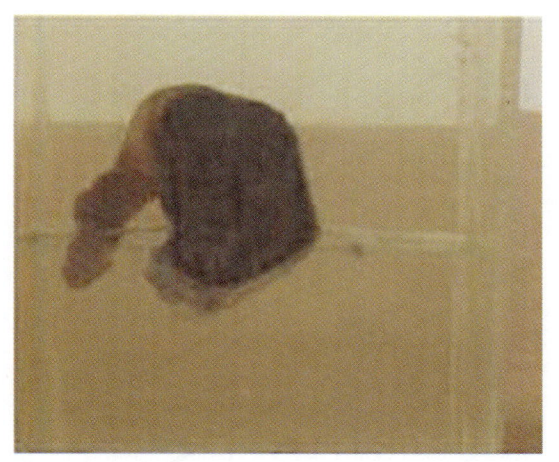

FIGURE 13.51 Ectopic Gestation

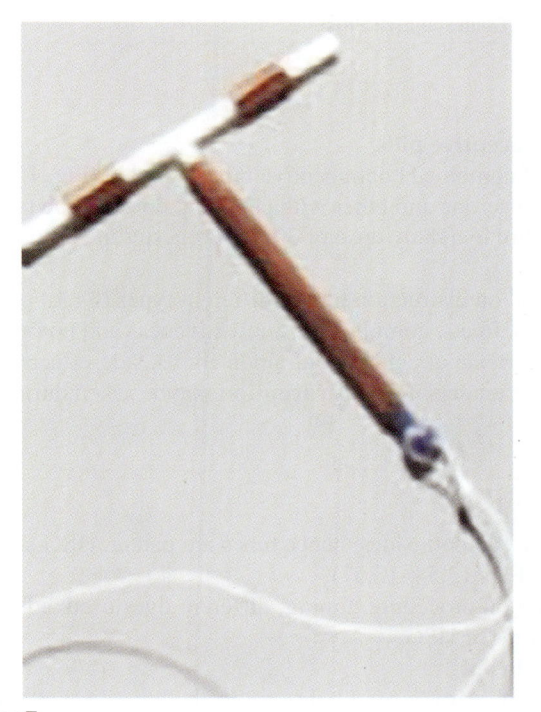

FIGURE 13.52 IUCD—Copper T

Introduced by withdrawal technique to avoid perforation.
Questions will be asked on contraindications, method of insertion, mode of action, advantages and disadvantages.
What are the different generations of IUCD? What are the other bio-active or medicated IUCD and their use?

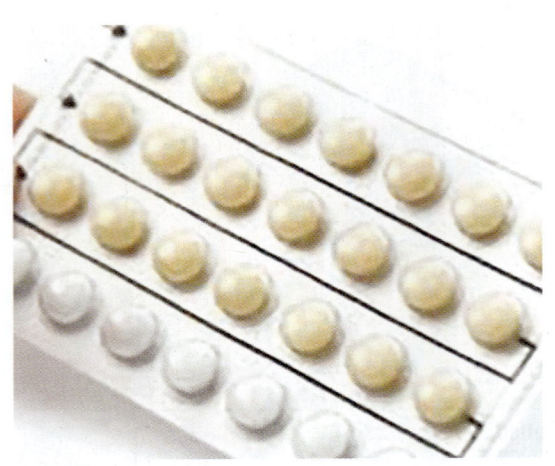

FIGURE 13.53 Combined Oral Contraceptive Pills

12. **Combined oral contraceptive pills**
    There are two types of combined contraceptive pills available (Fig. 13.53). One with fixed dose of oestrogen and progesterone and other with changing doses of the two hormones. Oestrogen used is ethinyl oestradiol in a daily dose of 30 µg. Progesterone used usually is nortestosterone derivative.
    Questions will be asked on instruction to use, different types of oral pills, mechanism of action, contraindications, side-effects, complications, effectiveness and non-contraceptive uses.
    Minipill—indications, mode of action, contraindications, side-effects, complications and its effectiveness and about **emergency contraception** maybe asked during viva examination.

HYSTEROSALPINGOGRAM

HSG shows free spill of dye on both sides, hence tubes are patent. HSG shows no spill of the dye and evidence of hydrosalpinx (Figs 13.54–13.57).

Questions will be asked on procedure, timing, different dyes used, advantages and disadvantages, indications and complications of HSG.

USG—anterior wall fibroid

USG picture shows uterus with hyperechoic area in the anterior wall. Hence anterior wall fibroid (Fig. 13.58).

Questions on fibroid will be asked.

USG—endometrial thickness

USG picture of uterus showing thickened endometrium (Fig. 13.59). Normal thickness of endometrium in reproductive age group is up to 10–13 mm.

Normal thickness in post-menopausal age group is 4 mm. Endometrial thickness is increased in conditions like endometrial hyperplasia, endometrial carcinoma.

HYSTEROSALPINGOGRAM 365

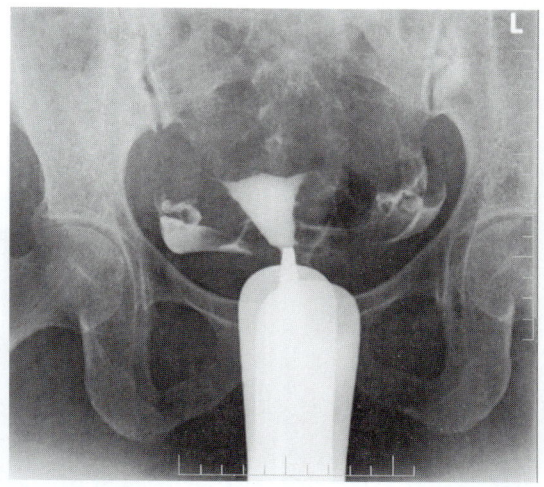

FIGURE 13.54 HSG Shows Free Spill

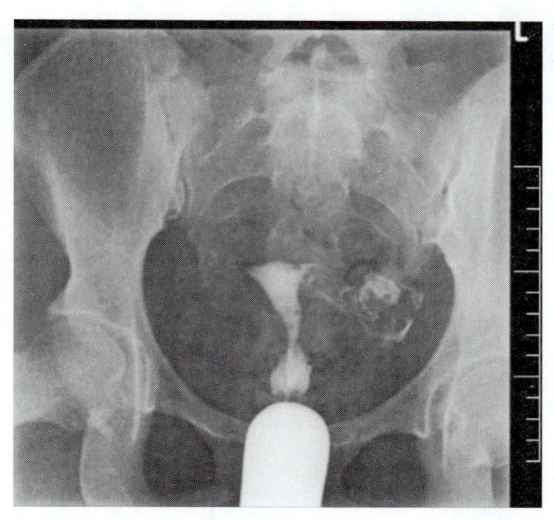

FIGURE 13.55 HSG Unilateral Block

Endometrial polyp has to be ruled out.

Investigations to be done—endometrial aspiration biopsy, which is a OP procedure/D&C/fractional curettage/hysteroscopy-directed biopsy.

Polycystic ovary
USG of ovary with multiple follicles arranged in the periphery—necklace pattern (Fig. 13.60). Questions on PCOD will be asked.

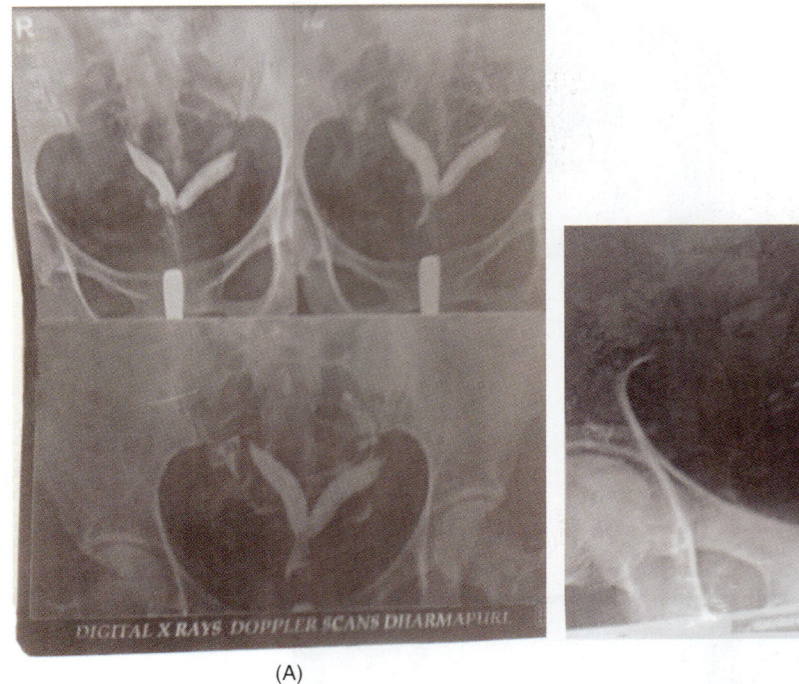

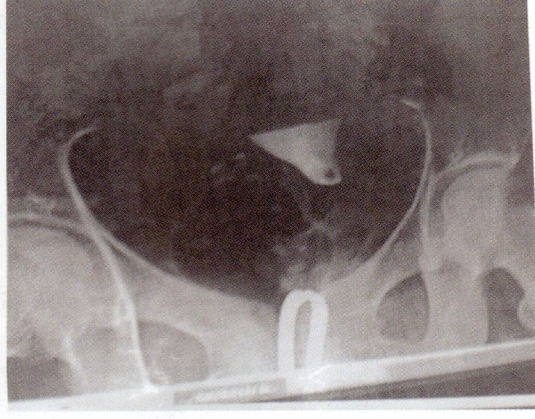

FIGURE 13.56
(A) Bicornuate Uterus (B) Bilateral cornual block.

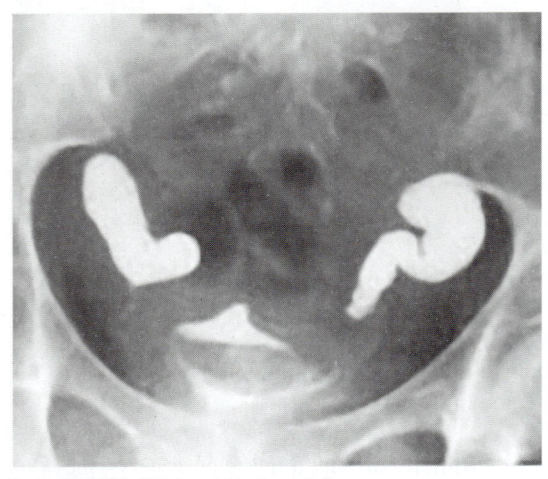

FIGURE 13.57 HSG Shows No Spill With Bilateral Hydrosalpinx

HYSTEROSALPINGOGRAM **367**

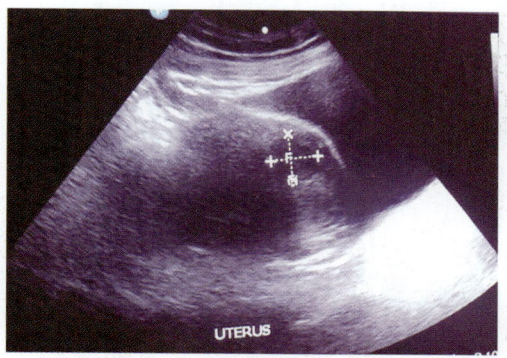

FIGURE 13.58 USG—Anterior Wall Fibroid

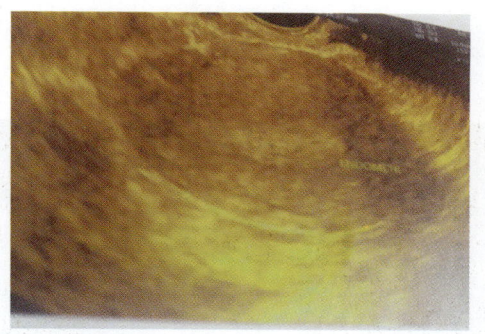

FIGURE 13.59 USG—Endometrial Thickness

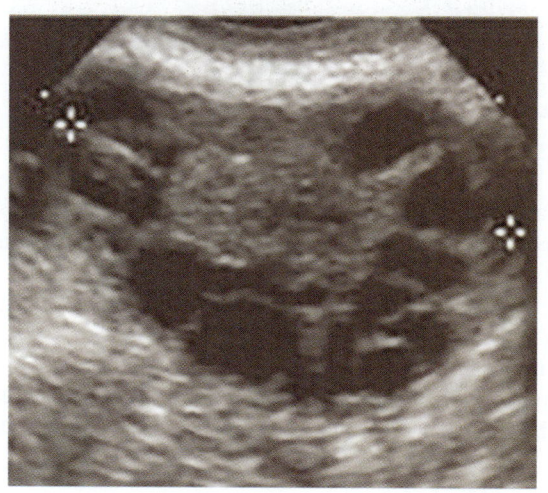

FIGURE 13.60 Polycystic Ovary

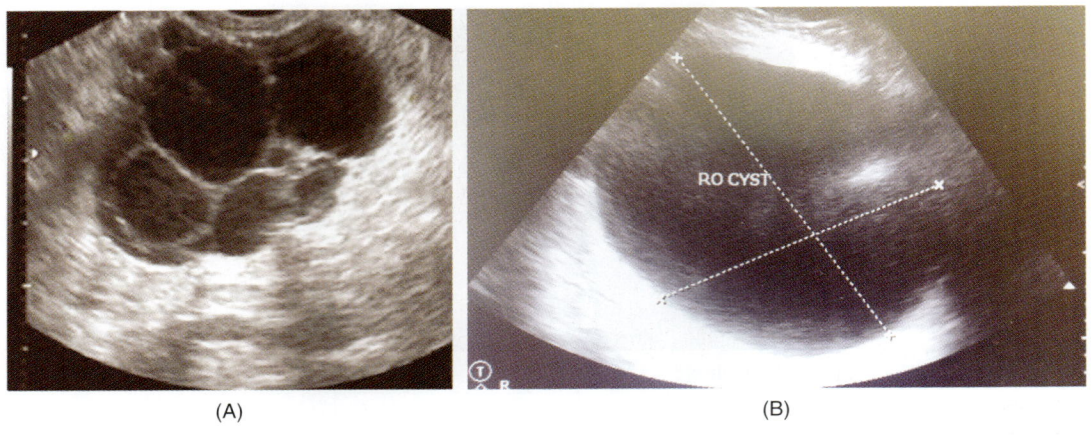

368 CASE 13 VIVA VOCE EXAMINATION IN GYNAECOLOGY

FIGURE 13.61
(A) Multiloculated ovarian cyst and (B) uniloculated ovarian cyst.

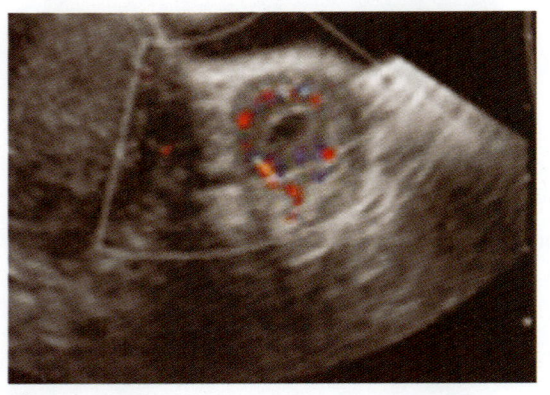

FIGURE 13.62 Ectopic Gestation

Multiloculated ovarian cyst and uniloculated ovarian cyst (Fig. 13.61)
Questions will be asked on USG criteria for benign and malignant ovarian tumours.

Ectopic gestation
USG shows adnexal gestational sac with vascularity—probably unruptured ectopic gestation (Fig. 13.62).

Criteria for medical management:
Sac size less than 4 cm; no cardiac activity; haemodynamically stable patient.
Question will be asked on signs and symptoms of ectopic, criteria for medical and surgical management of ectopic gestation.

Index

A

Abdomen pain, 220
Abdominal examination, 224–225, 243
    auscultation, 225
    inspection, 224
    mobility, 225
    palpation, 224
    percussion, 225
    tenderness, 225
Abdominal hysterectomy, 322, 339
    complications of, 252
Abnormal uterine bleeding (AUB), 241–252
    causes, 245
    endometrial pattern, types of, 248
    haematological test, 244
    investigations, 244–245
    management, 249–252
        hormonal treatment, 250
        non-hormonal treatment, 250
Abnormal vaginal discharge
    management, 236
    probable cause, 236
    types, 236
ABO incompatibility, 120
Abortion, 4, 12, 147, 151, 152, 193, 207, 209, 242, 272
Abruptio placenta, 4, 5, 29, 53, 64–66, 104, 114, 202
Abruption, 64
Acanthosis nigricans, 291
Acardiac foetus, 112
ACE inhibitors, 61
Activated prothrombin time, 58
Active management of third stage of labour, 39
Acute pelvic inflammatory disease (PID)
    stages, 238
    symptoms, 238
ADD-BACK therapy, 250
Addison's disease, 310
Adenomyosis, 219–221, 228, 241, 243, 245, 246, 267, 292, 358
    ovarian tumour, 221
Adnexal mass, 243
Adnexal swellings, 234
Adolescent, 249, 311
Adrenogenital syndrome, 302, 303
    treatment, 304
Allis forceps, 339, 340
Alloimmunisation, 119
Amenorrhoea, 3, 24, 37, 43, 49, 53, 71, 79, 87, 220, 251, 301, 304, 315, 316, 320
    causes, 220

    pathological, 220
    physiological, 220
    primary
        causes for, 302
        diagnosis, 301
        evaluation of, 305
        examination
            for breast development, 300
            gynaec, 300
            of axillary and pubic hair, 300
            of thyroid, 300
            per-rectal, 300
        investigations, 301
    secondary
        causes of, 310
        examination, 308
            abdominal, 308
            gynaec, 308
        investigations, 309
Amniocentesis, 119
Amniotic fluid index (AFI), 73, 153, 157
    measurements, 73
Amsel's criteria, 238
AMTSL (active management of third stage of labour), 39
Anaemia, 5, 16, 43–51, 55, 121, 224, 249, 316
    complicating pregnancy during labour, management of, 51
    in pregnancy
        FOGSI classification, 48
        ICMR classification of, 48
Androgen insensitivity syndrome, 300
Anencephalus baby foetus, 198
Anencephaly, 98
Anomaly scan, 32
Anovulation, 164, 218, 242, 289, 293, 297
Antenatal anaemia treatment, modality, 50
Antenatal care, routine investigations, 33
Antenatal foetal surveillance, 153
Antenatal period, precautions during, 121
Antenatal prophylaxis, 122
Antenatal tracing, 203
Anterior vaginal wall cyst, 260
Anti D administration, 120
Anti-coagulants, 242
    guidelines, 94
    therapy, 244
Anti-fibrinolytics, 250
Anti-hypertensive drugs, 61
Anti-oxidants, 61
Anti-phospholipid antibody syndrome, 151

Index

Anti-sperm antibodies, 294
APH (abruptio placenta, placenta previa), 44, 64, 114, 148, 181, 204
APLA syndrome, 61, 149, 157
ARM, 66, 74, 77, 113, 158
Arrhenoblastoma, 315, 316
ART. *See* Assisted reproductive technology (ART)
Artery forceps, 339, 340
Artificial rupture of membranes (ARM), 341
ASC. *See* Atypical squamous cells (ASC)
Asherman's syndrome, 183, 219, 249, 289, 294, 308, 309
Aspermia, 295
Assisted reproductive technology (ART), 107, 297
Asthenospermia, 295
Asymmetrical IUGR, 157
Atrial myxoma, 16
Atypical squamous cells (ASC), 278
AUB. *See* Abnormal uterine bleeding (AUB)
Auscultation, 28, 98
Ayre's spatula, 339, 340
Azoospermia, 293, 295

B

B-lynch
Babcock's forceps, 339, 340
Bacterial vaginosis, 221, 234, 235, 237, 238
    Amsel's criteria for diagnosis, 238
Benign tumours, 320
Bethesda system, 278
Bicornuate uterus, 268
Bilateral pedal oedema, 55
Bimanual examination, 243
Bimanual pelvic examination, 227, 229, 230
Binovular twins, 111
Biophysical profile, 73, 119, 152
Biopsy cervix, 235
Bishop score, 70–72
Bleeding, first trimester, 39
Blood dyskaryosis, 245
Blood pressure, 45
    measurement, 55
Blood sugar, 137
Blood transfusion, 51
Bonney's myomectomy clamp, 272
Breast carcinoma, 266
Breast-feeding, 164
    advantages of, 165
    contra indication for, 166
    problems faced in, 166
Breathlessness, 87
Breech, 98–104
Breech delivery, complications of, 103
Breech presentation, 98
    USG, as investigatory tool, 104
Bulb sucker, 192

C

Cachexia, 315, 316
Caesarean delivery, 82
Caesarean hysterectomy, 85
Caesarean in breech
    indications for, 104
Caesarean section, 63, 79–85, 93, 143, 165
    complications of, 85
    indications for, 82
    types of, 83
Caldwell and Moloy's classification of pelvis, 132
    according to shape, 132
Cancer cervix, 218, 230, 233, 275–286
Candidiasis, 221, 233–235
Caput succedaneum, 179
Carboprost, 192
Carcinoma endometrium, 277
Cardiac corrective surgery, 88
Cardiac failure, 74, 87, 88, 153
Cardiff count, 73, 152
Cardinal movements
    of head in vertex presentation, 38
Cardiovascular changes, during pregnancy, 90
Cardiovascular system, 89
    examination, 89
Cavaterm balloon therapy, 251
Cephalhaematoma, 179
Cephalopelvic disproportion (CPD), 125, 134
    abdomino-pelvic assessment
        Ian Donald method, 128
        Munro Kerr-Muller method, 128, 129
    basic investigations, 131
        cephalometry, 131
        MRI, 131
        USG, 131
    causes of, 126
    clinical methods of diagnosing, 127
        abdominal method, 127
        ian donald method, 128
    clinical pelvimetry, 130
    complications of, 133
    general examination, 126
    management of, 134
    medical history, 126
    obstetric examination, 127
    pre-requisites for assessing, 130
    surgical history, 126

trial of labour
    conduct of, 133
    failed trial labour, 133
    favourable and unfavourable sign of progression, 133
    indication and contraindication for, 133
    successful trial labour, 133
    termination, 133
Cervical dilatation, 103, 193, 213
Cervical fibroid, 269
Cervical intra-epithelial neoplasia (CIN), 276, 278, 280, 281
    diagnosis of, 280
        colposcopy, 280
    screening test for
        Bethesda system of reporting, 278
        liquid-based cytology (LBC), 278
        pap smear, 278
        visual inspection with acetic acid (VIA), 280
        visual inspection with Lugol's iodine (VILI), 280
    treatment of, 281
Cervical lymphadenopathy, 289
Cervical mucus, 236, 293
Cervical polyp, 39, 259, 361, 362
Cervical ripening, 12
Cervix, 164
    congenital infravaginal elongation, 259
    malignant lesions of, 282
        lymphatic drainage of, 282
    pre-invasive lesions of, management, 282
    trichomoniasis strawberry-appearance of, 237
Cervix cancer, 218, 230
    diagnosis
        differential, 277
        provisional clinical, 277
    examination
        bimanual pelvic, 277
        external genitalia, 277
        per rectal, 277
    investigation, 278
    malignant lesions of cervix, 282
        down-staging of, 283
        lymphatic drainage of, 282
        pathology of, 282
        risk factors for, 283
        spread of, 283
    management, 281
    pathology of, 282
    prevention of, 286
        primary, 286
        secondary, 286
    screening methods for, 278
        colposcopy, 278
        HPV testing, 278
        liquid-based cytology (LBC), 278
        visual inspection with acetic acid (VIA), 278
        visual inspection with Lugol's iodine (VILI), 278
    staging of, 283
    surgical management for, 284
        complications of, 285
        radiotherapy, 285
            brachytherapy, 285
            contraindications for, 286
            teletherapy, 286
Chorionicity, 111, 208
Chromosomal abnormalities, 32, 151
Chronic hypertension, 53, 60
Chronic inversion, 260
Chronic pelvic inflammatory disease (PID)
    signs, 239
    symptoms, 239
Classical caesarean, in modern obstetrics
    indications for, 85
Clitoromegaly, 225
Clubbing, 16, 18
Colonic cancer, 266
Colpocleisis, 264
Colpoperineorrhaphy, 263
Colporrhaphy, 263
Colposcopy, 235
Combined oral contraceptive pills, 364
Complaints noted, in chronological order, 8
    bleeding P/V, 8
    foetal movements, 8
    history, of present pregnancy, 8
Congenital cyanotic heart disease, 16
Congestive dysmenorrhoea, 219, 269
Conjoint twin, 112, 200
Contraception, 93
    history, 222
    in heart disease complicating pregnancy, 93
Contracted pelvis, 132
Coomb's test, 119, 122, 150
Cordocentesis, 119
Corpus luteum, 248
    cysts, 320
Couvelaire uterus, 202
    without cervix, 202
Couvelaire uterus, 202
Craniopagus, 200
Cryptomenorrhoea, 220, 299, 302
    treatment, 302
CTG tracing, 63, 75, 158, 203, 205
    abnormal, in labour, 203
    early deceleration, 203
    interpretation, 203
Cubitus valgus, 300
Curettage, 148

Cusco's speculum, 228, 339, 341
    advantage, 339
    disadvantage, 339
    examination, 228
Cushing's disease, 310
Cushing's syndrome, 300
Cyanosis
    central, 17
    peripheral, 17
Cyclical haematuria, 333
Cystocoele, 255, 257, 259, 345
Cystoglandular hyperplasia, 247

D

Daily foetal movement, 48, 59, 142, 152
Daily foetal movement count (DFMC), 72
Danazol, 250, 270
Dating scan, 32
Deaver's retractor, 339, 341
Decubitus ulcer, 219, 231, 257
    third degree prolapse, 257
    treatment, 262
Deep dyspareunia, 222
Delayed puberty, 222
Dermoid, 360, 361
    cyst, 360
Descent, 38
Diabetes, 138
    obstetric Doppler, 139
    specific investigations, 139
    USG, 139
Diagonal conjugate, 138
Dichorionic twins, 109, 110, 208
Digoxin, 93
Dilatation & curettage, 183, 244
Dinoprostone gel, 194
Diphtheria, 7
Direct Coomb's test (DCT), 122
Discordant twins, 110
Disposable cord clamp, 189
Disposal manual mucus sucker, 191
Disseminated intra-vascular coagulation (DIVC), 64, 65, 208
Diuretics, 64
Doderlein's lactobacilli, 236
Doppler velocimetry, 74, 153
Doyen's retractor, 194, 339, 341
DUB. *See* Dysfunctional uterine bleeding (DUB)
Ductus venosus, 59, 74, 119
Dysfunctional uterine bleeding (DUB), 241
    types, 245
Dysmenorrhoea, 218, 219, 221, 267, 290
    secondary, 219
    spasmodic, 219

Dyspareunia, 40, 41, 222, 267
Dyspepsia, 315
Dystocia dystrophy syndrome, 126

E

Early cord clamping, indications for, 39
Eclampsia, 53, 60, 63
    management, 63
Ecto cervix, 164
Ectopic gestation, 213, 241, 291, 361, 363
Eisenmenger's syndrome, 92
Embryo transfer (ET), 297
Emergency contraception, 364
Empty nest syndrome, 328
Encephalocoele, 199
Endocarditis prophylaxis, 92
Endocervical cancers, 282
Endocervical curettings, 248
Endocrine disorder, 149
Endocrine dysfunction, 60
Endometrial ablation, 250, 251
Endometrial aspiration, 244, 249
Endometrial carcinoma, 218, 228, 248, 268, 272, 326, 329
    risk factors for, 329
    treatment of, 329–330
Endometrial hyperplasia, 269
    causes, 248
Endometrial polyp, 361, 362
Endometriosis, 219, 228, 230, 243, 244, 267, 290, 292
Endometriosis-chocolate cyst, 267
Endometrium histopathology examination (HPE), 247
Enterocoele, 257
Epigastric/hypochondrial pain, 97
Epimenorrhoea, 218
Episiotomy, 40, 102, 187
    commonly used, 40
    definition, 40
    repair, 40
        advantages of mediolateral episiotomy, 41
        complications, 41
        first layer, 40
        indications, 41
        second layer, 41
        third layer, 41
    timing, 40
    types, 40
Episiotomy scissors, 187
Epsilon-aminocaproic acid, 250
Erythroblastosis foetalis, 120
    degree of manifestations, 121

ET. *See* Embryo transfer (ET)
Ethamsylate, 249, 250
External cephalic version (ECV), 103, 104, 117
    contraindications, 104
    indications, 104
External rotation, 39

F

Failed forceps, 134, 185
Failed trial labour, 133
False labour, 41
Female metal catheter, 345
Fertile period, 296
Fibrinolytic activity, 219
Fibroid, 100, 243, 360, 361
    polyp, 221, 261
Fibroid tumour *vs.* ovarian tumour, 268
Fibroid uterus, 223
    abdominal examination, 266
    bimanual pelvic examination, 267
    diagnosis, 267–268
    general examination, 266
    gynaec examination, 266
        infertility causes, 269
    investigations, 268
    management, 273
    medical management, 270
    menstrual history, 265
    myomectom, Indications for, 271
    pregnancy complications, 272
    pressure symptoms, 265
    rectal symptoms, 265
    red degeneration, 272
    speculum examination, 267
    symptoms, 269
    urinary symptoms, 265
FIGO classification system, 246
Fimbrioplasty, 297
First trimester, 39, 51, 109
Flexion, 38
Foetal anaemia, 119, 124
Foetal anomalies, 100
Foetal assessment, 48
Foetal cardiac activity, 207
Foetal distress
    causes for, 204
    signs, 205
Foetal growth restriction
    complications, 159
    management, 159
    symmetrical *vs.* asymmetrical, 158
Foetal heart, 98
Foetal lie, 81

Foetal macrosomia, 141
Foetal skull, 171, 177, 180
    areas of, 177
    clinical points, 180
    diameters, 178
        measurements and presentation, 178
    sutures and fontanelles, 177
Foetal wellbeing, assessment, 59
Foetomaternal haemorrhage, 117, 119, 120, 122
    calculation, 122
    conditions, 120
Foetoscope, 28, 190
Foley's catheter, 180
Follicular cyst, 320
Forceps, 79, 84
Forniceal palpation, 230
Fothergill's, 151, 223, 263
    operation Shirodkar's modification, 263
    stitch, 263
    surgery, 294
Fothergill's with PFR
    steps of
        amputation of cervix, 356
        anterior colporraphy, 357
        D&C-dilatation, 355
        Fothergill's stitch, 356
        lip formation, 357
        Mackenrodt's cut and clamped, 355
        posterior colpoperineorrhaphy, 357
        round ligament, 352
        steps of, 354
        vaginal wall reflected, 355
Fundal grip, 25, 26
Fundus, height, 24, 25
    conditions
        uterus is bigger than period of amenorrhoea, 24
        uterus is lesser than period of amenorrhoea, 24
    fundal grip, 25, 26

G

Gainesville classification, 238
Galactorrhoea, 300, 308
Gants's roll over test, 60
Gardnerella vaginalis, 233
Gartner's cyst, 259
General examination, 223–224
    anaemia, 224
    breast, 224
    build, 223
    nourishment, 223
    pedal oedema, 224
    stature, 224
    thyroid, 224

Genital prolapse, 218
  diagnosis, 259
  examination, 256–259
    abdominal, 256
    bimanual pelvic examination, 259
    general, 256
    gynaec, 256
    per rectal examination, 259
  investigations, 259
Genital tract
  defence mechanism, 236
  infections, 296
Genital ulcers, 290
Gestational age, 147
  determination of, 11
Gestational diabetes (GDM)
  change in gluconeogenesis, 140
  definition of, 139
  HbA1C-glycosylated haemoglobin, 141
  high risk factors, 139
  in past pregnancy, 138
  increased lipolysis, 140
  insulin resistance, 139
  management of, 143, 144
    Maternal, Foetal and Neonatal Complications, 140
  polyhydramnios, 145
    management, 145
  screening test, 140
    DIPSI criteria, 140
    NDDG criteria, 140
    OGCT, 140
    WHO criteria, 140
Gestational hypertension, 59
Gestrinone, 270
Glandular atrophy, 250
Glucose challenge test, 9, 150
Glycaemic control, 142
GnRH analogues, 243, 250
Granulosa, 316
Grave's disease, 17
Gravidogram, 29
Grips in breech, 99
Groove sign, 243, 318
Gynaec examination, 223, 225–231
  inspection, 225
  positions
    dorsal recumbent, 226
    lithotomy position, 226
    Sim's left lateral, 226
Gynaec surgeries, 347
Gynaecological problems
  at different age groups, 217

H

Haematocolpos, 302
Haematometra, 228, 263, 268, 300, 354
Haemoglobin, 58, 109
Haemoptysis, 87
Haemorrhoids, 107
Hand Doppler, 28, 190
HbA1C-glycosylated haemoglobin, 141
Head in breech, techniques to deliver, 102
  forceps for after-coming head, 103
  Marshall Burn's technique, 102
  Mauriceau-Smellie-Veit manoeuvre, 102
Heart disease, 87
  conduct of labour in complicating pregnancy, 92
  effect of pregnancy on, 91
  symptoms and signs, 90
Heavy menstrual bleeding (HMB), 218
Hegar's dilators, 182
HELLP syndrome, 55, 64
Hepatobiliary disease, 16
Hepatomegaly, 89, 225, 276
Hepatosplenomegaly, 121
Hereditary non-polyposis colorectal cancer (HNPCC), 316
Hereditary ovarian cancer, 326
Hirsutism, 300
  treatment of, 311
HMB. *See* Heavy menstrual bleeding (HMB)
HPV vaccine, 286
Huhner's test, 294
Human chorionic gonadotrophin (HCG), 297
Hybrid leiomyomas, 247
Hydralazine, 93
Hydrocephalus, 28, 132
  baby, 199
Hydrops foetalis, 148
  USG findings in, 120
Hydrops tubae profluens, 233, 234
Hydroureteronephrosis, 269
Hyperemesis, 8, 141
Hyperhomocysteinaemia, 150
Hyperoestrogenic state, 270
Hyperoestrogenism, 235
Hyperprolactinaemia, 219, 220, 291, 305, 307, 310, 311
  causes, 311
  treatment, 305, 311
Hypertensive disorders in pregnancy, 59
Hyperthyroidism, 219, 243
Hypogonadotropic hypogonadism, 305
  treatment, 305
Hypomenorrhoea, 218, 219, 251
  causes, 219
Hypospadias, 297

Hypothalamo pituitary axis (HPO) axis, 220
Hypothyroidism, 243, 289, 311
Hypoxia, 74
Hysterectomy, 256, 266, 281, 334, 339, 346
    indications for, 251
    routes of, 251
    types of
        Shauta Mitra vaginal hysterectomy, 284, 285
        Wertheim's hysterectomy, 284, 285
Hysterosalpingogram (HSG), 364
    anterior wall fibroid, 364, 367
    bicornual block, 366
    cornual block, 366
    criteria, for medical management, 368
    ectopic gestation, 368
    endometrial thickness, 367
    free spill of dye, 364, 365
    multiloculated ovarian cyst, 368
    no spill with hydrosalpinx, 366
    polycystic ovary, 365, 367
    unilateral block, 365
    uniloculated ovarian cyst, 368
Hysteroscope-guided resection, 251
Hysteroscopy, 243, 244, 268, 365
    indications for, 249

I

Ian Donald method, 128
Idiopathic thrombocytopenic purpura (ITP), 219, 244
Immunisation, 7, 167
    diphtheria, 7
Immunosuppressant drugs, 276
Incompetent os, 148, 150, 151, 182, 211
Indirect Coomb's test (ICT), 119, 122, 150
Indomethacin, 145
Induction of labour, 74, 119, 158, 181, 194
Infective endocarditis, 89, 91, 92
Infertility, 218, 239, 269, 289
    causes of, 294
    examination, 291
        abdominal, 291
        gynaec, 291
    female
        causes for, 294
        management, 297
    investigations, 292
        female partner, 293
        male partner, 292
    male
        aetiology of, 295
        factor evaluation, 295
        management, 296
    primary, 294
    secondary, 289, 291, 294
Infravaginal elongation, 221, 259, 343
Insemination, intra-uterine, 296, 297
Intermenstrual bleeding, 241, 269
Internal rotation, 38, 101
Intra uterine transfusion, 121
Intra-uterine death, 166
Intrapartum management, of twins, 112
Intrauterine contraceptive device, 233, 362
Intrauterine death, 117, 148
    previous, 148
Intrauterine transfusion, 121
Involution of uterus, 51, 163
Iron deficiency anaemia, 46–48
Isoimmunisation, 119
Isoprisinol, 270
ITP. See Idiopathic thrombocytopenic purpura (ITP)
IUCD-copper T, 362, 363

J

Jaundice, 16, 17, 45, 121
Johnson's formula, 29

K

Karyotyping, 150, 293
Kelley's forceps, 346, 347
Khanna's sling surgery, 263
Kleihauer Betke test, 122
Klinefelter's syndrome, 293
Knane's rule, 9
Kocher's forceps, 341, 342
Korotkoff, 20, 55

L

Lacerated perineum, 41
Lactation, 165
    indications for suppression, 166
    physiology, 165
Lactational amenorrhoea, 71
Laparoscopy, 223, 239, 266, 268, 285, 289, 293, 342
Laparotomy, 83, 201, 239, 266, 322, 330, 339
Last menstrual period (LMP), 7
    calculation, of EDD, 7
    Naegele's rule, 7
LBC. See Liquid-based cytology (LBC)
Leech Wilkinson's cannula, 342
Lefort's surgery, 263
Leiomyoma classification, 247
Leopold's manoeuvres—obstetric grips, 25

Leucorrhoea, 235
Levator ani, assessment of tone, 258
Levonorgestrel, 250
Liley's curve, 121
Liley's zone 1, 121
Liquid-based cytology (LBC), 278, 279, 280
Lochia, 163
    changes in, 163
Low birth weight (LBW), 44
LSCS procedure, 194–197
Lymphadenopathy, 224
Lymphatic drainage, 282

M

Mackenrodt's ligament, 261, 347, 354
Macroadenoma, 311
Macrosomia, 16, 72, 75, 108, 139, 141, 143
Magnesium sulphate, 194
Malarial parasite, 47
Malignant ovarian tumour, 225, 318
    chemotherapeutic agents in, 323
    fertility sparing treatment, 323
    management of, 322
    risk factors for, 321
Malpresentation, 100, 108
Manning's biophysical profile, 152
Marital history, 12, 222
Marshall and Bonney's test, 335
Mass descending, 221
Mathew Duncan dilator, 344, 345
Mayer-Rokitansky-Kuster-Hauser syndrome, 303
    treatment, 303
McCall culdoplasty, 263
McDonald's cerclage, 152
Mean arterial pressure (MAP), 60
Medroxyprogesterone acetate, 250
Megaloblastic anaemia, 46
Membranous dysmenorrhoea, 220
Menarche age, 222
Menopausal hormone therapy (MHT), 325
Menopause, 220, 235, 250, 321, 328
    hormone therapy benefits, 329
    management of, 329
    symptoms, 328
Menorrhagia, 183, 218, 241, 242, 265, 267, 269, 316
    causes, 219
        blood dyscrasias, 219
        endocrine causes, 219
        functional, 219
        systemic causes, 219
Menstrual history, 9, 222
    LMP, 7

    menstrual cycle, 9
    Naegele's rule, 9
Menstrual problems, 218–220
Mental retardation (MR), 299
Methylergometrine, 193
Metropathia haemorrhagica, 247
Metrorrhagia, 218, 241
    causes, 219
$MgSO_4$, 62
MHT. *See* Menopausal hormone therapy (MHT)
Microadenoma, 311
Micturition, 221, 275
    problems, 255
Mifepristone, 193
Miller—Kurzrok test, 294
Minipill, 364
Misoprostol, 115, 193
Modified biophysical profile, 59, 62, 71, 73, 119, 142, 152, 157
Moniliasis, 221, 234
    vaginal, 237
Monochorionic diamniotic, 110
Monochorionic twins, complications, 112
Monozygotic twin, 111
Moulding of head, 179
    degrees of moulding, 179
MR. *See* Mental retardation (MR)
Multiloculated ovarian cyst, 358, 368
Multiple pregnancy, 100
    antenatal management of, 111
    antenatal, foetal and intrapartum complications, 112
Mumps orchitis, 290
Munro Kerr Muller's method, 31
Myolysis, 266
Myoma screw, 346
Myomectomy, 14, 82, 149, 266, 271, 272
    complications, 272
    pre-requisites, 271

N

Naegele's rule, 9
Necrospermia, 295
Needle holder, 343, 344
Nitroglycerin, 93
Non-steroidal anti-inflammatory drug (NSAID), 249
Normocytic normochromic, 49
Nuchal translucency, 32, 109, 209
Nulliparous, 31, 218
    woman, 262
Nulliparous prolapse uterus
    surgeries, 263
Nutritional deficiency, 48

O

Obese, 138
Obstetric forceps, 183
Obstetric history, 222
  antenatal booking, 7
  foetal complications, of elderly primi, 5
  guidelines for, 3
  maternal complications in
    elderly primi, 4
    teenage pregnancy, 4
  patient's details, 3
  socioeconomic class, 5
  terminology in, 6
  WHO guidelines, 7
Obstetric vesicovaginal fistulas, 333
Oedema, 15, 18, 19, 22, 54–56, 61, 88, 108, 224, 315
  below knee, 55
  grading of, 55
  of abdominal wall, 56
OGCT test, 139, 140
OGTT test, 139, 143
Oligoasthenoteratozoospermia, 298
Oligohydramnios, 74, 76, 111
  management, 77
Oligomenorrhoea, 218, 290, 315
  causes, 219
Oligozoospermia, 296
Oophorectomy, 266
Optic funds examination, 58
Oral combined contraceptive pill, 242
Oral/insulin dose, 138
Ormeloxifene, 250
Osteoporosis, 271
Ovarian cyst, 359
Ovarian malignancy, 230
Ovarian tumours, 218, 244, 267, 316
  acute pain situations, 315
  causes, for ovarian cyst torsion, 321
  clinical differentiation, benign and malignant ovarian tumours, 318
  complaints, 315
  complications of, 322
  diagnosis, 319
  differential diagnosis, of mass abdomen, 320–321
  Doppler findings in benign and malignant ovarian mass, 320
  examination, 316
    abdominal, 317
    bimanual pelvic, 318
    general, 316
    per rectal, 319
    speculum, 318
  functional cysts of, 320
  history, 316
    family, 316
    menstrual, 316
    past obstetric, 316
    past medical, 316
  risk factors for, 321
  routine investigations, 319–320
Over-distended uterus, 109
Ovulation, 164
  induction, 289
Ovulatory dub, 248–249
Ovum forceps, 181
Oxytocin, 12, 66, 75, 92, 112, 133, 163, 192

P

Packed cell, 51
Pain
  coitus, 222
  causes, 220
  in abdomen at term, differential diagnosis of, 41
  menstruation, 269
Pallor, 108
Palpating mass, 224
Palpation, 98, 224, 289
  fundal grip, 98
  in suprapubic area, 81
  pelvic grip, 98
Papanicolaou system, 278
Papillary projections, 360
Papsmear, 223, 235, 244, 259, 278, 279, 328, 339
  test, 223
Paralytic ileus, 272
Parenteral iron preparations, 50
Partogram, 213
Past obstetric history, 242
Pawlik's grip, 25
PCOS. *See* Polycystic ovarian syndrome (PCOS)
Pedal oedema, 17, 19, 45, 108, 275, 316
Pedersen's hypothesis, 141
Pelvic assessment, 70
Pelvic floor repair (PFR), 262
Pelvic inflammatory disease (PID), 219, 233
  investigations, 239
    endo cervical smear, 239
    high vaginal swab, 239
  responsible organisms, 238
  treatment, 239
Pelvic kidney, 268
Pelvic Organ Prolapse Quantification (POPQ) system, 261
  stages, 262

Pelvis, 171
  brim, 172
  clinical importance, 176
  diameters, 175
  major and minor, 171
  outlet, 174
    curve of carus, 175
    waste space of Morris, 174
  plane, 174
  true and false, 172
Per rectal examination (P/R), 230
Percussion, 28
Perineal body, 258, 261
  integrity, 258
Perineal lacerations, 125
  degrees of, 42
Peritoneum, 164
Pessary
  disadvantages, 262
  indications, 262
  test, 262
Phenobarbitone, 122
Phototherapy, 122
Physical examination, 217
Physiological oedema, 18
  abdominal wall, 19
  above medial malleolus, 19
  below knee, 19
  dorsum of foot, 19
  reasons for, 18
  vulval, 19
PID. *See* Pelvic inflammatory disease (PID)
Pinard's foetoscope, 190
Placenta previa, 98
Placental sulphatase deficiency, 70
Plicating pubovesicocervical fascia, 350
Polycystic ovarian syndrome (PCOS), 307, 310
  clinical features, 310
  investigations, 310
  treatment, 311
Polycystic ovary, 365, 367
Polyhydramnios, 15, 24, 28, 74, 91, 98, 100, 108, 111, 118, 119, 121, 137, 138, 145
  management, 145
Polymenorrhoea, 218, 241, 269
  causes, 219
Post-coital bleeding, 255, 275, 325
Post-menopausal bleeding PV, 325
  causes for, 329
  diagnosis, 328
  evaluation of, 330
  examination
    abdominal, 327
    bimanual pelvic, 327
    general, 327
    inspection, of external genitalia, 327
    per rectal, 327
  history
    family, 326
    marital, 326
    menopausal, 326
    past menstrual, 326
  patient complaints, 325
  routine investigations, 328
Post-menopausal symptoms, 271
Post-operative problems, 80
Post-partum haemorrhage (PPH), 114, 272
  atonic, 114
  defined, 114
  management, 115
  primary, 114
  secondary, 114
  traumatic, 114
  types and predisposing factors, 114
Post-placental IUCD insertion forceps, 346, 347
Pouch of Douglas (POD), 230, 257
Pre-conceptional anaemia, 43
Pre-eclampsia
  basic pathology, 59
  complications, 64
  general management, 62
  high risk factors, 60
  mild and severe, 61
  predictors of, 60
  prevention, 61
  role of diuretics in, 64
Precocious puberty, 222
Pregnancy
  complaints, in chronological order, 8
  determination of gestational age, 11
  diagnosis, 32
  family history, 14
  foetal complications
    elderly primi, 5
    teenage pregnancy, 4
  general examination, 15
  history, present pregnancy, 8
  immunisation, 7
  lactational amenorrhoea
  marital history, 12
  maternal complications in
    elderly primi, 4
    teenage pregnancy, 4
  menstrual history, 9
  obstetric examination, 22
  past medical history, 14
  past obstetric history, 12
    abortion, 12

contraceptive history, 13
    in lower segment caesarean section, 13
    lactation, 13
    post-partum period, 13
    pre-term delivery, 13
    previous pregnancy, labour and delivery, 12
patient's details, 3
personal history, 14
physical examination, 14
present illness, history, 8
relevance, of history and diagnosis, 10
specific problems, based on low socioeconomic class, 5
summary, 32
surgical history, 14
terminology, 6
WHO guidelines, at specified intervals, 7
Premature ovarian failure, 312
    causes, 312
    diagnosis, 312
    treatment, 312
Pressure symptoms, 108
Primary amenorrhoea, 220, 222
Prolapse uterus
    anatomical classification, 259
    management, 262
    post-menopausal women
        causes, 261
Prolonged pregnancy
    complications of, 75
    induction of labour in, 74
    management of, 75
Prophylactic forceps, 184
Prophylactic oophorectomy, 266
Prothrombin time, 58
Pruritis, menstrual cycle, relation to, 233
Pseudo-clubbing, 17
Pubouretheralis, 261
Pubovaginalis, 261
Puerperal uterus, 163
Puerperium, early, care of, 177
Puerperium, normal, 180
Punch biopsy forceps, 345, 346
Purandare's abdomino cervicopexy, 263
Pyometra, 228, 268, 276

Q

Quintero's classification, 111

R

Radical vulvectomy, 256
Random blood sugar, 137
Rectocoele, 255, 257, 258
Rectum abdominopelvic resection, 256

Recurrent malpresentation, 148
Recurrent pregnancy loss (RPL), 147–153
Red degeneration, 29, 266, 270, 272
Reproductive tract infection, 218, 276
Respiratory system, 20, 89, 256
Restitution, 39
Rh antibody, 120
Rh isoimmunisation, 117, 119, 122
Rh negative pregnancy, management, 123
Rheumatic fever, 88
Ru 486, 270
Rubber catheter, 180
Rubin's cannula, 342
Rupture uterus, 201
    management, 83
    symptoms and signs of, 83

S

Sacrocolpopexy, 264
Sacrospinous colpopexy, 264
Saline infusion sonography, 268, 293
Salpingitis, 291
Sarcomatous degeneration, 270
Scar dehiscence, 83
Schiller's test, 280
Schroeder's disease, 247
Secondary amenorrhoea, 220, 307–312
Secretory endometrium, 248
cystoglandular hyperplasia, 248
Senile vaginitis, 277, 327
Sertoli-Leydig cell tumour, 316
Serum fibrinogen, 58
Sex cord stromal tumours, 221, 267, 316
Sexual dysfunction, 290, 297
Sexually transmitted infections (STI), 275
Sheehan's syndrome, 308, 310
Shirodkar's sling surgery, 263
Sickle cell anaemia, 44
Sim's speculum, 181, 342, 343
    advantage, 342
    disadvantage, 342
    examination, 227
Skull sutures, 177
    areas of, 177
Socioeconomic class, 218
    higher, 218
    lower, 218
Socioeconomic status, 218
Spasmodic dysmenorrhoea, 219, 269
Speculum examination, 234, 243, 267, 318, 327, 335
Spina bifida, 143, 256
Splenomegaly, 89, 225
Sponge holding forceps, 182

Spontaneous abortion, 147
Spontaneous conception, 147
STI. *See* Sexually transmitted infections (STI)
Stillbirth, 139
Stress incontinence, 217, 255, 325
Sub-acute bacterial endocarditis, 16
Suction cannula, 186
Superficial dyspareunia, 222
Supraclavicular node, 317

T

T-sign in monochorionic diamniotic twins, 109
Tachycardia, 20, 80, 84, 205
Tamoxifen therapy, 325
Tanners staging, 300, 301
TCRE. *See* Transcervical resection of endometrium (TCRE)
Teratospermia, 295
Testicular feminization syndrome, 299, 300, 303
Tetanus/diphtheria vaccine (Td), 7
Thalassaemia, 44
Theca cell tumour, 221, 267, 316
Theca lutein cysts, 320
Thelarche, 301
Third degree prolapse, 257
Thrombophilias, 60, 151
Thyroid disorder, 149
Thyroid dysfunction, 241
Thyroid enlargement, 20
Thyroid function test, 244
Thyrotoxicosis, 89
Torsion, 221, 225, 239, 266, 269, 321, 322
Total abdominal hysterectomy (TAH) with bilateral salpingo-oophorectomy, 348
    steps of, 348–351
        bladder pushed down, 353
        Mackenrodt's ligament, 354
        ovarian ligament, 352
        uterine artery, 353
        uterovesical fold, 352
        vault closed, 354
Tranexamic acid, 249, 250, 270
Transcervical resection of endometrium (TCRE), 251
Trial forceps, 185
Trichomonas vaginalis, 235
Trichomoniasis, 221, 233, 237
Triple dysmenorrhoea, 220
True labour pains *vs.* false labour pains, 41
Tubal carcinoma, 277
Tubal factor, 269
Tubal patency, 293, 342
    tests for, 293
        hysteroscopy, 293

        saline infusion sonography, 293
        salpingoscopy, 294
Tubectomy, 93, 339
Tuberculosis, 320
Tuberculous endometritis, 310
Tuboplasty, 342
Turner's syndrome, 208, 299, 304
Twin gestation, management of, 113
Twin reversed arterial perfusion (TRAP), 112
Twin-to-twin transfusion syndrome (TTTS), 112

U

Umbilical cord cutting scissors, 191
Umbilical grip, 25, 26
Uretherocoele, 257
Urethral diverticula, 259
Urethral syndrome, 328
Uric acid, 58, 139
Urinary incontinence, 333
    diagnosis, 335
    examination, 334
        abdominal, 334
        bimanual pelvic, 335
        external genitalia, 334
        general, 334
        Marshall and Bonney's test, 335
        speculum, 335
    excoriation of vulva, 335
    history, 333
        family, 334
        medical, 334
        menstrual and marital, 333
        obstetric, 333
        surgical, 334
    investigations, 336
    patients complaints, 333
USG
    Crown-rump length (CRL), 207
    ectopic gestation, 211
    fluid in pouch of Douglas, 244
    foetal cardiac activity, 207
    gestational sac, 206
    hydrops foetalis, 120–122
    incompetent os, 211
    missed abortion, 208
    nuchal translucency, 209
    placenta previa, 211
    T Sign, 210
    twin peak sign, 210
    vesicular mole, 209
    yolk sac, 206
Uterine anomalies, 100, 150

Uterine contraction, 29, 39, 132, 193, 203
Uterine curette, 183, 344
Uterine fundus, 259
Uterine prolapse, 221, 231
Uterine sarcoma, 268
Uterine sound, 182, 248, 343
Uterosacral ligament, 244, 263
Uterovaginal prolapse, 259
Uterus with ovarian cyst, 359
UV fold of peritoneum, 194

V

Vagina
    agenesis, 299, 302
    curdy white discharge, 234
    trichomonas infection, 234
Vaginal birth after caesarean (VBAC), 83
    advantages and disadvantages, 85
    monitoring during, 84
    pre-requisites, 83
Vaginal discharge, 221
    bimanual examination, 234
    culture medium
        Feinberg Whittington medium, 235
        Saboraud's medium, 235
        Thayer Martin medium, 235
    examination, 234
    investigations, 235
    pelvic inflammatory disease, role of, 238–239
Vaginal hysterectomy, 262, 263, 284, 339, 345, 347
    complications, 263
    with PFR, steps of, 347
        anterior vaginal wall, reflected, 347
        bladder, pushed up, 348
        clamp-tubes, ovarian and round ligaments, 350
        Mackenrodt's ligaments, 350
        perineal skin, 351
        plicating pubovesicocervical fascia, 350
        posterior colpoperineorrhaphy, 351
        Pouch of Douglas, 349
        uterosacral ligaments, 349

Vaginal pH, 235
Vaginismus, 290
Vanishing twin, 109
Varicose veins, 20, 21, 107
Varicosity, 108
Vasodilators, 93
Vasopressin, 272
Vault prolapse surgery, 264
Ventouse (vacuum extractor), 187
Vesicovaginal fistula, 333
Vesicular mole, 200, 201
VIA. *See* Visual inspection with acetic acid (VIA)
Vibroacoustic stimulation test (VAST), 73
VILI. *See* Visual inspection with Lugol's iodine (VILI)
Virchow's node, 224
Visual inspection with acetic acid (VIA), 278
Visual inspection with Lugol's iodine (VILI), 278
Vomiting, 107
Von Willebrand's disease, 245
Vulsellum, 248, 343, 344
Vulval dystrophy, 233
Vulval oedema, 56
Vulval-curdy white discharge, 237
Vulvovaginitis, 290

W

Ward Mayo's vaginal hysterectomy, 262
Warfarin, 94
Weight gain, 15, 54, 107, 142
Wertheims hysterectomy, 334
Whiff test, 235
Wrigley's outlet forceps, 184

Z

Zone (Liley's), 121
Zuspan regime, 63
Zygosity determination, 111
Zygosity of twins, 111